A Color Handbook of

Small Animal Emergency and Critical Care Medicine

Elizabeth A Rozanski
DVM, DACVIM (Internal Medicine), DACVECC
Tufts University, North Grafton, Massachusetts, USA

John E Rush
DVM, MS, DACVIM (Cardiology), DACVECC
Tufts University, North Grafton, Massachusetts, USA

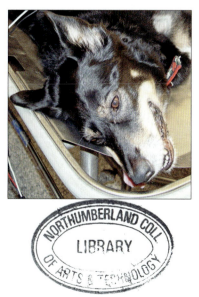

MANSON PUBLISHING/ THE VETERINARY PRESS

This book is dedicated to the memory of Jeff Proulx, DVM, DACVECC.

For full details of all Manson Publishing titles please write to:
Manson Publishing Ltd, 73 Corringham Road, London NW11 7DL, UK.
Tel: +44(0)20 8905 5150
Fax: +44(0)20 8201 9233
Website: www.mansonpublishing.com

Commissioning editor: Jill Northcott
Project manager: Ayala Kingsley
Copy editor: Joanna Brocklesby
Proof reader: John Forder
Book design and layout: Ayala Kingsley, diacriTech
Colour reproduction: Tenon & Polert Colour Scanning Ltd, Hong Kong
Printed by: New Era Printing Co Ltd, Hong Kong

5DW	5% dextrose in water	CV system	cardiovascular system
ACD	acid–citrate–dextrose	CVD	central vestibular disease
ACE	angiotensin-convering enzyme	CVP	central venous pressure
ACR	anticoagulant rodenticide	DC	direct current
ACT	activated clotting time	DEA	dog erythrocyte antigen
ACTH	adrenocorticotropic hormone	DIC	disseminated intravascular coagulation
ALP	alkaline phosphatase	DKA	diabetic ketoacidosis
ALT	alanine aminotransferase	DOCP	desoxycorticosterone pivolate
aPTT	activated partial thromboplastin time	DPL	diagnostic peritoneal lavage
ARDS	acute respiratory distress syndrome	ECG	electrocardiogram
		EEG	electroencephalogram
ARF	acute renal failure	EMD	electromechanical dissociation
ASA	American Society of Anesthesiologists	EMG	electromyography
		FCE	fibrocartilagenous embolism
AST	aspartate aminotransferase	FDP	fibrin(ogen) degradation products
AT	antithrombin	FeLV	feline leukemia virus
ATP	adenosine triphosphate	FFA	free fatty acid
AV	atrioventricular	FFP	fresh frozen plasma
BMBT	buccal mucosal bleeding time	FiO_2	fraction of inspired oxygen
bpm	beats per minute	FIP	feline infectious peritonitis
BPH	benign prostatic hypertrophy	FIV	feline immunodeficiency virus
BUN	blood urea nitrogen	FLUTD	feline lower urinary tract disease
cAMP	cyclic adenosine monophosphate	FP	frozen plasma
CBC	complete blood count	Fr	French gauge
cGMP	cyclic guanosine monophopshate	ga	gauge
CHF	congestive heart failure	GABA	gamma aminobutyric acid
CNS	central nervous system	GDV	gastric dilatation–volvulus
CO_2	carbon dioxide	GFR	glomerular filtration rate
COP	colloid osmotic pressure	GGT	gamma-glutamyl transpeptidase
CPA	cardiopulmonary arrest	GI	gastrointestinal
CPDA-1	citrate–phosphate–dextrose–adenine	HGE	hemorrhagic gastroenteritis
		hpf	high-power field
CPR	cardiopulmonary resuscitation	IM	intramuscularly (used in describing dosages of medication)
CRF	chronic renal failure		
CRH	corticotropin-releasing hormone	ITP	immune-mediated thrombocytopenia
CRI	continuous rate infusion		
CRRT	continuous renal replacement therapy	IV	intravenously (used in describing dosages of medication)
CRTZ	chemoreceptor trigger zone	IVIG	intravenous immunoglobulin
C-section	Cesarean section	IVP	intravenous pyelography
CSF	cerebrospinal fluid	MAH	malignancy-associated hypercalcemia
CT	computed tomography		

MRI	magnetic resonance imaging	U	units
NCPE	noncardiogenic pulmonary edema	UO	urethral obstruction
NPO	*non per os* (nothing by mouth)	US	United States
NSAID	nonsteroidal anti-inflammatory drug	V–Q	ventilation–perfusion
OHE	ovariohysterectomy		
$PaCO_2$	partial pressure of arterial carbon dioxide		
PaO_2	partial pressure of arterial oxygen		
PCV	packed cell volume		
PEG	percutaneous endoscopic gastrostomy		
PES	primary epileptic seizure		
PGF_2	Prostaglandid F_2		
PIVKA	proteins induced by vitamin K absence or antagonism		
PO	*per os* (by mouth)		
PPN	partial parenteral nutrition		
pRBC	packed red blood cells		
PT	prothrombin time		
PTE	pulmonary thromboembolism		
PTH	parathyroid hormone		
PTH-rP	parathyroid hormone related protein		
PTT	partial thromboplastin time		
PU/PD	polyuria/polydipsia		
PVD	peripheral vestibular disease		
RER	resting energy requirement		
RES	reactive epileptic seizure		
SaO_2	arterial oxygen saturation		
SC	subcutaneously (used in describing dosages of medication)		
SES	structural epileptic seizure		
SI	small intestinal		
SIRS	systemic inflammatory response syndrome		
SpO_2	arterial oxygen hemoglobin saturation		
SVT	Supraventricular tachycardia		
TBSA	total body surface area		
TLI	trypsin-like immunoreactivity		
TPN	total parenteral nutrition		
TT	thrombin time		

Emergency and critical care is one of the fastest growing fields of veterinary medicine. Veterinarians engaged in emergency veterinary medical practice must be able to recognize and manage a dizzying array of diseases. Virtually every life-threatening disease can present for emergency evaluation, and the emergency clinician must be prepared to successfully manage all cases. This requires a strong working knowledge of many specialty areas, including internal medicine, neurology, cardiology, oncology, anesthesia, and many other fields. The emergency clinician must be prepared to make a quick assessment or diagnosis, and then follow these decisions with action regarding surgery, diagnostics, and medical interventions. The appropriateness of these actions can mean the difference between life and death for the animal.

In contrast, the critical care veterinary clinician often has a good working knowledge of the primary disease, and some therapy has typically been initiated by the time the critical care veterinarian becomes involved. The criticalist is required to recognize subtle changes in the clinical course of animals, often in a stressful 24-hours-a-day environment, and to take corrective action before severe systemic disease becomes irreversible. Clinical decisions regarding seemingly small items, such as fluid therapy, antibiotics or analgesics, can have a profound impact on patient outcome. The best criticalist uses a combination of years of experience, a solid understanding of pathophysiology of all organ systems, and acute clinical acumen.

This manual is intended to complement comprehensive textbooks of emergency and critical care medicine, and other texts which provide the required fundamental basics of pathophysiology, pharmacology, surgery, or internal medicine. Certain diseases occur commonly, and certain predictable dilemmas arise in the intensive care unit. Some diseases or clinical problems can be best demonstrated or described with accompanying illustrations. The main aim of the book is to discuss management of the common clinical conditions and scenarios that we encounter in our clinical practice, with the hope that these will also be common dilemmas for the reader. There can be many successful approaches in clinical medicine, especially in a rapidly developing field like emergency and critical care, and our biases in the medical and surgical approach to certain diseases will undoubtedly show. We have included figures or illustrations for situations where an image can do greater justice to the topic than a lengthy textual description and have highlighted key information in tabular form. The aim is to bring this information into a small manual which might be a ready resource for clinicians actively engaged in the field. We hope that you will find this manual on the counter or desk more often than on the bookshelf.

PART I

Emergency medicine

Overview of emergency medicine

Emergency medicine represents an exciting and developing field in veterinary medicine. Success in emergency medicine requires a strong knowledge base in all areas of medicine and surgery and the ability to make decisions in an expedient fashion.

Triage refers to the evaluation of patients in order to determine urgency of further therapy and to help prioritize cases for care by the veterinarian and the technician (1). Triage may occur initially over the telephone or may occur when a patient is presented to the animal hospital. 'Telephone triage' may be very difficult to perform safely. In many daytime practices and emergency hospitals, clients frequently call for advice on whether or not a situation is an actual emergency. In practice settings, where the clients are well known to the receptionists or technicians, it may be easier to determine the ability of a client to recognize an emergency in their pet. In general, the safest advice is 'if the client thinks it is an emergency then the pet should be seen'. However, it may be possible to help the client over the phone.

Any animal that has collapsed, is having difficulty breathing, or has suffered a major trauma should obviously be seen immediately without the need to ask further questions. Otherwise, basic questions regarding signalment, past medical history, and clinical signs exhibited by the pet should be asked. It is important to maintain control of the conversation politely but firmly. The receptionist/technician should try to verify the stability of the major body systems (cardiovascular, respiratory, and neurological).

Ideally the emergency policy of the practice should be well understood among all employees and be well explained to the clients prior to the development of an emergency situation. For example, some practices always (24 hours a day) want to see their own emergencies, while other hospitals elect to refer some emergencies to other facilities, depending on the time of day and the activity level in the hospital.

Appropriate triage of the patient presented to the animal hospital is an important job for the veterinary technician in all types of veterinary hospitals. All animals that are presented for emergency care should be evaluated by a technician for stability within moments of arrival. Some

I Triage protocol.

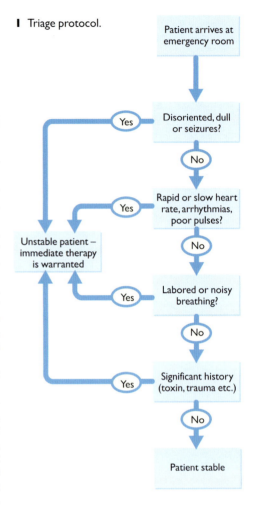

emergency conditions require immediate therapy to prevent the death of the patient. The patient should be rapidly evaluated for stability of the major body systems. A brief ('capsule') history from the owner should also be obtained. A triage should generally be able to be completed within 2–3 min of patient arrival.

The ABCs (airway, breathing, circulation) should be immediately assessed. The technician should try to follow a systematic approach to triage to ensure that no step is overlooked and to help with efficiency. The breathing pattern and effort should be evaluated. Any animal appearing to have difficulty breathing requires immediate further therapy. Loud or noisy breathing often suggests upper airway obstruction, such as may occur with laryngeal paralysis. Short, shallow breathing suggests pleural space disease, such as pleural effusion or pneumothorax. Labored breathing often indicates low oxygen levels (hypoxemia) that may occur with pneumonia or CHF. The cardiovascular system may be evaluated by checking the mucous membrane color and capillary refill time, heart rate, and the pulse quality.

The neurological status of the pet should also be evaluated. A typical dog or cat should be alert and oriented to his environment. Any mental depression suggests that further evaluation is indicated. The bladder of any male cat with abnormal behavior should be palpated for possible obstruction. Finally, the capsule history from the owner should be evaluated for any historical complaints that would require rapid therapy (such as the ingestion of rat poison or other toxins).

After triage, patients should be assigned to either the 'stable' or 'not stable' category. Patients that are stable should be cared for using the standard approach at the specific veterinary hospital.

Patients that are unstable should have immediate care begun (**2**).

Patients with signs of cardiovascular instability (tachycardia, weak pulses, prolonged capillary refill time), should be immediately placed on a treatment table and given supplemental oxygen. An intravenous catheter should be placed and blood samples should be collected for analysis (ideally a CBC, biochemistry profile, and urinalysis) but minimally a PCV/total solids/glucose/azo-stik. Shock fluid therapy may be begun if there is no concern about cardiogenic shock.

Patients with respiratory instability should be administered supplemental oxygen and kept in a quiet environment. Pets (particularly cats) are intolerant of stresses when respiratory distress is present so testing should be kept to a minimum. Animals demonstrating mental depression should be evaluated for metabolic causes and placed in a cage where their mental status can be easily assessed. Some animals that appear depressed may be weak from other causes, such as anemia or hypoglycemia.

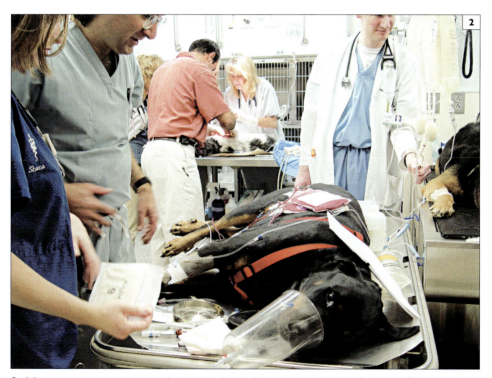

2 A busy emergency service may have several critical patients to treat simultaneously. Personnel should be available and the room equipped and fully stocked.

CHAPTER 1

Shock

- **Hypovolemic shock**

- **Sepsis/septic shock**

- **Cardiogenic shock**

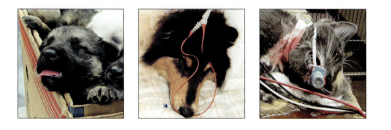

Shock, or ineffective oxygen delivery, may result from a variety of causes. Classically, in veterinary medicine, shock is divided into hypovolemic, septic, and cardiogenic shock. The common feature of these is the failure to adequately deliver sufficient oxygenated blood to meet the cellular needs. Animals assessed as unstable during triage will often be in shock. While each patient should be individually assessed, a flow chart may help to guide the clinician in determining the class of shock (3).

Hypovolemic shock

Hypovolemic shock develops when there is inadequate circulating blood volume to deliver oxygen effectively to the tissues. Hypovolemic shock results from either blood loss or progressive interstitial dehydration leading to intravascular depletion.

Successful treatment is aimed at restoring deficits and correcting the initial cause of the loss. Hypovolemic shock is considered the most common type of shock detected in animals. Estimates for the volumes of blood loss that may be tolerated vary depending on the patient. Certainly, a young healthy dog will tolerate blood loss significantly better than an older pet. Healthy dogs may tolerate up to a 40% loss of blood volume, or approximately 35–40 ml/kg.

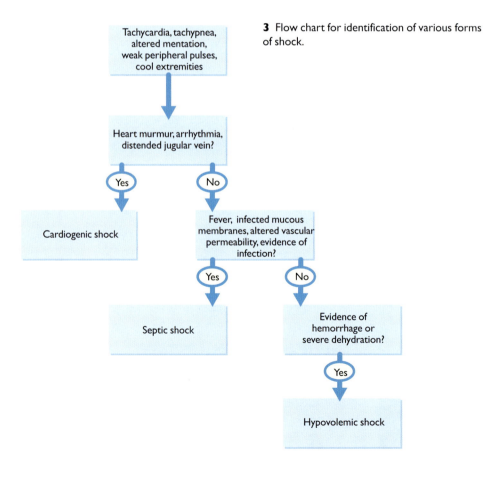

3 Flow chart for identification of various forms of shock.

The treatment approach to hypovolemic shock requires several steps:

1. Rapid placement of at least one short, large-bore intravenous catheter. Recommended sizes of catheter are 25–50 mm (1–2 inch), 14–16 ga in dogs >20 kg (>44 lb); 16–18 ga in dogs 10–20 kg (22–44 lb); and 18–20 ga in dogs <10 kg (<22 lb) and cats. If need be, placement may be facilitated by performing a mini or full cut-down. In most cases, the jugular and/or the cephalic vein should be used. The most skilled individual should initially secure venous access; afterwards, less experienced individuals should attempt to place second and third lines.

2. Administration of a volume and type of fluid to restore adequate perfusion. Estimates of the blood volume for cats and dogs are 90 ml/kg and 60 ml/kg respectively. Commonly, due to low cost and widespread availability, crystalloid fluids (e.g. lactated Ringer's solution, 0.9% NaCl) are initially chosen. Multiple (up to four) boluses of 10–20 ml/kg are administered over 10–15 min and the effect on clinical signs (e.g. heart rate, respiratory rate, mucous membrane color, and pulse quality) are observed. If desired, resuscitation may be undertaken with colloids (e.g. dextrans, etherified starch) with boluses of 2–5 ml/kg repeated q10–20 min until a good response is observed. In very large dogs, or those with concurrent head injury or pulmonary contusion, fluid resuscitation with hypertonic saline (7.5%) may be performed. Hypertonic saline is dosed at 4–6 ml/kg as a rapid bolus and then ideally followed with 5–15 ml/kg of colloid to prolong the effect of the hypertonic saline. In cases of severe hemorrhagic shock, transfusion with packed red blood cells or whole blood is indicated.

3. The underlying cause for the hypovolemia must be aggressively identified and corrected. Surgical intervention is often warranted, and will be more successful if performed as soon as the pet is stable enough for surgery.

For more complete details, see also Chapter 15: Fluid therapy for critical care patients.

Hypotensive resuscitation is a specific form of therapy for hypovolemic shock from hemorrhage. The goal of this therapy is to maintain blood pressure in a range that is adequate for perfusion to vital organs but not so high as to 'blow off' developing clots. In people, this form of therapy is linked with operative control of hemorrhage, so this may not be directly applicable to dogs and cats. However, it may be prudent to carefully titrate fluid therapy and patient manipulations to avoid disrupting any forming clot. Coagulopathy may develop by dilution of clotting factors with crystalloids and colloids, particularly in the face of ongoing hemorrhage.

Hypovolemic shock is very rewarding to treat. It is essential to continually reassess the patient to ensure adequate volume status. Animals that have significant ongoing losses, such as severe vomiting, diarrhea, PU/PD, or hemorrhage are particularly challenging.

Two specific scenarios may be used to highlight the therapeutic approach in hypovolemia.

CASE 1
Signalment
A 40 kg (88 lb) Labrador Retriever has been hit by a car. It presents to the veterinary hospital about 20 minutes after the accident.

Initial physical examination
- Dull but responsive, increased respiratory rate but no increased effort, heart rate 180 bpm, weak pulses.
- Initial test results: PCV 45%, total solids 54.0 g/l (5.4 g/dl).
- Chest radiographs document a small cardiac silhouette, vena cava, and liver.
- Ultrasonographic examination of the abdomen reveals a large volume of effusion.
- Abdominocentesis confirms hemoabdomen.

Recall that the low presenting total solids is a strong indictor of hemorrhage in a trauma patient.

Assessment
Hypovolemia due to hemorrhagic shock from trauma.

Initial fluid resuscitation
Half of the calculated shock dose of fluid should be infused.

Shock dose = 90 ml/kg/hr (40 kg × 90 ml/kg) = 3600 ml

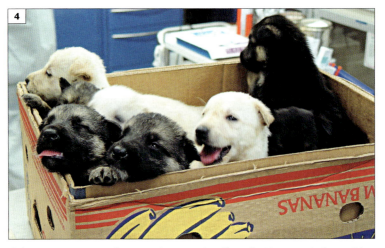

4 It is not uncommon for entire litters to be affected with parvoviral enteritis.

Thus 1.5–2 l of a balanced crystalloid solution should be infused over 15–30 min. If an improvement in heart rate and other cardiovascular parameters is observed, then the infusion rate should be decreased. However, if no improvement is detected, then the remaining 50% should be infused, and thought should be given to supplemental colloid therapy (such as etherified starch) or blood transfusion. Failure to stabilize and persistent hypovolemia suggest ongoing hemorrhage. In some cases, an exploratory celiotomy is warranted to control the source of hemorrhage. Abdominal wraps are frequently used and may be beneficial provided respiratory impairment is not present.

CASE 2
Signalment
A 12-week-old mixed breed puppy, weight 5 kg (11 lb), has had vomiting and bloody diarrhea for 3 days, and is now collapsed. It is not vaccinated against parvovirus.

Physical examination
- 12–15% dehydrated, collapsed, heart rate 180 bpm, respiratory rate 30 breaths/min, temperature 36.7°C (98°F), very weak pulses.
- Initial laboratory tests: PCV 42%, total solids 74.0 g/l (7.4 g/dl), blood glucose too low to measure, examination of the blood smear documents profound leukopenia.

Assessment
Profound dehydration leading to hypovolemia, suspect underlying parvoviral infection (**4**).

Initial fluid resuscitation
This includes restoring intravascular volume, correcting hypoglycemia, and providing for ongoing losses. Immediate therapy for hypoglycemia should include an intravenous bolus of 0.5–1 ml/kg of 50% dextrose diluted in a 1:3 ratio with a crystalloid. The shock dose of fluids is 90 ml/kg × 5 kg = 450 ml of crystalloid. Since the puppy is also profoundly dehydrated, the entire 450 ml should be infused over 30–45 min. If the puppy is improved, he should be continued on a rate designed to replace deficits, and provide for maintenance needs and ongoing losses (see also Chapter 15: Fluid therapy for critical care patients). However, if he is not improved, an additional bolus of fluids, either another 200–250 ml of crystalloid or 50–75 ml of a colloid is warranted.

Sepsis/septic shock

Septic shock refers to patients with evidence of systemic inflammation, infection, and hypotension that is refractory to fluid resuscitation. Sepsis, severe sepsis, and septic shock are terms that have been used to define a continuum of systemic response to infection. In 1992 a consensus was reached to apply specific definitions for these terms as they relate to people with critical illness. Since systemic inflammation associated with an infectious process is also a common cause of critical illness in veterinary medicine, these definitions have been extrapolated for use in dogs and cats.

SIRS is a systemic response to a severe insult and consists of changes in two of more of the following criteria:
- Heart rate (tachycardia).
- Respiratory rate (tachypnea).
- Temperature (fever or hypothermia).
- White blood cell count (leukocytosis or leukopenia or >3% bands).

The cause of SIRS does not have to be bacterial, and can originate from viral, protozoal, or fungal infections as well.

Sepsis describes a condition in which systemic inflammation (SIRS) occurs along with evidence of infection. In addition to the changes listed above, these patients must have either a positive microbiological culture, histological evidence of infection, or intracellular bacteria visualized on cytology. Other abnormalities that are frequently found in dogs or cats with sepsis include hypoglycemia, hyperbilirubinemia, hypoalbuminemia, and thrombocytopenia. Coagulation times including the PT and the aPTT may be prolonged in those animals developing DIC. During the initial stages of sepsis, compensatory mechanisms ensure adequate oxygen delivery to tissues despite changes in vascular resistance.

Septic shock develops when compensatory mechanisms are overwhelmed. Tissues are no longer adequately perfused, and oxygen delivery cannot be maintained despite aggressive fluid resuscitation. In veterinary medicine, little is known about the true incidence of septic shock. Cats with systemic inflammation in general are much more susceptible to profound hypotension that is difficult to correct.

Successful treatment of septic shock is based on restoration of oxygen delivery through the use of fluid therapy, antibiotics, identification of an underlying cause, and vasopressors.

FLUID THERAPY

Due to changes in vascular permeability and losses through cavitary effusions, hypoalbuminemia is common in septic shock and can be profound. As crystalloids may contribute to peripheral edema in states of reduced colloid osmotic pressure, colloids such as etherified starch (e.g. hetastarch) (10–20 ml/kg/day in the dog, 5–10 ml/kg/day in the cat) are frequently added. While fresh frozen plasma can be used for the correction of a coagulopathy, it should not be considered a significant source of albumin except in very small patients. Recombinant bovine purified hemoglobin solution (Oxyglobin®), acts as an oxygen-delivering colloid and may improve oxygen delivery in animals with septic shock. Caution must be employed when administering Oxyglobin® to cats, as those with occult cardiomyopathy or cats that have been aggressively resuscitated with crystalloids may experience volume overload as a result of its administration. Additionally, Oxyglobin® is currently only licensed for use in dogs. The exact volume of fluids to administer can be difficult to determine in the patient with sepsis. Monitoring of CVP can be helpful if a central line has been placed (jugular or saphenous in cats). Animals with reduced CVP (<5 cmH$_2$O) and reduced urine production may require additional fluid therapy for volume support while those with CVP >10–12 cmH$_2$O should have the fluid rate either stopped or markedly decreased. Urine output should be closely monitored, and the total volume of fluids administered should be compared with the volume of fluid produced (via urine, drains, vomit) several times per day.

ANTIBIOTICS

Coupled with fluid support, and the search for an underlying cause, antibiotics are vital in successful therapy for sepsis. While awaiting bacterial culture and sensitivity testing results, broad-spectrum antibiotics are warranted. Antibiotics should be effective against Gram-positive, Gram-negative, and anaerobic organisms. Commonly used combinations include ampicillin–gentamicin or cefazolin–enrofloxacin–metronidazole. In patients with suspected nosocomial infection, antimicrobials should be effective against known endemic pathogens.

IDENTIFICATION OF AN UNDERLYING CAUSE

Rapid identification and correction of an underlying source of sepsis are vital to successful outcome. Thoracic and abdominal radiographs are useful, as is abdominal ultrasonography (**5**). Collections of septic fluid should be drained and the source eliminated. Pyometra should be excluded in every intact female dog. Common sources of sepsis in cats and dogs include pneumonia (dogs more frequently than cats), septic peritonitis, urosepsis, pyometra, and pyothorax. Surgical therapy (where warranted) should be undertaken as soon as the patient is stable enough to tolerate the intervention (**6**).

VASOPRESSORS

A vasopressor should be added when hypotension persists despite adequate and aggressive fluid administration as evidenced by a CVP > 8–10 cmH$_2$O. Traditionally, dopamine has been the first-line pressor agent used for the treatment of hypotension in the intensive care unit. Administered at a dose of 5–10 µg/kg/ min, dopamine stimulates β_1 receptors and acts as a positive inotrope. At doses >10 µg/kg/ min, α_1 effects predominate and vasoconstriction occurs. In cases where dopamine fails to restore blood pressure, other pressors can be used until the desired effect is achieved. If hypotension persists despite dopamine therapy, then another pressor, such as norepinephrine (noradrenaline) can be added (0.5–3 µg/kg/min). No studies exist comparing the efficacy of various pressors in critically ill animals, and the choice of drug is often based on individual preference and personal experience.

Studies in people investigating effects of sepsis on adrenal gland function and cortisol production suggest that some patients with septic shock may have reduced cortisol production, and an abnormal response to the ACTH stimulation test. One study investigating adrenal gland dysfunction in dogs admitted to an intensive care unit found no evidence of adrenal insufficiency, however more studies are warranted to determine if adrenal gland dysfunction contributes to the hypotension seen in this species.

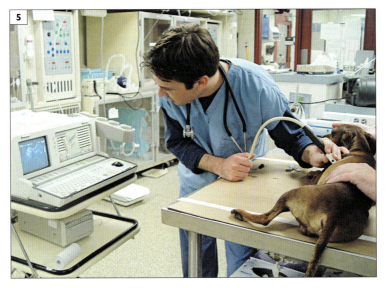

5 Using ultrasound in the ER.

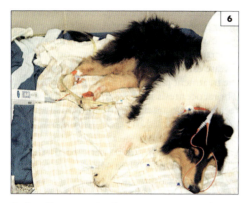

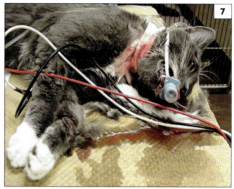

6 A collie recovering from surgery to repair a septic abdomen. Note the nasal oxygen providing supplemental oxygen. This dog was suffering from SIRS and had acute lung injury.

7 A cat following unsuccessful CPR. The cat had developed respiratory distress earlier in the day and was presented agonally. There is a large amount of pulmonary edema which has drained from the endotracheal tube. Post-mortem examination confirmed severe hypertrophic cardiomyopathy and death from cardiogenic shock.

Cardiogenic shock

Cardiogenic shock is present when the heart fails, as a pump, to deliver an adequate amount of blood and oxygen to the body, which results in hypoperfusion of organs and tissues. The heart can fail to generate adequate stroke volume and cardiac output due to reduced contractile (systolic) function, impaired myocardial diastolic function, severe valvular disease, pericardial or other constraint to cardiac filling, or severe cardiac arrhythmia. Dilated cardiomyopathy is the most common cause of reduced contractile function leading to cardiogenic shock. In cats, hypertrophic cardiomyopathy is the predominant cause of severe diastolic dysfunction leading to cardiogenic shock (7). Valvular disease severe enough to cause cardiogenic shock is uncommon in the cat but can be seen in dogs with advanced chronic valvular disease, especially those with rupture of a chorda tendinae or papillary muscle. Diseases that can cause constraint or limitation to cardiac filling sufficient to result in cardiogenic shock include pericardial effusion with tamponade, constrictive pericarditis, and tension pneumothorax. Ventricular tachycardia and severe bradycardia, such as third degree AV block, are the most common arrhythmic causes of cardiogenic shock. Finally, myocardial dysfunction resulting from overdose of certain drugs, such as beta-blockers and calcium channel blockers, can cause or contribute to shock.

Cardiogenic shock is recognized by the presence of clinical and laboratory findings of hypoperfusion in the absence of hypovolemia, sepsis, neurological, or other noncardiac disorders. Typical clinical findings are similar to those seen in other forms of shock and include muscular weakness, mucous membrane pallor, delayed capillary refill time, weak arterial pulses, cool limbs, elevated blood lactate, metabolic acidosis, azotemia, oliguria, hypotension, and decreased mental acuity. Dyspnea and tachycardia are often noted. Hypothermia may exist and is particularly common in cats with cardiogenic shock. The effect of hypothermia on the sinus node may blunt the expected clinical finding of tachycardia. Unlike in other forms of shock, the jugular vein is often distended and/or thoracic radiographs will document evidence of CHF, such as pulmonary edema or pleural effusion. CVP and/or pulmonary capillary wedge pressure are typically elevated in animals with cardiogenic shock, unless cardiogenic shock is accompanied by concurrent volume depletion. Cardiac arrhythmia is usually easily identified as severe bradycardia or tachycardia with abnormal arterial pulse quality.

Cardiopulmonary resuscitation

KEY POINTS
- A well executed CPR (cardiopulmonary resuscitation) attempt has a higher chance of success than a badly executed one (**8**).
- Animals often have severe underlying disease prior to arrest, rather than sudden ventricular fibrillation as may affect people.

DEFINITION/OVERVIEW
CPR is a set of procedures and pharmacological interventions designed to increase oxygen delivery to the heart and the brain during cardiac arrest (**9**). The ultimate goal of CPR is to restore spontaneous, effective cardiac and respiratory efforts. CPA (cardiopulmonary arrest) is present when there is a sudden and unexpected cessation of heart function and/or when cardiac pumping failure results in loss of consciousness and eventual respiratory arrest. Respiratory arrest develops when ventilatory failure leads to a loss of consciousness that, unless corrected, rapidly leads to combined CPA.

ETIOLOGY AND RISK FACTORS
Common rhythm disorders identified at the time of CPA in dogs and cats include asystole, ventricular fibrillation, sinus bradycardia, and EMD (electromechanical dissociation). The arrhythmia may be the result of primary cardiac disease (e.g. dilated cardiomyopathy) or severe systemic disease which has lead to cardiac instability (e.g. trauma, pancreatitis). Thromboembolic disorders, such as PTE or thromboembolic disease to the coronary arteries, are other possible causes of sudden, otherwise unexplained CPA.

Factors which often contribute to CPA include hypoxemia or cellular hypoxia due to respiratory disease and/or poor tissue perfusion, hypovolemia or fluid overload, narcotics administered for analgesia or other anesthetic agents, acidosis, anemia, CNS depression leading to reduced ventilatory drive from disease or drugs, coagulopathy, electrolyte disturbance, and myocardial disease.

A pre-existing cardiovascular, respiratory, or CNS disorder is typically present in dogs and cats with spontaneous CPA. Following CPR in any individual case, it can be informative to review the factors present before arrest (e.g. disease of heart, brain, or lungs) that led to CPA, and determine whether any of them might have been managed differently. It is useful to review these factors, and learn from the arrest, in order to better recognize and treat contributing CPA risk factors in future cases and be better able to avoid CPA in future cases. A prevented CPA is always preferable to a successful CPR effort.

DIFFERENTIAL DIAGNOSES
The differential diagnoses for CPA include seizure disorders and syncope.

DIAGNOSIS
CPA is identified by combined lack of respiratory and cardiac activity with loss of consciousness. Cardiac arrest is confirmed by a lack of arterial pulses, absence of cardiac sounds on auscultation, and/or ECG findings indicative of cardiac arrest (i.e. ventricular fibrillation, asystole, and so on). Isolated respiratory arrest is present when failed ventilatory effort leads to agonal breathing and then loss of consciousness, although cardiac function is present and arterial pulses are palpable.

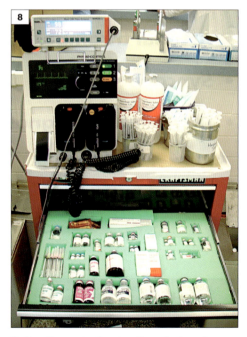

8 A well organized and well stocked crash cart, combined with practice sessions with key employees, can make a huge difference in the outcome of CPR.

9 Algorithm for cardiopulmonary resuscitation.

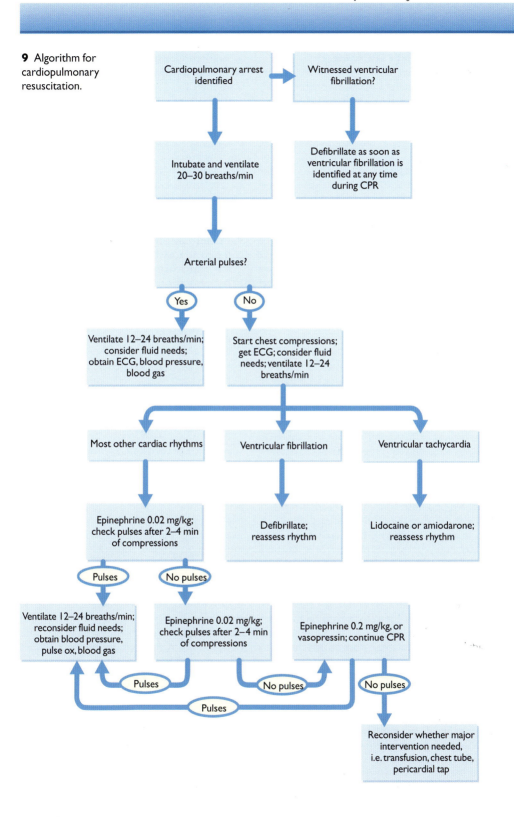

MANAGEMENT / TREATMENT
Airway
Once agonal breathing or loss of consciousness is identified the first step is to intubate. Obstructions to the airway are usually immediately apparent during endotracheal intubation, and in cases of fixed upper airway obstruction (i.e. due to a large mass) a slash tracheotomy may be required. The endotracheal tube should have the cuff filled in order to ensure adequate manual ventilation, and the endotracheal tube should (eventually) be secured in place to prevent dislodgement as the animal is turned for defibrillation or other maneuvers. Suctioning of the airway may be required for animals with massive edema, and animals can be briefly tipped into a head-down vertical position, with brief chest compressions, in order to help drain edema fluid from the airway.

Breathing
Manual ventilation is immediately initiated at a rate of 20–30 breaths/min for the first minute with 100% oxygen, and then the rate is reduced to between 12 and 24 breaths/min. Immediate adjustments to the rate or effort of manual or mechanical ventilation can be made following assessment of the amount of pressure required to fill the lungs and the degree of rise and fall of the thorax. Inadequate filling of the endotracheal cuff is a common cause for inadequate rise of the chest wall with low pressure, and pneumothorax should be a differential diagnosis if increases in ventilatory pressure develop during CPR.

Respiratory alkalosis from excessive ventilation should be avoided. Manual or mechanical ventilation should be continued until long after the onset of spontaneous respiratory efforts. Following CPA, most animals will not have *effective* respiratory drive or ventilatory effort at the time that they first start to breathe on their own or start to chew on the endotracheal tube. It is advised that a very low dose of diazepam or a narcotic be given to permit ongoing intubation, and that manual or mechanical ventilation be continued for at least 20 min following the onset of spontaneous efforts at ventilation. The authors *do not* recommend use of acupuncture points and do not recommend cessation of ventilation in order to determine whether the animal is able to breathe using its own effort at any time during the CPR effort. All animals that eventually recover will breathe on their own, and to stop ventilation and watch for spontaneous effort only contributes to hypoxemia and tissue compromise.

Circulation, drugs, and fluids
Lack of palpable femoral or lingual pulse, and/or lack of cardiac sounds should rapidly confirm the presence of cardiac arrest. Following intubation, initiation of breathing, and confirmation of cardiac arrest, efforts at cardiac compression should be initiated. CPR is ideally performed with the animal in right lateral recumbency to facilitate venous return to the heart.

- In small dogs the hands are placed lower on the chest, over the heart, and compression of the heart is initiated at a rate of 70–90 compressions/min.
- In some small-breed dogs more effective cardiac compressions can be achieved using one hand on either side of the thorax, instead of two hands on top of the thorax with the table as the base to press against.
- In cats the heart can often be stabilized and compressed using a single hand with the thumb on one side of the thorax and three fingers on the other side of the chest.
- For medium- to large-breed dogs both hands are usually placed higher on the chest wall and the chest and heart are compressed between the table and the hands.

The more dorsal hand location in large-breed dogs is based on the recognition that effective compressions may occur from either the cardiac pump mechanism (direct cardiac compression) or the thoracic pump mechanism (increase in intrathoracic pressure forces blood out of the chest cavity and valves prevent retrograde flow). It is suspected that direct cardiac compression can be achieved in cats and small-breed dogs; however the thoracic pump mechanism may be more important for large-breed dogs. Some authors recommend dorsal recumbency with compression of the sternum during CPR for medium- to large-breed dogs; however, the authors have not found this technique to be more effective and have not adopted it in their institution. The duty cycle, or duration of compression to relaxation, should be approximately 50:50 with equal time devoted to each phase.

A large number of adjunctive CPR procedures have been proposed and include techniques such as interposed abdominal compression, active-compression–decompression CPR, simultaneous ventilation and chest compression, and a number of other interesting techniques. It is still acceptable, and it is the authors' routine practice, to employ standard CPR and to make no serious attempt to coordinate the chest compressions and the ventilations.

Successful cardiac compression is documented by palpation of femoral or lingual arterial pulses (**10**). If pulses are not identified then CPR efforts should be evaluated and adjusted. Possible interventions to restore pulses include adjustment of compression effort or rate, adjustment of hand position to higher or lower on the thorax, administration of epinephrine and/or vasopressin, administration of crystalloids or colloids, and open-chest CPR for manual cardiac compression. The temptation to stop chest compression to check on the cardiac rhythm should be resisted as each stoppage of CPR leads to a rapid (3–5 s) drop in blood pressure and it requires 25–45 s of CPR before blood pressure returns to the prior CPR-effected level. Hand position and compression effort can be adjusted prior to the identification of a cardiac rhythm; however the authors recommend ECG evaluation prior to administration of drugs or initiation of open-chest CPR in most cases.

Ventricular fibrillation is only effectively treated with electrical DC defibrillation. Defibrillation should be attempted as soon as the rhythm is identified, as any delay in defibrillation rapidly reduces the chance of a successful conversion. Epinephrine should *not* be routinely administered prior to defibrillation. Proposed initial energy settings for external defibrillation are 2–4 J/kg body weight. Energy required for internal defibrillation during open-chest CPR is much lower with a recommended dose of 5–50 J. An initial defibrillation effort should be followed by evaluation of the cardiac rhythm, and an immediate repeat shock at the same energy should be attempted if ventricular fibrillation persists. If this fails to result in conversion then a higher energy setting (increased by 20–50%) is selected, defibrillation is performed, and if unsuccessful then chest compression and CPR are continued with subsequent administration of epinephrine, vasopressin, or other therapies for 2–3 min before another attempt at defibrillation.

Asystole is recognized by a total lack of cardiac activity. Asystole is treated with continued cardiac compression and administration of epinephrine.

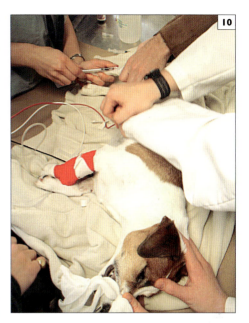

10 Cardiopulmonary resuscitation often requires a number of individuals and several simultaneous actions. In this dog, one person is performing ventilation with an Ambu bag, another is checking for femoral arterial pulses, one is performing chest compressions, and another is drawing blood to check for correctable abnormalities in serum electrolytes, pH, or blood glucose. An ECG is being recorded, the dog has just received a dose of epinephrine intravenously, and intravenous fluids are being administered to restore recent blood loss.

EMD is recognized as an electrocardiographically identifiable rhythm that is not accompanied by palpable arterial pulses (11). EMD can be the result of inadequate venous return to the heart due to hypovolemia, cardiac tamponade, or tension pneumothorax, or it may result from severe acidosis, myocardial hypoxia, or severe myocardial dysfunction, hypoxia, or ischemia. EMD due to myocardial disease is rarely reversible, however efforts to identify and treat hypovolemia, pleural or pericardial space disease, metabolic or respiratory acidosis, and severe electrolyte imbalance can often be rewarding. Sodium bicarbonate may be useful in animals with EMD or asystole and known pre-existing acidosis or hyperkalemia, and calcium administration can be used in animals with known or documented hypocalcemia or hyperkalemia. Sinus bradycardia can be treated with atropine, and if this is ineffective then epinephrine can be administered.

Ventricular tachycardia that develops during the course of CPR should be assessed for heart rate and the presence of a pulse-generating rhythm. Ventricular tachycardia at a rate <200 bpm that results in arterial pulses should generally not be treated, as the resulting rhythm might be asystole. If the rate during ventricular tachycardia starts to rise to >240 bpm then the chance of ventricular fibrillation increases and the likelihood of effective pulses decreases so administration of lidocaine or amiodarone is recommended.

Epinephrine

Epinephrine has long been a recommended therapy for dogs and cats with CPA. The positive inotropic and chronotropic effects of epinephrine stimulate cardiac contractile function via β-receptors, and epinephrine stimulates α-receptors to create vasoconstriction and increases in blood pressure. It may be that the α-mediated effects of epinephrine are more important than the β-mediated effects in some cases. The increase in blood from vaso-constriction leads to improved coronary and cerebral blood flow. The enhanced vasoconstriction seen with higher doses of epinephrine (0.2 mg/kg) compared with standard doses (0.02 mg/kg) has resulted in a debate about the relative merits of high-dose vs. low-dose (standard-dose) epinephrine administration. High-dose epinephrine (0.2 mg/kg) is associated with myocardial injury and myocardial calcium overload leading to reduced function in the post-CPR timeframe. It also increases the risk for epinephrine-induced ventricular fibrillation. For these reasons, most authors currently recommend use of standard-dose epinephrine initially (0.02 mg/kg). If this dose is ineffective then epinephrine administration can be repeated every 2–3 min with dose escalation until the desired response is achieved.

Vasopressin

New research supports the use of vasopressin (antidiuretic hormone) during CPR to improve vascular tone and blood pressure. The proposed dose in dogs is 0.8 U/kg IV. Further research is required in order to determine whether epinephrine, vasopressin, or a combination of the two drugs is most useful for CPR.

Fluids

Routine administration of large volumes of crystalloid fluids during CPR may not be required for successful outcome. In fact, animals known to have pre-existing cardiac failure, respiratory failure with pulmonary edema or infiltration, or CNS edema formation may be adversely affected by administration of large volumes of crystalloid or colloid fluids during CPR. Prior to administration of fluids during CPR, some effort should

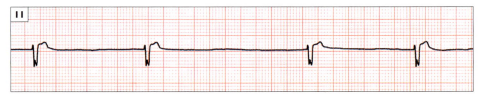

11 ECG obtained from a dog during the course of cardiopulmonary resuscitation. There are defined QRS-T complexes but there were no corresponding arterial pulses, leading to a clinical diagnosis of EMD, also referred to as pulseless electrical activity (PEA).

be made to consider the role of edema formation in the underlying disease process, the serum albumin level, and whether the animal is hypovolemic or in a state of overhydration at the time of CPA. Fluid administration is clearly appropriate for animals with known hypovolemia. Crystalloid fluids or colloids can be useful in normovolemic animals that develop loss of effective circulating volume due to fluid pooling in venous structures shortly after CPR. The volume of fluid returning to the heart is easily assessed during open-chest CPR based on palpation of cardiac filling during the diastolic phase of manual compression, however this can be very difficult to evaluate during closed-chest CPR.

Open-chest cardiac compression

Open-chest CPR can result in significantly greater increases in cardiac output when compared with closed-chest CPR. However, there is little evidence that open-chest CPR will improve outcome. In addition, open-chest CPR leads to a huge resource and personnel utilization and creates an entirely new set of complications not seen with closed-chest CPR. There are certain clinical settings where early open-chest CPR is indicated or preferred and these include CPA associated with tension pneumothorax, large-volume pleural effusion, flail chest, diaphragmatic hernia, and cardiac tamponade. If the decision has been made that the owner wishes to proceed to open-chest CPR if closed-chest CPR is unsuccessful then the clinician is advised to make this decision early, in the first 5 min after closed-chest CPR is initiated. A step-by-step description of open-chest CPR is beyond the scope of this chapter, however the following advice is offered based on observation of multiple efforts by a variety of individuals:

- The incision made is often too far forward and this can make it difficult to grasp the heart – the incision must be at either the fifth or sixth intercostal space.
- Entry to the thorax in a somewhat uncontrolled fashion often leads to lung lobe laceration, therefore care is advised for this step.
- It can be difficult to grasp and incise the pericardium, an essential step for good open-chest CPR, and laceration of the myocardium, coronary artery, or atrium may occur when this incision is made in a poorly controlled fashion.

- The heart should be compressed in an apical to basilar fashion in order to maximize the effectiveness of compressions.
- The individual performing cardiac massage should make a conscious effort to assess cardiac filling during diastole to assess the need for more fluids. In addition, the degree of cardiac tone and vigor of contraction can be assessed which allows for feedback to others participating in CPR relative to inotropic state and the need for inotropic therapy. In most cases, the author finds that a component of active diastolic filling with increased cardiac tone will precede the onset of effective systolic contractile function.

Post-resuscitation care

A critical factor in successful CPR is the effort of those involved in post-resuscitation care. A repeated episode of CPA is common, and to avoid a repeat arrest it is usually essential to identify at least one major contributing factor to the arrest and eliminate this factor. Possible examples of risk factors that could be corrected include some of the following:

- Pleural space disease is corrected by centesis.
- Anemia is treated with transfusion.
- Respiratory failure is managed with mechanical ventilation.
- Narcotics are reversed and then either discontinued or used in lower doses.

Serial monitoring is recommended in the first 24 hours with techniques such as continuous ECG monitoring, pulse oximetry, serial blood lactate and blood gases, blood pressure, urine output and/or CVP measurement, and end-tidal CO_2 until extubated. Infusions of positive inotropes, like dopamine or dobutamine, are indicated for animals with hypotension or myocardial depression.

PROGNOSIS

The outcome from CPR efforts in veterinary patients may appear to be rather poor as only 2–20% of cases will survive to hospital discharge. The author's experience is that a 5–7% survival to hospital discharge is a reasonable expectation for dogs and cats.

Congestive heart failure in the dog

12 Algorithm for congestive heart failure.

KEY POINTS

- Thoracic radiographs are essential to definitively diagnose congestive heart failure (CHF) (**12**).
- For CHF, high doses of furosemide, either as a bolus or as a CRI, are often effective.
- In severe CHF, either sodium nitroprusside or intubation and intermittent positive pressure ventilation may be successful.

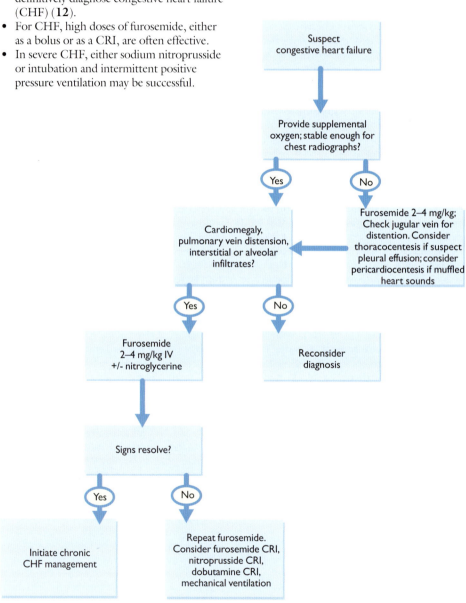

DEFINITION / OVERVIEW

CHF may be defined as the presence of fluid accumulation in the lungs (pulmonary edema), pleural space (pleural effusion), abdominal cavity (ascites), or pericardial sac (pericardial effusion) due to cardiac dysfunction. Cardiogenic fluid accumulation only occurs in dogs with elevated diastolic ventricular and/or atrial filling pressures. Left-sided CHF develops in dogs with elevated left heart filling pressures and leads to pulmonary edema with or without small-volume pleural effusion. Right-sided CHF occurs in dogs with elevated right heart filling pressures and is manifest as ascites with or without pleural effusion. Most dogs with large-volume pleural effusion have biventricular heart failure with elevated right and left heart filling pressures.

ETIOLOGY AND RISK FACTORS

The most common causes of CHF in the dog are acquired chronic valvular disease and dilated cardiomyopathy. Acquired chronic valvular disease, or endocardiosis, primarily affects the mitral valve, although up to one third of affected dogs have both mitral and tricuspid regurgitation. Pericardial effusion is also a cause of CHF, usually in large-breed dogs. Dogs with congenital heart disease may also develop CHF, as can dogs with bacterial endocarditis and a variety of uncommon cardiac disorders.

Large- and giant-breed dogs are predisposed to dilated cardiomyopathy. The condition has also been recognized in Cocker Spaniels. Small and medium-size breeds of dogs are predisposed to chronic valvular disease. CHF is more usual in middle-aged to older dogs, but can develop as a result of congenital disease; dilated cardiomyopathy can be seen within the first few years of life. In general, there is a slight predisposition for the development of CHF in male dogs.

PATHOPHYSIOLOGY

CHF develops after ventricular diastolic filling pressures rise to abnormally high levels. This elevated pressure is transmitted back to the venous system and the elevated capillary pressures lead to fluid exudation into the interstitium and edema formation. Left-sided CHF, most commonly observed as pulmonary edema in dogs (13), often develops after the left ventricular or left atrial filling pressures rise above 15–20 mmHg. Right-sided CHF, recognized as ascites and/or pleural effusion, develops in most dogs once right heart filling pressures rise above 10–12 mmHg. In some dogs, chronic left heart failure leads to elevations in pulmonary arterial pressures and biventricular heart failure develops. Biventricular heart failure is identified as combined pulmonary edema, pleural effusion, and ascites.

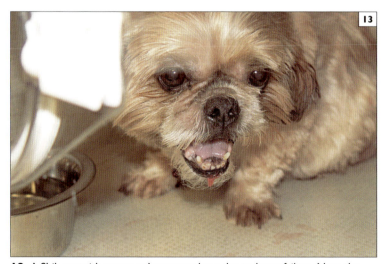

13 A Shih-tzu with severe pulmonary edema due to heart failure. Note the expectorated pulmonary edema.

CLINICAL PRESENTATION
Historical signs
Cough is the most common presenting complaint for dogs with CHF. Additional historical complaints for dogs with CHF may include tachypnea or dyspnea, syncope, lethargy or exercise intolerance, abdominal distention, anorexia, and weight loss. While some dogs have slow development of clinical signs, it is common for clinical signs to appear more acutely.

Physical examination findings
Dyspnea, cough, and ascites may be noted. Femoral arterial pulses are often weak and the jugular vein is typically distended above the bottom third of the neck in dogs with right-sided or biventricular heart failure. Pulmonary crackles are often present on auscultation in dogs with pulmonary edema, and dogs with pleural effusion may have dull lung sounds ventrally. CHF in the dog is often associated with an S3 gallop (14). A murmur of mitral or tricuspid valve regurgitation is the most frequent murmur noted on auscultation, and the murmur is often loud in dogs with chronic valvular disease and soft in dogs with dilated cardiomyopathy. Arrhythmias with pulse deficits, mucous membrane pallor, or delayed capillary refill time may also be noted. Some dogs with CHF have a recent unplanned weight loss.

DIFFERENTIAL DIAGNOSES
Differential diagnoses include collapsing trachea, pneumonia, chylothorax, various forms of primary or metastatic neoplasia, diaphragmatic hernia, and bronchitis. In the author's practice, bronchitis is an infrequent diagnosis in mature to older large-breed dogs, and dilated cardiomyopathy with mild CHF should be a key differential in this setting.

DIAGNOSIS
CHF can be reliably diagnosed based on a few key clinical findings. It is worth noting that echocardiography alone is generally not sufficient to diagnose CHF, and auscultation of the lungs for pulmonary crackles is also an unreliable method for diagnosing CHF.

Radiography
The key findings on thoracic radiographs (15) that can lead to a diagnosis of CHF are:
- Cardiomegaly.
- Pulmonary venous distention.
- Caudal vena cava distention.
- Perihilar pulmonary infiltration.

In dogs, the first radiographic evidence of left-sided CHF is an interstitial pattern, which can be difficult to distinguish from the aging pulmonary interstitial changes that are seen in many dogs. Resolution of this interstitial pattern following furosemide administration can be a method for distinguishing the two clinical entities. As CHF progresses, a bronchial pattern may be noted in many medium- to large-breed dogs; this is followed by overt alveolar flooding, which results in radiographic air bronchograms. Pleural effusion or ascites is usually evident in dogs with biventricular or right-sided CHF.

Additional testing
Additional diagnostic testing that is recommended for dogs suspected of having CHF includes an ECG and an echocardiogram. Baseline laboratory testing, including a CBC and serum biochemistry profile with electrolytes, is also recommended.

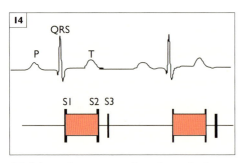

14 Schematic representation of auscultation findings commonly noted in dogs with CHF. The first and second heart sounds are the normal heart sounds (S1 and S2), with S1 occurring shortly after the onset of the QRS complex and S2 occurring near the end of the T wave. The S3 gallop, present in early diastole, is the result of rapid cessation of passive diastolic ventricular filling and is often heard in dogs with dilated cardiomyopathy or in dogs with chronic valvular disease at the onset of CHF. The gallop is best noted using the bell of the stethoscope. The systolic murmur of mitral regurgitation is depicted by the red band between S1 and S2.

Electrocardiogram

Findings from the ECG are not specific for CHF but can include a left atrial or left ventricular enlargement pattern, conduction disturbances, such as bundle branch block, and cardiac arrhythmias are common (16). Supraventricular arrhythmias are often present in dogs with chronic valvular disease, while atrial fibrillation and/or ventricular arrhythmias are more common in dogs with dilated cardiomyopathy.

Serum biochemistry

Modest elevations of BUN or creatinine may result from prerenal azotemia due to inadequate cardiac output or prior diuretic administration, elevated liver enzymes may be noted due to chronic passive hepatic congestion, and mild hypoproteinemia is common in dogs with ascites.

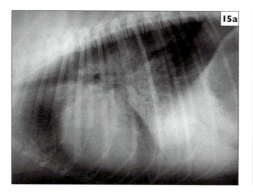
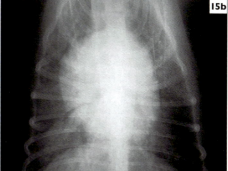

15 Lateral (15a) and dorsoventral (15b) thoracic radiographs obtained from a dog with chronic valvular disease leading to mitral regurgitation and left-sided CHF. There is moderate generalized cardiomegaly with left atrial enlargement. The perihilar interstitial and alveolar pulmonary infiltrate is characteristic of cardiogenic pulmonary edema in dogs.

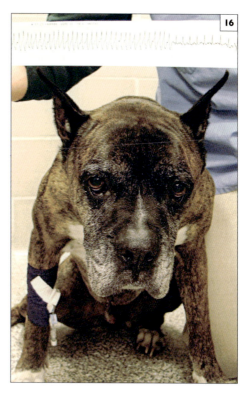

16 Boxer with cardiomyopathy and a serious ventricular tachycardia. The ventricular arrhythmia resolved and sinus rhythm was present following treatment with sotalol.

Echocardiography

The key echocardiographic finding to confirm a diagnosis of cardiogenic pulmonary edema in dogs is dilation of the left atrium. In dogs suspected to have right-sided CHF, dilation of the right atrium should be easily visualized, except in dogs with pericardial effusion. A variety of additional findings may be present and are usually specific to the type of heart disease that has led to CHF (**17, 18**).

MANAGEMENT / TREATMENT
Initial emergency management

Emergency management of CHF usually comprises oxygen therapy, high doses of diuretics, and nitrates. Thoracocentesis should be performed in dogs with pleural effusion that is of sufficient volume that it likely contributes to dyspnea. Dogs with large-volume ascites may benefit from abdominocentesis, especially if the ascitic fluid is limiting respiratory effort or lung volume. Cage rest is indicated, and supplemental oxygen can be administered through a number of methods.

Furosemide

Furosemide is the most commonly used diuretic in dogs and it can be administered in high doses, up to 4 mg/kg IV every hour, until relief of dyspnea is evident. There is recent enthusiasm for administration of furosemide via a CRI. A CRI of furosemide can be dosed at 0.1–1 mg/kg/hr. Injectable furosemide is diluted to a concentration of 10 mg/ml in either 5% dextrose in water or 0.9% NaCl.

Nitroglycerine

Nitroglycerine (glyceryl trinitrate) can be administered transcutaneously to the inner surface of the ear pinna, the inguinal region, or even smeared directly onto the oral mucous membranes. The 2% paste formulation can be dosed at 6–12 mm (0.25–0.5 inch) of paste for every 5 kg (11 lb) body weight.

Additional treatment

When these initial measures for emergency management of CHF are ineffective then sodium nitroprusside, dobutamine, or mechanical ventilation can be used.

Sodium nitroprusside

The most effective drug for dogs with severe pulmonary edema refractory to standard treatment is sodium nitroprusside. This drug is used for 1–3 days while other therapies for management of CHF are being initiated. Sodium nitroprusside is administered as a CRI at 1–5 µg/kg/min in 5% dextrose in water. Blood pressure measurement is desirable as a dramatic drop in blood pressure is possible and systolic blood pressure <70–90 mmHg should be avoided.

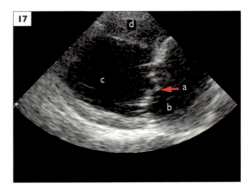

17 Two-dimensional echocardiogram obtained from the right parasternal long axis view from a dog with chronic valvular disease. The mitral valve is thickened and prolapses (a) beyond the mitral valve annulus. There is enlargement of the left atrium (b) and ventricle (c). Right ventricle = d.

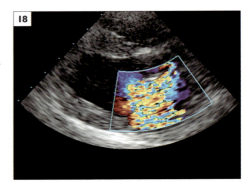

18 Color-flow Doppler echocardiogram obtained from the right parasternal long axis view from a dog with chronic valvular disease (same dog as in **17**). The turbulent flow of blood back into the left atrium is indicative of mitral regurgitation.

Other side effects include GI signs, and cyanide intoxication is possible for dogs treated at higher doses for >24 hours.

Dobutamine

Dobutamine at 1–10 µg/kg/min is recommended for dogs with refractory CHF associated with decreased cardiac function, such as with dilated cardiomyopathy. An initial CRI at 1–2 µg/kg/min is titrated upwards every 30 min until adequate clinical response or side effects are

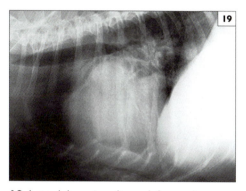

19 Lateral thoracic radiograph from a dog with persistent cough due to advanced chronic valvular disease and severe left atrial enlargement.

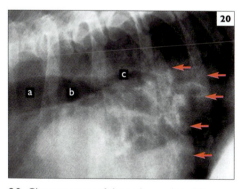

20 Close-up view of the radiograph in **19**. There is marked cardiomegaly and the considerably enlarged left atrium (arrowheads) causes dorsal displacement of the trachea (a) and carina (b), and compression of the mainstem bronchus (c).

noted. Side effects can include sinus tachycardia, supraventricular or ventricular tachyarrhythmias, and GI side effects.

Mechanical ventilation

In selected cases, mechanical ventilation can be a very successful adjunct to the other therapies. Mechanical ventilation with use of positive end-expiratory pressure should be considered in any dog judged to be at imminent risk for CPA. It allows for control of the airway and avoidance of respiratory failure leading to respiratory arrest while other therapies are being performed. Positive end-expiratory pressure is useful in helping to clear pulmonary edema. Mechanical ventilation requires adequate equipment in addition to ventilator skills and a significant commitment of time and resources.

Long-term management

For chronic management of CHF, exercise limitation, dietary sodium restriction, diuretic therapy, and ACE inhibitors usually form the backbone of therapy. Cough, often due to left atrial enlargement, may be a troublesome long-term management concern (**19, 20**).

PROGNOSIS

With the exception of easily correctable congenital defects, the prognosis for dogs with CHF is always guarded. Many dogs respond well to initiation of medications and dietary recommendations, while others fail to respond or encounter repeated side effects or bouts of CHF. To some degree, the dedication of the owner and the owner's financial means can play a big role in the outcome for dogs with CHF. While a 2-year survival is possible for some dogs with chronic valvular disease, a 6-month to 1-year survival might be more typical once CHF has developed.

In dogs with dilated cardiomyopathy the survival is often shorter than that of dogs with mitral regurgitation due to chronic valvular disease. In one study, the median survival was only 2 months, and several studies have identified a particularly short survival time for Doberman Pinschers. Still, with dedicated owners who are willing to make several adjustments to therapy, survival beyond 6 months is possible for many dogs with dilated cardiomyopathy. For dogs with CHF due to uncorrectable congenital heart disease the long-term survival is often only a few months with medical therapy alone.

Congestive heart failure in the cat

KEY POINTS
- Cats with severe pulmonary edema due to CHF are unstable and prone to stress. Stressful maneuvers, such as phlebotomy and catheter placement, should be delayed for several hours.
- The radiographic location of pulmonary edema can be variable in cats with CHF.
- Many cats with CHF can survive well beyond 1 year following initiation of successful management.
- ACE inhibitors are indicated for cats with CHF.
- Ultrasonography in the emergency room can be useful to identify the presence of pleural effusion or left atrial enlargement.

DEFINITION / OVERVIEW
CHF can be defined as the presence of fluid accumulation in the lungs (pulmonary edema), pleural space (pleural effusion), abdominal cavity (ascites), or pericardial sac (pericardial effusion), due to cardiac failure. Cardiogenic fluid accumulation occurs in cats with elevated diastolic ventricular and/or atrial filling pressures. Left-sided CHF develops in cats with elevated left heart filling pressures and leads to pulmonary edema with or without a small to moderate volume of pleural effusion and, rarely, pericardial effusion. Right-sided CHF occurs in cats with elevated right heart filling pressures. Most cats with large-volume pleural effusion have biventricular heart failure with elevated right and left heart filling pressures.

ETIOLOGY AND RISK FACTORS
Common causes of CHF in the cat are hypertrophic (21), restrictive, or dilated cardiomyopathy and, less frequently, congenital heart disease, such as ventricular septal defect, patent ductus arteriosus, and mitral or tricuspid valve dysplasia. Endocarditis is an uncommon cause of CHF. Some cats with heartworm disease will develop right-sided CHF.

Breeds at increased risk for hypertrophic cardiomyopathy include Maine Coon cat, Norwegian Forest cat, Persian, and American Short Hair cat. Middle-aged, male cats are predisposed to hypertrophic cardiomyopathy, and surveys of cats with hypertrophic cardiomyopathy indicate that affected cats have a higher median weight than unaffected cats. Recent corticosteroid administration, especially long-acting formulations of prednisone (prednisolone), can precipitate CHF in otherwise compensated individuals. Trauma, intravenous fluids, and recent surgery or anesthesia with ketamine can also predispose to the development of CHF.

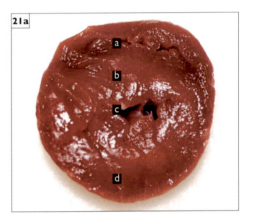

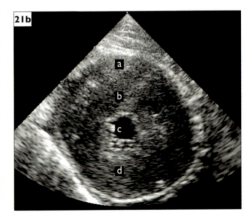

21 Necropsy specimen (**21a**) and two-dimensional echocardiogram (**21b**) demonstrating a short-axis cross-section of the heart from a cat with CHF due to hypertrophic cardiomyopathy. There is marked hypertrophy of the interventricular septum (b) and left ventricular free wall (d), and the left ventricular internal lumen (c) is decreased in size. Right ventricle = a.

PATHOPHYSIOLOGY

The pathophysiology of CHF in cats is similar to that described for CHF in the dog. CHF develops following a rise in ventricular diastolic filling pressures, which is transmitted back to the pulmonary veins or systemic veins. This leads to elevated capillary pressures and edema formation. Left-sided CHF is most commonly seen as pulmonary edema in cats, although a small to moderate volume of pleural effusion develops in some cats. Right-sided CHF is clinically observed as ascites and/or pleural effusion in cats. Biventricular heart failure leads to pleural effusion with or without pulmonary edema and small-volume ascites. Large-volume ascites of cardiogenic origin in cats is uncommon.

CLINICAL PRESENTATION
Historical signs

The history provided in most cats with CHF is acute illness of 1–3 days' duration. Dyspnea is recognized by some owners; however, lethargy, reduced food intake, and limited interaction with family members (e.g. hiding in the closet) are the predominant abnormalities noted in many cases. Overt dyspnea in some cats is not apparent until the travel to or visit at the veterinarian. Additional possible historical complaints for cats with CHF are syncope, intermittent open-mouth breathing, reduced exercise tolerance before open-mouth breathing, abdominal distention, and, occasionally, weight loss in cats with pleural effusion or ascites.

Cough is an uncommon presenting complaint for cats with CHF. Feline asthma, heartworm, or lungworm should be considered as more likely diagnoses in cats with cough.

Physical examination findings

Dyspnea is often the most prominent initial finding on initial evaluation of cats with CHF. Harsh lung sounds with pulmonary crackles are typically present in cats with pulmonary edema. Cats with pleural effusion of cardiogenic origin often have muffled lung sounds on the ventral thorax, hepatomegaly, and jugular vein distention. Femoral arterial pulses are often weak and mucous membranes can be pale or cyanotic. Rectal temperature is often low.

Auscultation of the heart can be an important contributor to the diagnosis of CHF as a soft murmur, a gallop, or arrhythmia is often present (22). Cardiac murmurs in most feline heart disease are best transmitted to the sternal border. A loud (IV/VI or louder) murmur in a young cat with CHF is often an indicator of congenital heart disease.

DIFFERENTIAL DIAGNOSES

Differential diagnoses include:
- Idiopathic chylothorax.
- Feline asthma.
- Bronchitis.
- Lymphosarcoma and other primary or metastatic neoplasia.
- Heartworm disease.
- Lungworm.
- Pneumothorax.
- Pulmonary contusions.
- Diaphragmatic hernia.

DIAGNOSIS

As described for dogs, certain clinical findings are strongly indicative of CHF (see CHF in the dog).

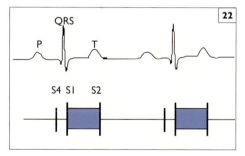

22 Schematic representation of typical auscultation findings from a cat with cardiomyopathy. The first and second heart sounds are normal (S1 and S2), with S1 occurring shortly after the onset of the QRS complex and S2 occurring near the end of the T wave. The S4 gallop is present in late diastole, after the P wave, and is the result of atrial contraction of blood into a stiff and hypertrophied ventricle.

The gallop is often heard best using the bell of the stethoscope. Many cats have a soft, systolic cardiac murmur near the left or right sternal border and the murmur is depicted by the blue band between S1 and S2.

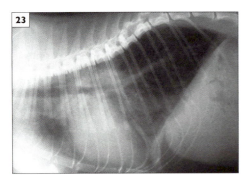

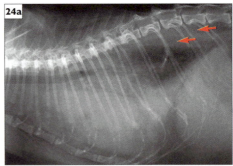

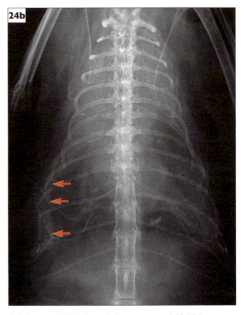

23 Lateral thoracic radiograph from a cat with hypertrophic cardiomyopathy and CHF. There is an interstitial to consolidating alveolar infiltrate in the perihilar lung fields and the pulmonary vasculature is engorged, findings that are typical of cardiogenic pulmonary edema. Cardiomegaly is evident and the liver is also enlarged.

Radiography

Thoracic radiographic findings that are typically present in cats with CHF include cardiomegaly and pulmonary infiltrates.

- Cardiomegaly is most readily identified on the dorsoventral radiographic view with reduced cardiothoracic index due to atrial enlargement. In cats with left-sided CHF both pulmonary arteries and veins become distended.
- Perihilar pulmonary infiltration, commonly noted in dogs with cardiogenic pulmonary edema, is a less consistent finding for cats (**23**).
- Pulmonary edema can develop in the perihilar region, or in the ventral lung fields, or edema may be noted to have a patchy distribution in one or more lung lobes. A bronchial pattern is uncommon in cats with CHF and should instead lead to consideration of asthma, lungworm, or heartworm.
- Pleural effusion is identified by pleural fissure lines, lung lobe retraction from the chest wall, partial collapse of the cranial lung lobes, and loss of the cardiac silhouette (**24**). The caudal vena cava may become distended, however the presence of pleural effusion can obscure observation of the cava and hepatomegaly may be a more reliable radiographic indicator of CHF.

24 Lateral (**24a**) and dorsoventral (**24b**) thoracic radiographs obtained from a cat with biventricular CHF. Cardiomegaly is present; this is difficult to confirm, however, due to silhouetting of the heart in the pleural effusion. On the lateral thoracic radiograph the caudal lung lobes are partially collapsed and retracted away from the spine (arrowheads). The liver is enlarged. On the dorsoventral view the cranial lungs lobes are nearly completely collapsed due to pleural effusion and the lungs are retracted away from the chest wall (arrowheads). There are several rib fractures that can be appreciated on the dorsoventral view in the right caudal thoracic wall just to the left of the arrowheads, and these fractures likely resulted from increased respiratory effort associated with dyspnea.

The combination of interstitial to alveolar pulmonary infiltrates and small-volume pleural effusion is strongly suggestive of a diagnosis of CHF.

Additional testing
Additional diagnostic testing recommended in cats with presumptive CHF includes blood pressure, an ECG, and an echocardiogram. Baseline laboratory testing, including a CBC and serum biochemistry profile with electrolytes, is also recommended, and thyroid testing is recommended for cats >6 years of age.

Electrocardiography
Common electrocardiographic findings include evidence of atrial enlargement with a P wave >0.2 mV or a left ventricular enlargement pattern. Cats with a deep S wave in lead II should have multiple leads obtained to determine whether a right axis shift or left anterior fascicular block pattern is present. Common cardiac arrhythmias include ventricular and/or atrial premature depolarizations, and atrial fibrillation; third degree AV block is common in older cats and those with hyperthyroid heart disease. Mild elevation of BUN or creatinine may be identified but this is more common after initiation of medical treatment. Elevated liver enzymes, especially AST or ALT, may be noted due to chronic passive hepatic congestion.

Ultrasonography
Ultrasonography can be very useful in the emergency setting to confirm the presence of either pleural effusion or significant atrial enlargement. Moderate to marked left atrial enlargement is virtually always present in cats with cardiogenic pulmonary edema (**25**, **26**). The concentric hypertrophy present in cats with hypertrophic cardiomyopathy, the most common cause of heart failure in cats, is also relatively easy to identify via echocardiography. Echocardiography is the best tool to determine the specific cause of cardiac disease and to rule in or rule out cardiac disease as the cause of the clinical signs.

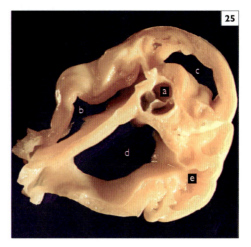

25 Necropsy specimen demonstrating a short-axis cross-section of the heart from a cat that died of CHF due to hypertrophic cardiomyopathy. The aorta (a) and semilunar valves are evident in the center, with the enlarged right atrium (b) and right ventricle (c) above the aorta, and the markedly enlarged left atrium (d) and left auricular appendage (e) below the aorta.

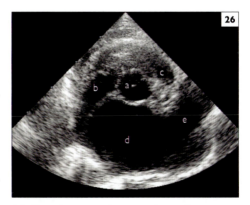

26 Two-dimensional echocardiographic image from the right parasternal short-axis plane of the aorta (a) and left atrium (d). The image is from a similar orientation as in the necropsy specimen in **25**. There is marked enlargement of the left atrium and left auricular appendage (e). Right atrium = b, right ventricular outflow tract = c.

MANAGEMENT / TREATMENT
Emergency management

Emergency management of CHF in cats can be one of the most challenging emergencies faced by a veterinarian; however, successful management can be very rewarding. Oxygen therapy, appropriate doses of furosemide, nitrates, and thoracocentesis for cats with moderate to large volumes of pleural effusion are the key treatment approaches in most cases (27). Limited stress is a crucial aspect of emergency care for dyspneic cats suspected to have CHF.

Once a diagnosis of CHF is suspected, cats should be given 4 mg/kg furosemide IM or IV by direct medial saphenous vein injection and placed in an oxygen cage. Transcutaneous nitroglycerine (glyceryl trinitrate) can be used and is administered as 3–6 mm (0.125–0.25 inch) of the 2% paste formulation applied to the inner pinna, inguinal region, or oral membranes q6–8hr.

Blood should *not* be drawn, an intravenous catheter should *not* be placed, and if radiographs have not yet been obtained then it is advised that 1–3 hours of initial treatment and oxygen cage stabilization be allowed before radiography is attempted. Cats are very susceptible to stress-induced deterioration of dyspnea, especially when they have first arrived in a new and unfamiliar environment. Once dyspnea is improved then it is safer to place an intravenous catheter and perform additional testing. Empiric thoracocentesis is not recommended for cats with pulmonary crackles; however, thoracocentesis prior to radiography may be appropriate for a cat with dull lung sounds ventrally, a distended jugular vein, and hepatomegaly, that is breathing with shallow respirations at an expanded lung volume. Additionally, cats that have had pleural effusion in the past are likely to develop it again.

Furosemide can be repeated at 4 mg/kg IV every hour until relief of dyspnea is evident.

Additional treatment

In cats that fail to respond to initial management then additional treatment approaches can include a CRI of furosemide, intravenous enalaprilat or sodium nitroprusside. Although some cats with CHF have physical evidence of dehydration (based on abnormal skin tent), elevated PCV or total solids, or azotemia, fluid therapy is *not* warranted in a cat with CHF.

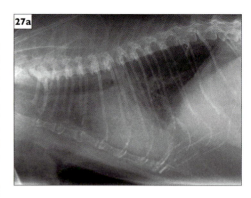

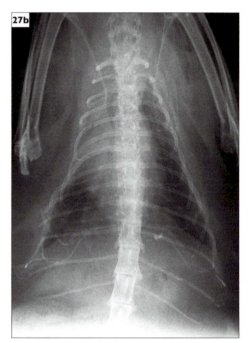

27 Lateral (**27a**) and dorsoventral (**27b**) thoracic radiographs of the cat in **24** after having thoracocentesis and treatment for CHF for several days. There is a dramatic reduction in the volume of pleural effusion and the lung lobes are more fully expanded. The liver has decreased in size.

Furosemide

Furosemide can be diluted to a concentration of 10 mg/ml in 0.9% NaCl or 5% dextrose in water and administered via a CRI at 0.2– 1 mg/kg/hr.

Enalapril

Enalapril is usually considered to be more effective as a chronic medication for CHF and is not indicated in an emergency setting. However, the authors have seen some cats with severe pulmonary edema respond favorably to 0.25–0.5 mg enalaprilat administered intravenously.

Sodium nitroprusside

This is useful for cats that fail to respond to initial intravenous doses of furosemide. A CRI of nitroprusside is administered at a dose of 0.5–3 µg/kg/minute in cats. To limit stress, blood pressure measurement is commonly not performed as long as the cat appears to be resting comfortably.

Dobutamine

Dobutamine can also be used in cats but, due to frequently observed toxicities of vomiting and seizures, the drug is usually reserved for echocardiographically confirmed systolic dysfunction. The dose of dobutamine usually employed in cats, a dose lower than that recommended in dogs, is 1–3 µg/kg/min, and the duration of dobutamine infusion is usually limited to <24 hours in cats to avoid side effects.

Mechanical ventilation

As described for dogs, mechanical ventilation can be used in cats with pulmonary edema when CPA seems imminent.

PROGNOSIS

The prognosis for cats with CHF can be difficult to predict. Some cats with severe, life-threatening pulmonary edema can respond very well to treatment and may live for 3 years or longer. In other cases CHF is the proximate cause of death at the time of the first hospitalization. Other cats respond poorly or experience side effects of medications and short-term survival or euthanasia is the result. As with dogs, in some cases the dedication and financial means of the owner can play a big role in the outcome for cats with CHF. Cats with pleural effusion and those with more severe left atrial enlargement appear to have a reduced survival.

Cardiac arrhythmias

KEY POINT

- Correct identification of the arrhythmia is required for proper treatment and so that an appropriate prognosis can be given.

DEFINITION / OVERVIEW

Cardiac arrhythmia can be defined as any arrhythmia that is not considered normal for a healthy member of the species. All normal cardiac rhythms originate from the sinus node. In addition to sinus rhythm, sinus arrhythmia and second degree AV block can be normal rhythms in the dog. Sinus bradycardia is often observed in healthy large-breed dogs at rest, and sinus tachycardia is seen with excitement or exercise. In cats, sinus rhythm and sinus tachycardia are considered normal cardiac rhythms. Sinus arrhythmia and sinus bradycardia can be seen in cats at rest but these rhythms are rarely seen in healthy cats in a hospital environment.

ETIOLOGY AND RISK FACTORS

Cardiac arrhythmias can result from primary cardiac disease or from a wide variety of diseases or metabolic disturbances. Hypovolemic shock in the dog often leads to microscopic regions of myocardial necrosis and ventricular arrhythmias. Hypoxemia, acidosis, electrolyte disturbances, coaguloapthy, CNS disorders, hypovolemia, and a number of other disease processes can cause or contribute to cardiac arrhythmias.

Animals with underlying cardiac disease are at risk for development of cardiac arrhythmias. Severe systemic disease often results in ventricular arrhythmias in the dog, while the majority of cats with ventricular arrhythmias have underlying myocardial disease.

PATHOPHYSIOLOGY

Cardiac arrhythmias are of concern for their effects on cardiac output. Bradycardia can lead to weakness, lethargy or exercise intolerance, and long pauses in the cardiac rhythm decrease blood flow to the brain and can cause syncope. Tachycardias also can decrease cardiac output, with decreases in cardiac output of 20–50% or more for many supraventricular and ventricular arrhythmias. Some arrhythmias are markers for animals at risk for cardiac arrest, including third degree AV block, sinus bradycardia in critically ill dogs, and rapid ventricular arrhythmias.

28 Algorithm for tachycardia.

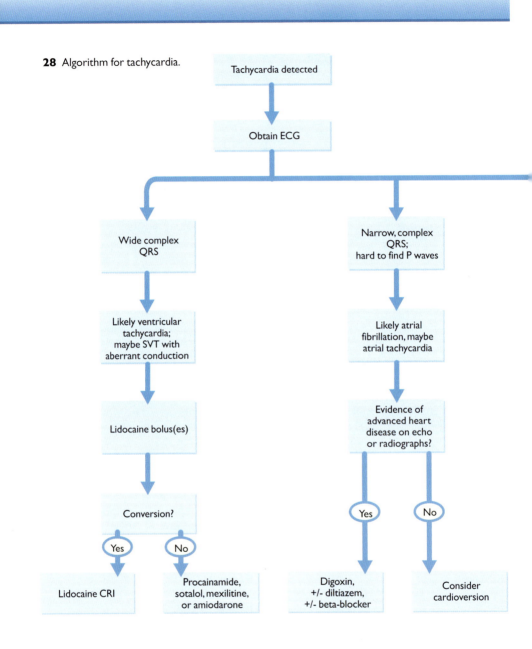

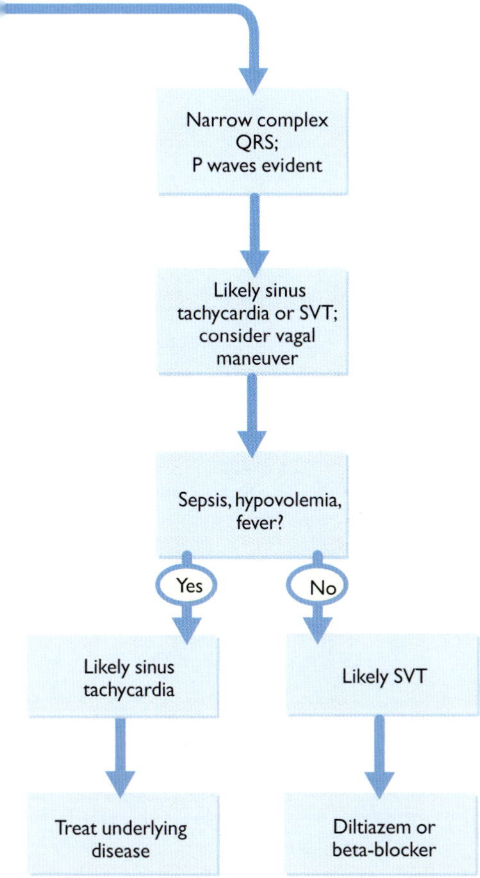

Flowchart

Narrow complex QRS; P waves evident

↓

Likely sinus tachycardia or SVT; consider vagal maneuver

↓

Sepsis, hypovolemia, fever?

— Yes → Likely sinus tachycardia → Treat underlying disease

— No → Likely SVT → Diltiazem or beta-blocker

CLINICAL PRESENTATION
Historical signs
The history in dogs with cardiac arrhythmia usually reflects the systemic disease which leads to cardiac arrhythmia (i.e. vomiting, hemoabdomen, and so on). Animals with primary cardiac disease may have a history of collapse, dyspnea, tachypnea, cough, weakness, abdominal distention, or reduced capacity for exercise.

Physical examination findings
Identification of a tachycardia (**28**), a bradycardia (**29**, overleaf), or an irregular cardiac rhythm is essential to raise a clinical suspicion for arrhythmia and trigger the decision to obtain an ECG. Animals with tachycardias often have pulse deficits, identified by auscultation of some heart beats that are not translated into palpable arterial pulses. Arterial pulses can be weak or of variable intensity in dogs with low cardiac output, however dogs with bradycardia often have very strong arterial pulses.

A cardiac murmur or gallop is often present in dogs and cats with underlying cardiac disease. Cardiac auscultation might also allow identification of variable intensity of the heart sounds. Severe arrhythmias lead to severe reduction of cardiac output with attendant mucous membrane pallor or delayed capillary refill time. Evidence of CHF with tachypnea, dyspnea, pulmonary crackles, jugular distention, or ascites may be present. In animals with systemic disease as the cause of cardiac arrhythmia, the physical examination findings often reflect the disease.

DIFFERENTIAL DIAGNOSES
The ECG is the key diagnostic tool to differentiate the various cardiac arrhythmias. Multiple ECG leads, including chest leads, can be useful to identify P waves and distinguish between ventricular and supraventricular arrhythmias.

29 Algorithm for bradycardia.

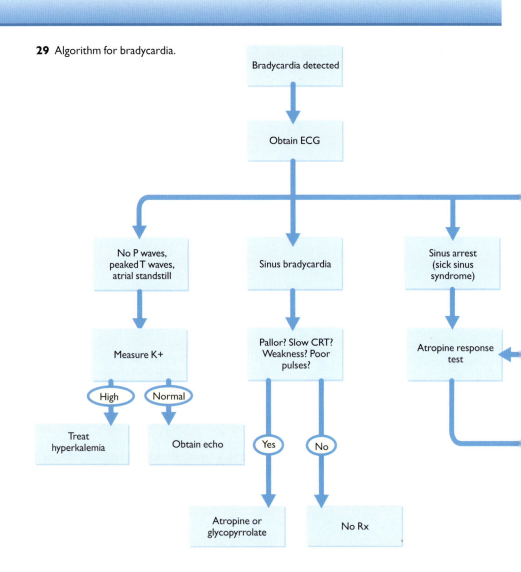

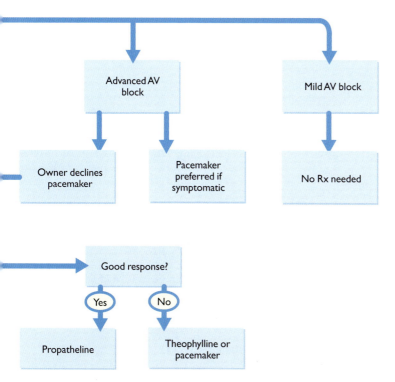

Advanced AV block

Mild AV block

Owner declines pacemaker

Pacemaker preferred if symptomatic

No Rx needed

Good response?

Yes

No

Propatheline

Theophylline or pacemaker

DIAGNOSIS

In animals suspected of having cardiac arrhythmia in association with cardiac disease the routine diagnostic testing includes an ECG, an echocardiogram, and thoracic radiographs. Baseline laboratory testing, such as a CBC, biochemistry profile, and urinalysis, is usually indicated to rule out concurrent systemic disease. Blood pressure measurement can be helpful to identify hypertension or hypotension. Thyroid testing is recommended for cats >6 years of age and dogs that are currently on thyroid supplementation, as excess thyroid supplementation can contribute to arrhythmia. Additional testing, such as blood gas analysis, abdominal radiographs or ultrasonography, or other specialized testing may be appropriate based on whether other underlying diseases are suspected.

DIAGNOSIS, MANAGEMENT, AND TREATMENT OF SPECIFIC CARDIAC ARRHYTHMIAS

Normal sinus rhythm

Diagnosis

P-QRS-T complexes are seen in a regular fashion at a normal heart rate for the species (30).

Management

No therapy is required for this normal rhythm.

Sinus arrhythmia

Diagnosis

The heart has a slow to normal rate with cyclic irregularity of rhythm that often results in speeding of the heart on inspiration and slowing of the heart on expiration (31). The P-QRS-T complexes are usually normal, although cyclic variations of the P wave, identified as a wandering sinus pacemaker, may be present. Sinus arrhythmia is normal in dogs and may be pronounced in animals with upper respiratory obstruction or certain neurological conditions.

Sinus bradycardia

Diagnosis

Normal P-QRS-T complexes at a rate <60 bpm in the dog and <140 bpm in the cat (32). Sinus bradycardia can be associated with high vagal tone, head trauma, electrolyte disturbances, hypothermia, and certain drugs (beta-blockers, sedatives).

Management

No treatment is required unless evidence of low cardiac output is present. If needed, a parasympatholytic (i.e. atropine) or sympathomimetic (i.e. epinephrine) can be administered. The primary cause should be treated if one is identified.

Sinus tachycardia

Diagnosis

Sinus tachycardia is recognized by P-QRS-T complexes that are at a rate that is higher than accepted as normal for the species (**33**). Sinus tachycardia is present in most normal dogs with a heart rate >160 bpm; in giant-breed dogs a heart rate >140 bpm, in toy breeds a heart rate >180 bpm, and in puppies a heart rate >220 bpm qualify as sinus tachycardia. A heart rate >240 bpm on an ECG from a cat is indicative of sinus tachycardia. A vagal maneuver may cause transient slowing of the sinus rate with sinus tachycardia. Abrupt termination of an arrhythmia in response to a vagal maneuver is most consistent with a diagnosis of supraventricular tachycardia. Sinus tachycardia is the appropriate response to stress and situations that result in hypotension and/or low cardiac output, pain, excitement, fever, hypotension, and shock.

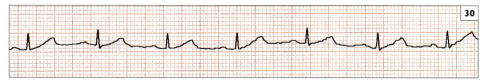

30 Sinus rhythm. Lead II ECG obtained at 50 mm/s and I cm/mV from a normal cat. The heart rate is 180 bpm and the rhythm is sinus rhythm.

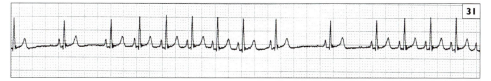

31 Sinus arrhythmia. ECG obtained using a transthoracic lead system at 25 mm/s from a cat with neurological disease which has resulted in increased intracranial pressure. The heart rate is normal to slow (approximately 140 bpm) with speeding of the heart rate during inspiration and slowing of the heart rate during expiration. These findings are typical of respiratory sinus arrhythmia.

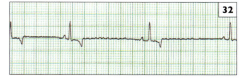
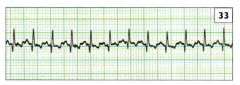

32 Sinus bradycardia. ECG obtained using a transthoracic lead system at 25 mm/s and I cm/mV from a dog with a recent onset seizure disorder. Normal P-QRS-T complexes are present, indicating sinoatrial node origin with normal AV conduction, but the heart rate is slow at 55–60 bpm. These findings are indicative of sinus bradycardia.

33 Sinus tachycardia. Lead II ECG obtained at 25 mm/s and I cm/mV from a dog with septic shock due to pyometra. The P-QRS-T complexes occur in a regular distribution and the heart rate is elevated at 200 bpm.

Management

Treatment should be directed at the underlying cause for sinus tachycardia (e.g. fluids for shock, analgesics for pain). When sinus tachycardia persists and no underlying cause is evident then one should search for unrecognized causes of patient instability, such as inadequate fluid resuscitation, fluid overload, or sepsis.

Supraventricular premature depolarizations and supraventricular tachycardia

Diagnosis

Supraventricular arrhythmias result from premature impulses originating in the atria or AV junctional tissue. For emergency management, the various causes of supraventricular arrhythmia (automatic atrial tachycardia, re-entry arrhythmias, junctional tachycardia) can usually be considered together.

Supraventricular premature depolarizations can be identified as an irregular rhythm with a premature QRS-T complex that is relatively normal in configuration and morphology (34). The ectopic P wave may be identified before the QRS, buried in the QRS, or buried in the previous T wave. The PR interval of the supraventricular beat is usually different from a normal PR interval.

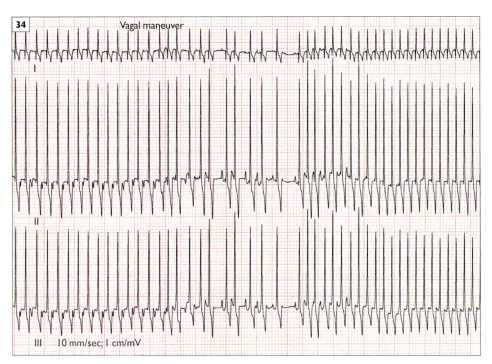

34 Supraventricular tachycardia. Lead I, II, and III ECGs obtained at 10 mm/s and 1 cm/mV from a dog with supraventricular tachycardia. The cardiac rhythm is supraventricular tachycardia at the beginning of the ECG tracing. During carotid sinus massage, noted as a vagal maneuver, there is an abrupt change in the cardiac rhythm, with sudden slowing that allows identification of P waves with differing morphology and then two clear sinus conducted beats before the rhythm returns back to supraventricular tachycardia.

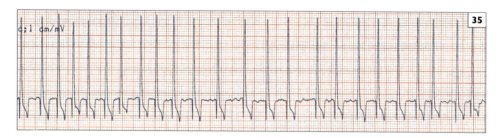

ECG signs of supraventricular tachycardia include a rapid arrhythmia that is often sustained or paroxysmal (i.e. starts and ends abruptly). The R-R interval is often very regular in sustained supraventricular tachycardias. Ectopic P waves may present and may be seen before the QRS, buried in the QRS, or in the ST segment or T wave. The QRS-T complex morphology is usually normal unless there is aberrant ventricular conduction.

Supraventricular arrhythmias are associated with chronic valvular and myocardial heart diseases, digitalis intoxication, and various pulmonary diseases. Some sustained supraventricular arrhythmias result from an abnormal connection between the atria and ventricles, an accessory pathway, that results in a re-entrant arrhythmia.

Management
Infrequent supraventricular premature depolarizations often do not require treatment, however frequent supraventricular depolarizations may respond to digoxin, beta-blockers, and calcium channel blockers. Supraventricular tachycardia may be abruptly terminated with a vagal maneuver (carotid or ocular pressure) in some cases; in most cases, however, there is no change with vagal maneuver. Digoxin is useful for dogs with concurrent supraventricular tachycardia and CHF. Procainamide, beta-blockers and calcium channel blockers can also be useful in long-term management. For emergency management of supraventricular tachycardia, intravenous diltiazem and the short-acting beta-blocker esmolol can be effective. Finally, cardioversion using an ECG-synchronized cardioverter/defibrillator can be useful to terminate sustained supraventricular tachycardias.

35 Atrial fibrillation. Lead II ECG obtained at 25 mm/s and 1 cm/mV from a dog with dilated cardiomyopathy. The heart rate is fast at 160–200 bpm and the rhythm is irregularly irregular. There are undulations in the baseline, f waves, and there is beat-to-beat variation in the height of the QRS complexes. These findings are consistent with atrial fibrillation, and the tall R wave in lead II is compatible with left ventricular enlargement.

Atrial fibrillation
Diagnosis
ECG findings include a rapid, irregularly irregular ventricular rhythm with no defined P waves (**35**). There are irregularly occurring baseline undulations (f waves) that have no relation to the QRS-T complexes. The QRS-T complexes often have fairly normal morphology, however there can be beat-to-beat variation in the height of the QRS. Atrial fibrillation is often seen in giant-breed dogs with cardiomyopathy and is less frequently seen in cats with cardiomyopathy and dogs with advanced chronic valvular disease. Atrial fibrillation can also be seen as an uncommon rhythm disturbance in large-breed dogs with severe systemic illness and no appreciable underlying cardiac disease.

Management
Treatment is usually directed toward slowing the ventricular response to atrial fibrillation. Digoxin is usually initiated, with either a beta-blocker or calcium channel blocker added later if needed, to slow the ventricular response to 160 bpm or less by reducing the number of impulses reaching the ventricles. In selected dogs without significant underlying heart disease, conversion from atrial fibrillation to sinus rhythm may be desirable. In these cases, quinidine may be administered or cardioversion can be attempted.

Ventricular arrhythmias

Diagnosis

Ventricular premature depolarizations are recognized as premature, wide QRS complexes with a morphology that is typically very different from the sinus-conducted beats (**36**). There is usually a large T wave in the opposite direction to the QRS complexes and there is usually a loss of the normal ST segment isoelectric shelf. When ventricular arrhythmias have multiple morphologic patterns there is often widespread myocardial disease. Ventricular tachycardia is present when a series of ventricular premature depolarizations, three or more in number and at a rate >160 bpm, break the underlying cardiac rhythm. When ventricular arrhythmias occur at rates between 60 bpm and 160 bpm they are more appropriately referred to as accelerated ventricular rhythms or idioventricular tachycardia.

Ventricular arrhythmias can be associated with significant underlying cardiac disease or they can be present in animals with minimal cardiac disease but severe systemic, traumatic, or metabolic disorders. Ventricular arrhythmias are commonly seen in dogs with GDV, trauma, splenic mass, pancreatitis, acidosis, electrolyte disorders, hypoxia due to pulmonary disease, and a variety of other disorders. Certain drugs and anesthestic agents can also predispose to the development of ventricular arrhythmias.

Management

Many ventricular arrhythmias do not require treatment. Isolated ventricular premature beats, no matter how frequent, pose little risk of death and usually cause only a modest negative impact on cardiac function. Repetitive (longer than 10 s) and/or rapid (faster than 180–200 bpm) arrhythmias often justify treatment. When there is underlying cardiac disease the treatment is usually lifelong, while animals with arrhythmias associated with systemic disease may only require treatment for a few days or weeks.

Lidocaine is still the drug of choice when an injectable anti-arrhythmic drug is required. Initial 2 mg/kg boluses of lidocaine can be given

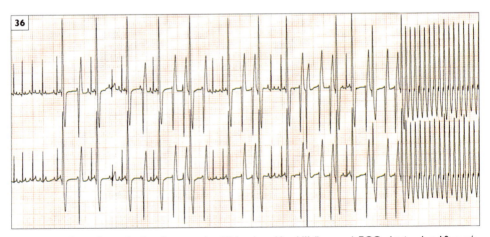

36 Ventricular tachycardia. Simultaneous lead II (top) and lead III (bottom) ECG obtained at 10 mm/s and 1 cm/mV from a dog. The initial sinus rhythm at the beginning of the tracing (heart rate 120 bpm) is interrupted by ventricular premature depolarizations. The ventricular premature complexes have more than one morphological appearance which is usually indicative of arrhythmia origin and/or disease in more than one region of the ventricle. Near the end of the strip the rhythm changes to ventricular tachycardia at a rate of 260 bpm, and this rhythm continued for longer than 30 s (remainder of the tracing not shown). Ventricular tachycardia lasting for more than 30 s is classified as sustained ventricular tachycardia.

up to a total dose of 8 mg/kg. When this is effective, a CRI of lidocaine can be initiated at 40–75 µg/kg/min. Other options for both short-term and long-term management of ventricular arrhythmias include procainamide, quinidine, beta-blockers, sotalol, and amiodarone. Underlying disorders, such as hypoxemia, electrolyte disturbances, coagulopathy, or hypovolemia, which might be contributing to arrhythmia formation, should be identified and treated.

Ventricular fibrillation
Diagnosis
Ventricular fibrillation is an irregular and disorganized ventricular activity that reduces cardiac output to zero and results in immediate CPA. It is identified by a lack of recognizable QRS-T complexes, which have been replaced with chaotic undulations in the baseline of the ECG (37).

Management
Ventricular fibrillation can only be effectively treated with countershock using a defibrillator.

Sinoatrial arrest
Diagnosis
The heart rate is slow or normal and there is a pause in the cardiac rhythm for longer than two P-P intervals without demonstrable atrial activity (38). Sinus arrest can be seen in brachycephalic breeds, animals with high vagal tone, and is common in middle-aged to elderly Cocker Spaniels, West Highland White Terriers and Miniature Schnauzers. These animals often present for syncope or seizure. In classic 'sick sinus syndrome', pronounced sinus bradycardia alternates with periods of sinus or supraventricular tachycardia.

Management
Permanent pacemaker implantation is usually the preferred therapy for dogs that are symptomatic with syncope, however medical management can be effective for a period of time in many dogs. If there is a good response to an atropine response test then propantheline is often effective; in other dogs sustained-release theophylline can reduce the frequency of syncope.

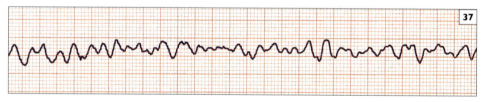

37 Ventricular fibrillation. Lead II ECG obtained from a dog at the time of CPA. There is no organized atrial or ventricular activity. The chaotic baseline undulations are typical of ventricular fibrillation.

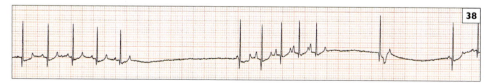

38 Sinus arrest. Lead III ECG obtained at 25 mm/s and 1 cm/mV from a dog with syncope. The rhythm at the beginning of the tracing is a junctional arrhythmia, followed by a 2 s pause in the cardiac rhythm with no P waves (i.e. sinus arrest). Sinus arrest ends with a junctional escape beat and then four complexes of sinus rhythm are again followed by sinus arrest, one junctional escape complex, and then a return to the original junctional rhythm. The combination of these findings is compatible with the clinical diagnosis of sick sinus syndrome.

Atrial standstill

Diagnosis

Atrial standstill is recognized by an absence of P waves (**39, 40**). Common clinical associations are severe hyperkalemia and atrial myopathy. Additional ECG signs of hyperkalemia can include bradycardia, flattening or loss of the P waves, ST-T segment depression or elevation, tented or peaked T waves, and eventually widening of the QRS complex. Persistent atrial standstill is a rare disorder in dogs, seen in Springer Spaniels and a few other breeds, and is identified by absence of P waves and a normal serum potassium.

Management

Hyperkalemia should be treated. Dogs with persistent atrial standstill usually benefit from pacemaker implantation.

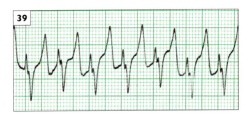

39 Atrial standstill. Lead II ECG obtained at 25 mm/s and 1 cm/mV from a cat with urethral obstruction and a serum potassium of 9.3 mmol/l. There are no identifiable P waves, which is consistent with a diagnosis of atrial standstill. The heart rate is approximately 150 bpm. The T waves are tall and the QRS morphology is abnormal with a deep S wave in lead II.

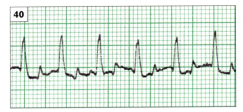

40 Lead II ECG obtained at 25 mm/s and 1 cm/mV from the same cat as in **39**, after the urethral obstruction was relieved and treatment of hyperkalemia had been initiated. The heart rate has risen to 180 bpm, the QRS complex has a more normal morphology, the T wave alterations are less pronounced, yet the P waves are still difficult to define.

First degree atrioventricular block

Diagnosis

Conduction is delayed through the AV node causing lengthening of the P-Q (R) interval beyond 0.13 s in a dog or longer than 0.9 s in a cat (**41**). First degree AV block can be normal in large-breed dogs and can be a result of treatment with certain medications, such as digoxin, calcium channel blockers, and some anesthetic agents.

Management

No treatment is indicated, however drugs that might further delay AV conduction may lead to more advanced AV block.

Second degree atrioventricular block

Diagnosis

Some atrial impulses are blocked at the AV node and therefore some P waves are not followed by a QRS-T complex (**41, 42**). Second degree AV block is further divided into Mobitz type I (Wenkebach) with progressive prolongation of the P-R interval before the block, and Mobitz type II, where the P-R interval is constant prior to the blocked P wave. Mobitz type I second degree AV block can be normal in the dog and is associated with high vagal tone. Mobitz type II second degree AV block is a more advanced degree of block and is usually associated with disease of the AV junction or His bundle. Digitalis intoxication is a common cause of first or second degree AV block.

Management

Anticholinergic drugs or sympathomimetic drugs may speed AV conduction and abolish the block. In most cases treatment is not necessary. Some dogs with Mobitz type II second degree AV block require therapy as outlined for third degree AV block.

Third degree atrioventricular block or complete heart block

Diagnosis

Third degree AV block results from an anatomic or persistent physiological interruption in impulse conduction through the AV node. No P waves are conducted through to the ventricle, and the dominant rhythm is supplied by a junctional or ventricular escape rhythm (**43**). Third degree AV block is usually associated with advanced disease of the conduction system, such as degeneration,

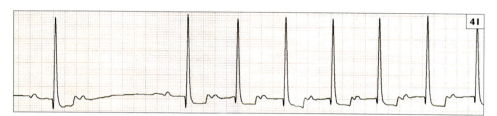

41 First and second degree AV block. Lead II ECG obtained at 50 mm/s and 1 cm/mV from a dog following treatment with digoxin. The PR interval is prolonged at 0.18 s, indicative of first degree AV block. The second P wave, immediately after the T wave of the first P-QRS-T complex, is also blocked and this is an example of second degree AV block.

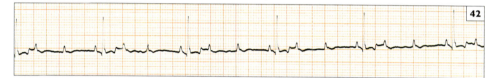

42 Second degree AV block. Lead II ECG obtained at 25 mm/s and 1 cm/mV from a dog with syncope. Two out of every three P waves are blocked at the AV node. The conducted P waves have a consistent relationship with the subsequent QRS complex and a normal P-R interval. These findings are consistent with Mobitz type II, or high-grade, second degree AV block.

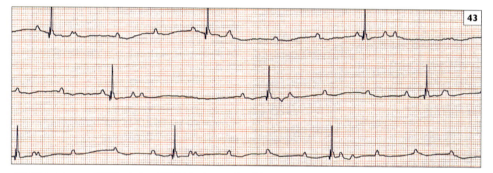

43 Third degree AV block. Lead II ECG obtained at 50 mm/s and 1 cm/mV from a dog with syncope. The P waves occur in a regular fashion, and the QRS-T complexes also occur in a regular fashion. However the P-R interval is inconsistent and there is no relationship between the P waves and the QRS-T complexes. The QRS-T complexes are suspected to originate from either a junctional escape rhythm or a ventricular escape rhythm high in the interventricular septum.

fibrosis, inflammation, thrombosis, or neoplasia. The heart rate is slow (usually <50 bpm) and there is no consistent association between the P waves and the QRS-T complexes.

Management

There is really no effective medical therapy for anatomical disruption leading to third degree AV block. In emergency situations, the ventricular rate can sometimes be increased by administering sympathomimetic drugs. Anticholinergic drugs are typically not effective at increasing heart rate or improving AV conduction. The treatment of choice is an implantable pacemaker, and temporary cardiac pacing may be indicated for animals with severely symptomatic bradycardia and those with CHF.

carries a better prognosis. Many cats will develop signs of CHF shortly after an episode of arterial thromboembolism.

In dogs with arterial thromboembolism the clinical signs often develop more slowly and posterior paresis, often with less severe pain than is seen in cats, is the main presenting complaint.

PHYSICAL EXAMINATION FINDINGS

The diagnosis is often clear based on clinical signs and physical examination findings alone. Loss of femoral arterial pulses is usually the key clinical finding to lead the clinician away from diagnoses of orthopedic or neurological disease in dogs. Other physical findings seen in affected animals can include a cardiac murmur or gallop, cardiac arrhythmia, and dyspnea or tachypnea if heart failure has developed. In dogs the underlying systemic disease that led to arterial thromboembolism may dominate the physical examination and clinical picture.

DIFFERENTIAL DIAGNOSES

Differential diagnoses for arterial thromboembolism include intervertebral disc disease, osteoarthritis, myopathy, and other disorders that might cause transient limb weakness. It is possible for cats to have clinical signs of arterial thromboembolism that last for only a few minutes, however this is uncommon and most cats with repeated transient limb weakness do not have arterial thromboembolism.

DIAGNOSIS

If the diagnosis is in question after the physical examination, blood sampled from the affected limb will usually have a lower blood glucose and higher lactate than blood sampled from an unaffected peripheral vein. Blood pressure as measured by Doppler is absent in the affected limbs. Ultrasonography of the distal aorta and angiography can also be performed if the diagnosis remains in question.

Other routine testing recommended for animals with arterial thromboembolism includes a CBC, chemistry profile, thoracic radiographs, urinalysis, and, in cats, echocardiography is indicated. Coagulation abnormalities can also be observed in cats with arterial thromboembolism, and coagulation testing is usually appropriate in dogs. Elevation of FDPs or D-dimers may be seen in affected dogs. Elevation of BUN, creati-

nine, AST, or ALT can be seen. Oliguric renal failure is an uncommon complication resulting from either arterial thromboembolism at the renal level or hypotension or reperfusion-related renal failure. Reperfusion can lead to serious hyperkalemia and metabolic acidosis.

Echocardiography sometimes documents another thrombus in the left ventricle, left atrium, or, most commonly, in the left auricular appendage (54). In a dilated left atrium there is often spontaneous, swirling hyperechoic 'smoke', which is judged to be an indicator of cats at risk for arterial thromboembolism. Contrast angiography can be useful to help identify the exact location of the thrombus, especially if surgical or catheter embolectomy is planned (55).

MANAGEMENT / TREATMENT

Many therapies have been attempted to restore perfusion to the rear limbs, cause dissolution of the thrombus, or inhibit further enlargement of the thrombus. Supportive care and nursing efforts are important in the management of arterial thromboembolism. Hypothermic cats should be gently warmed, yet direct warming of affected limbs that have lost autoregulatory control should be avoided. Cats should not be excessively heated to the point of panting due to limited cardiopulmonary reserves. Physical therapy to the affected limb(s) is indicated once pain is controlled. Narcotics, such as buprenorphine or fentanyl, are indicated to control discomfort.

Vasodilators

Vasodilators have been advocated for animals with arterial thromboembolism, since experimental studies have documented that simple ligation of the terminal aorta in cats does not result in clinical signs of arterial thromboembolism. Substances elaborated by the thrombus are thought to lead to vasoconstriction of collateral vessels which, if opened, could improve blood flow to affected tissue. Use of these vasodilating drugs (e.g. acepromazine or hydralazine) can lead to reduction in blood pressure, which may be a more important predictor of blood flow to tissues at risk.

Thrombolytic drugs

The role for thrombolytic drugs in the management of arterial thromboembolism in dogs and cats is still unclear. In contrast to heparin, thrombolytic drugs have the ability to dissolve a thrombus once it has lodged. Thrombolytics are relatively contraindicated in cases known to have an intracardiac thrombus. The use of tissue plasminogen activator and streptokinase has been described in cats, and the authors have recently had some favorable experiences with urokinase for cats with arterial thromboembolism. For all

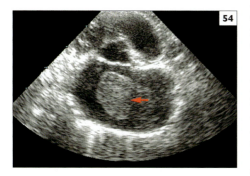

54 Two-dimensional echocardiogram from a right parasternal short axis view in a cat with arterial thromboembolism. There is a large thrombus (arrow) in the left atrium.

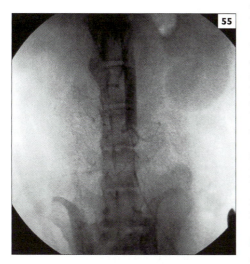

55 Angiogram from a dog in ventrodorsal recumbency following placement of a catheter into the distal aorta from the left femoral artery. There is an abrupt termination of the contrast in the distal aorta just caudal to the kidneys. This finding is characteristic of arterial thromboembolism of the terminal aorta.

thrombolytic drugs, bleeding complications are possible and complications resulting from reperfusion injury (hyperkalemia and metabolic acidosis) can be life-threatening. Based on studies in human patients, early thrombolytic administration is key to saving the at-risk tissue; that is the tissue that has not yet died after arterial thromboembolism but still has reduced blood flow and is at risk of permanent loss. Based on this information, it is recommended that if thrombolytic drugs are to be used then they should be initiated immediately, ideally within 2–4 hours after the onset of clinical signs.

Heparin

Heparin is often used to prevent further enlargement of the thrombus. While several doses of heparin have been proposed, a high dose of heparin (200–300 U/kg q6–8hr SC) is recommended once arterial thromboembolism has been diagnosed. Heparin can be administered subcutaneously or intravenously, and an initial intravenous bolus of heparin can be followed by a CRI of heparin (10–20 U/kg/hr). Ideally, a baseline aPTT is obtained and serial aPTTs are obtained q6–24hr if a CRI is used. Heparin is usually continued until the time of hospital discharge or until coumadin (warfarin sodium) therapy has been initiated for at least 72 hours.

Surgical treatment

Surgical thrombolectomy can be attempted for removal of the thrombus. Although there is little published on the use of thrombolectomy, the dogma is that cats with arterial thromboembolism treated with thrombolectomy do poorly in the peri-operative period.

Preventative medication

Prevention of repeated episodes of arterial thromboembolism can be attempted with a number of medications, including aspirin, coumadin and low molecular weight heparins.

PROGNOSIS

Arterial thromboembolism to the front limb carries a better prognosis for complete or near complete return of function when compared with rear limb arterial thromboembolism. Cats with arterial thromboembolism affecting a single limb are reported to have a better outcome than cats with multiple limb arterial thromboembolism. Cats with weak pulses to the rear limbs appear to have a better prognosis than cats with no pulses to the rear limbs. Cats with a low rectal temperature (<37.2°C [<99°F]) have a worse prognosis than cats with a more normal body temperature. Up to 50% of cats that are not euthanized will live to hospital discharge, and of those discharged from the hospital it is more likely that they will succumb to CHF than that they will die or be euthanized for repeated arterial thromboembolism. There is less information published on the clinical outcomes for dogs with arterial thromboembolism, however the authors' experience indicates this is a disease that has a high mortality.

Syncope

KEY POINTS
- Syncope is a clinical sign and the underlying cause must be sought.
- Animals with syncope and bradycardia are usually best treated with pacemaker implantation.
- Diagnostic testing for syncope may be frustrating and costly as the cause can be elusive.

DEFINITION / OVERVIEW
Syncope is a more common cause of emergency presentation in dogs than in cats. Syncope is defined as a sudden, transient loss of consciousness with spontaneous recovery. Syncope is an alarming occurrence for an owner and can be a warning sign that occurs before sudden death. In other disease processes, such as vasovagal syncope, syncope can occur repeatedly and never result in sudden death. Syncope is a clinical sign of an underlying disease and diagnostic testing is indicated to search for the cause of syncope.

ETIOLOGY
Causes of syncope include bradyarrhythmias, tachyarrhythmias, low cardiac output due to a variety of cardiac diseases or drugs, hypoglycemia, hypoxia, and hyperviscosity syndromes. Hypotension due to hypovolemia or inadequate vascular tone (e.g. due to vasodilators) can also result in or predispose to syncope. Dogs with chronic valvular disease can experience syncope, often at the time of the original occurrence of CHF, and the etiology of syncope in these cases can be elusive. Paroxysmal coughing can cause syncope (tussive syncope or 'cough-drop syndrome') and one of the most common causes of syncope is a vagally mediated reflex that leads to bradycardia and hypotension, termed vasovagal or neurocardiogenic syncope.

PATHOPHYSIOLOGY
Syncope develops when the CNS is deprived of blood flow, leading to reduced delivery of oxygen and other metabolites, and the result is a loss of consciousness. In most dogs with arrhythmic collapse, a pause in the cardiac rhythm of 7–12 s is required before syncope is seen (**56, 57**).

CLINICAL PRESENTATION
Historical signs

The owner complaint for most animals with syncope will be seizure, collapse, or fainting. Differentiating syncope from a seizure episode can be difficult, however a careful history can help in making the distinction. A seizure typically has a pre-ictal period or aura, the ictus or actual seizure, and a post-ictal period. During the ictal event, most animals lose consciousness, have tonic/clonic limb motions, facial chomping, and hypersalivation. In contrast, the classic syncopal event rarely has an aura or prior warning, and urination or defecation occurs somewhat less frequently with syncope compared to with a seizure.

Dogs and cats with syncope typically collapse and lose consciousness, however syncopal animals rarely have facial chomping or hypersalivation. Syncopal animals may struggle when recovering from the event, but they usually do not have classic tonic/clonic limb motion. Syncopal animals may become limp during the event, or they may extend the head back into a position of opisthotonus.

A seizure often lasts 1–2 min or longer, while syncope in animals often lasts <30 s. The post-ictal period is usually longer after a seizure (minutes to hours) while animals with syncope are often awake and have close to normal mentation within 30 s to 2 min of the event. The time needed for recovery from a syncopal episode can be much longer for large- and giant-breed dogs, especially those with arrhythmias that may not have completely resolved after the initial collapse. The complaint of an event following exercise or excitement is more commonly found in dogs with syncope than with seizure, however this association is a less reliable historical finding in cats.

Physical examination findings

The physical examination can be normal in animals presented for syncope. If cardiovascular disease is the underlying cause of syncope then arrhythmia, a cardiac murmur or gallop, dyspnea, tachypnea, pulmonary crackles, ascites, or jugular vein distention may be noted. When cardiac arrhythmia is the cause of collapse then an irregular heart rhythm and/or pulse deficits may be present. When syncope occurs due to a systemic disease, the physical examination may reflect the primary disease (e.g. pale mucous membranes and brisk arterial pulses with anemia). The neurological examination is usually normal in animals with syncope.

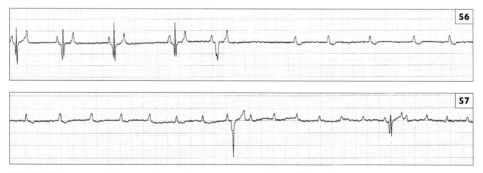

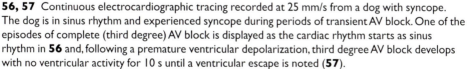

56, 57 Continuous electrocardiographic tracing recorded at 25 mm/s from a dog with syncope. The dog is in sinus rhythm and experienced syncope during periods of transient AV block. One of the episodes of complete (third degree) AV block is displayed as the cardiac rhythm starts as sinus rhythm in **56** and, following a premature ventricular depolarization, third degree AV block develops with no ventricular activity for 10 s until a ventricular escape is noted (**57**).

DIFFERENTIAL DIAGNOSES

Differential diagnoses for syncope include:
• Seizures.
• Narcolepsy.
• Catalepsy.
• Collapse due to muscular weakness.

DIAGNOSIS

Syncope is a clinical finding and a specific cause for syncope must be sought in every case. Establishing the cause of syncope can be challenging and in up to 50% of cases a specific cause for syncope is never discovered. Confirmation of a cardiac cause for syncope requires simultaneously documenting the syncope and a hemodynamically cardiac arrhythmia such as a profound bradycardia or very rapid tachycardia.

Routine initial testing of animals with syncope often includes a cardiac and neurological examination, a CBC, serum biochemistry profile, urinalysis, thoracic radiographs, and an ECG. Anemia can contribute to the development of vasovagal syncope, and hypoglycemia can cause either seizure or syncope. Hypoxemia can also predispose to syncope so pulse oximetry or arterial blood gas evaluation may be useful if dyspnea is present.

Radiography

Thoracic radiographs are indicated to search for cardiac enlargement, CHF, intrathoracic mass lesions, and other underlying diseases.

Echocardiography

Cardiac causes of syncope that are best identified with echocardiography include pulmonic or subaortic stenosis, pericardial tamponade, dilated or hypertrophic cardiomyopathy, congenital cardiac defects associated with polycythemia and cyanosis, and cardiac mass lesions or thrombi. Dogs with chronic valvular disease and mitral and/or tricuspid regurgitation often have syncope, although the cause of syncope is rarely evident on echocardiography. Echocardiography can also assist in diagnosis in dogs with pulmonary hypertension including animals with heartworm disease or PTE.

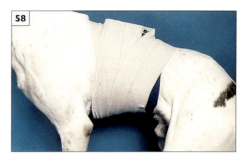

58 Application of a continuous ambulatory (Holter) ECG recorder to a dog. The ECG leads are bandaged and the recorder is securely attached to the body.

Electrocardiography

Syncope will rarely occur at the time a screening ECG is obtained, however a cardiac arrhythmia that could account for syncope (e.g. ventricular tachycardia, sinus arrest) might be identified. In many cases, a screening lead II ECG will not provide a definitive diagnosis and further testing is required.

A cardiac event recorder is useful to search for an arrhythmic cause in dogs with infrequent syncope. Event recorders can be attached to the animal for several days to a week or longer. The event recorder continuously records a loop of ECG and, after activation of a button, the loop is saved for subsequent evaluation and ECG analysis to determine whether cardiac arrhythmia was temporally related to syncope. A recent study identified a high diagnostic yield for cardiac event recording, although this high rate of yield has not matched the experience of this author.

Continuous ambulatory (Holter) ECG recording is also useful to search for arrhythmic causes of syncope (**58**). For a Holter monitor recording, the electrocardiograph leads are attached and an ECG recording device saves the ECG for an entire 24 hours for subsequent analysis. The analysis of the Holter recording may provide a definitive cause for syncope, however the animal may not experience a syncopal event during the recording. In one veterinary study, Holter recordings were useful in establishing a diagnosis in 42% of cases.

Additional testing

If a cause is not evident based on the above testing, additional tests that can help establish a cause include abdominal ultrasonography, ECG recording during a vagal maneuver, or advanced imaging, such as MRI or CT scanning, if neurological disease remains a differential diagnosis.

MANAGEMENT / TREATMENT

Since syncope is a sign of a disease and not a specific diagnosis, the therapy needs to be directed toward the underlying disease. Permanent pacemaker implantation is indicated for most animals with bradycardia (59, 60, 61).

Drug therapy can be attempted for dogs with sinus arrest or AV block, especially when pacemaker implantation is not an option, based on financial limitations or owner wishes. Anticholinergic drugs (e.g. propantheline bromide), sympathomimetic drugs (e.g. terbutaline), and theophylline or aminophylline are useful in selected cases to increase the heart rate and/or improve conduction across the AV node. Tachyarrhythmias are usually treated medically.

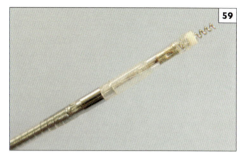

59 A close-up picture of a transvenous endocardial pacing lead that can be actively fixed into the myocardium of the right ventricle.

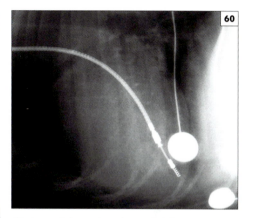

60 Lateral thoracic radiograph following permanent pacemaker implantation in a dog. The endocardial lead originates in the right jugular vein and courses through the right atrium, across the tricuspid valve and is implanted into the apex of the right ventricle. The three circular metallic densities are external electrodes and leadwires on the outer chest wall, which are connected to an ECG monitoring device.

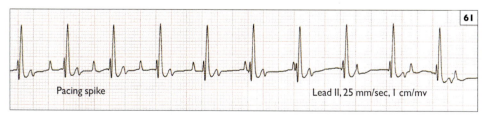

Pacing spike   Lead II, 25 mm/sec, 1 cm/mv

61 ECG recorded at 25 mm/s following pacemaker implantation into a dog with third degree AV block and syncope. The paced rhythm is recognized by the presence of a high-frequency pacing spike at the beginning of the QRS complex. Third degree AV block is still present as there is no association between the P waves and the paced QRS-T complexes.

Syncope that develops in dogs with CHF can result from cardiac arrhythmias, abnormal baro-receptor function, and drug-induced hypo-tension. Digoxin is useful for eliminating syncope in many dogs with chronic valvular disease and syncope of uncertain cause. Dogs with chronic valvular disease and concurrent respiratory disease may respond favorably to either theo-phylline or antitussive drugs.

Vasovagal syncope, sometimes diagnosed in young Boxers, may respond to metoprolol (Lopressor). When syncope is associated with an underlying disease process that results in hypovolemia, anemia, or hypoglycemia, treat-ment of the underlying disease will often eliminate syncope.

PROGNOSIS

Prognosis for animals with syncope is usually related to the prognosis for the underlying disease.

CHAPTER 3

Respiratory emergencies

- **Respiratory distress**

- **Upper airway obstruction**

- **Pneumonia**

- **Feline asthma**

- **Pulmonary thromboembolism**

- **Noncardiogenic pulmonary edema**

- **Pneumothorax**

- **Pyothorax**

- **Pulmonary neoplasia**

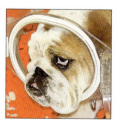 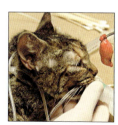 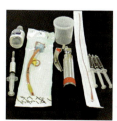 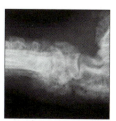

Respiratory distress

The general approach to a case of respiratory distress is illustrated in **62**.

KEY POINTS

- Respiratory difficulty may be life-threatening.
- Abnormalities in the upper airways, the lower airways, the pulmonary parenchyma, or the pleural space may result in respiratory distress.
- Hypoxemia and hypercarbia define respiratory and ventilatory failure.

SUPPLEMENTAL OXYGEN

Normal room air contains approximately 21% oxygen. Increasing the inspired oxygen fraction will often relieve the hypoxemia. Methods to provide supplemental oxygen include flow-by (**64**), nasal oxygen (**63, 65**), oxygen hood (**66**), or oxygen cage (**67**). In rare cases, supplemental oxygen may be provided by a mechanical ventilator (**68**).

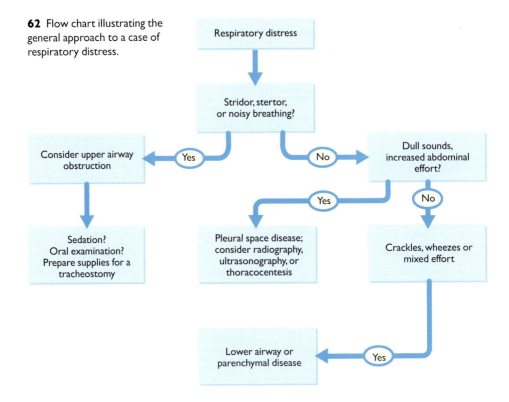

62 Flow chart illustrating the general approach to a case of respiratory distress.

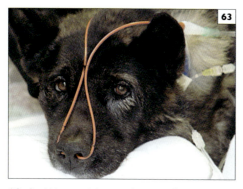

63 An Akita receiving nasal oxygen for treatment of hypoxemia.

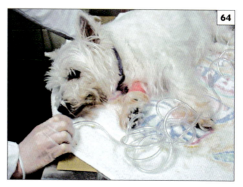

64 A West Highland White Terrier with pulmonary fibrosis receiving flow-by oxygen.

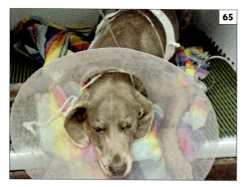

65 Nasal oxygen in a Weimeraner recovering from pulmonary contusions.

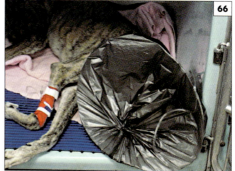

66 An inexpensive oxygen hood may be constructed from an Elizabethan collar and plastic wrap. This Greyhound was intolerant of nasal oxygen, but comfortable with an oxygen hood.

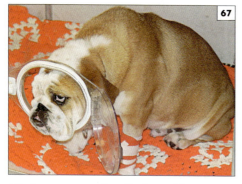

67 An oxygen cage is well tolerated by most animals, but when the cage is opened to administer treatment, the oxygen content rapidly equilibrates with room air.

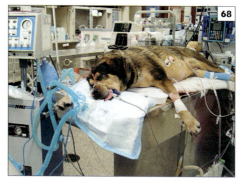

68 A dog receiving mechanical ventilation following surgery to remove a thymoma associated with myasthenia gravis, hypoventilation, and aspiration pneumonia.

Upper airway obstruction

KEY POINTS
- Upper airway obstruction is usually recognized by noisy breathing.
- Tracheostomy may be life-saving when airway obstruction is severe.
- Anxiety or stress will increase air flow rates and magnify effects of obstruction.

DEFINITION / OVERVIEW
Upper airway obstruction may develop from any condition that decreases the air flow rate through the mouth and upper airways. Airway obstruction may be life-threatening and should be promptly addressed.

ETIOLOGY AND RISK FACTORS
Airway obstructions can be fixed or dynamic and may be chronic or may develop acutely. Any anxiety or stress will increase the flow limitation and increase the degree of obstruction. Brachycephalic breeds, like Pugs and Bulldogs, are particularly predisposed to upper airway obstruction. Airway obstruction in these breeds is due to a combination of stenotic nares, elongated soft palate, everted laryngeal saccules, and, possibly, laryngeal collapse or tracheal hypoplasia. Neoplasia of the larynx or caudal oropharynx may result in airway obstruction. Foreign objects may acutely lodge in the airway and cause obstruction. Dynamic obstruction may result from laryngeal paralysis. Extra-airway cellulitis, abscessation, or neoplasia may also cause obstruction. Allergic reactions, while rare, may result in upper airway obstruction.

Upper airway obstructions are uncommon in cats but may develop from neoplasia, granulomatous change, or nasopharyngeal polyps.

PATHOPHYSIOLOGY
Any flow limitation in the airway may trigger an increased respiratory rate and effort, in order to attempt to overcome the obstruction. Increased flow rates may result in airway swelling and worsen the obstruction. Gradually developing airway obstructions may be well tolerated until a critical point is reached. The underlying cause of the obstruction may have more specific underlying pathophysiology.

CLINICAL PRESENTATION
Animals presented as emergencies with upper airway obstruction will be anxious and have noisy breathing. A stridor or stertor may be heard. Referred upper airway sounds may be auscultated in the chest. Animals may be acutely affected if a foreign object or infectious cause is present. Animals may be febrile or cyanotic. They will often appear frantic due to air hunger.

DIFFERENTIAL DIAGNOSES
Differential diagnoses include other causes of respiratory distress, such as pleural space disease or pulmonary infiltrates.

DIAGNOSIS
A presumptive diagnosis may be made based upon clinical presentation. Evaluation under anesthesia (69) is required to both confirm the diagnosis and to either relieve the obstruction or perform a tracheostomy. It is essential to be efficient in induction of general anesthesia, and additionally have all potentially needed supplies close at hand. The underlying diagnosis may reflect anatomic abnormalities, foreign objects, mass lesions, or dynamic flow limitation.

The underlying prognosis can differ substantially depending on the cause, thus knowledge of the source of the obstruction is prognostic.

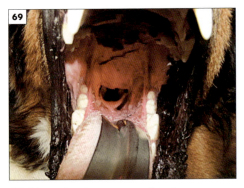

69 Normal canine anatomy of the larynx. Intrinsic motion should be assessed under a light plane of anesthesia, with either thiopental or propofol. Doxapram (1–2 mg/kg IV) may be used to stimulate respiration and improve detection of abnormal function.

MANAGEMENT / TREATMENT
Management is directed at reducing the obstruction to air flow. In some cases, sedation with low doses of acepromazine or butorphanol may be warranted. Supplemental oxygen is helpful in reducing the sensation of dyspnea. Tracheostomy may be life-saving (**70**). More specific treatment is directed at the underlying cause (**71**) and may include soft palate resection, arytenoid lateralization, or chemotherapy. In rare cases, permanent tracheostomy is required to permit adequate ventilation.

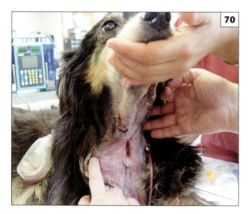

70 A tracheostomy was placed in this dog to secure an airway following severe bite wounds.

Pneumonia

KEY POINTS
- Pneumonia may develop following aspiration of gastric contents, or following viral infection.
- Broad-spectrum antibiotic therapy is warranted pending bacterial culture and sensitivity testing.
- Pneumonia is rare in cats; pulmonary infiltrates usually represent CHF.

DEFINITION/OVERVIEW
Pneumonia represents an inflammation of the lung parenchyma. Inflammation results in V–Q mismatching and subsequent hypoxemia. Clinical signs of infection are common. Pneumonia may be mild or rapidly life-threatening.

ETIOLOGY
Pneumonia often develops in dogs following aspiration of gastric contents. Aspiration may occur due to vomiting or regurgitation, laryngeal paralysis, or following general anesthesia. Dogs with megaesophagus are particularly prone to aspiration pneumonia (**72**). Pneumonia may also develop following tracheobronchitis (kennel cough) or following a viral infection. In endemic regions, infection with dimorphic fungi (e.g. blastomycosis, histoplasmosis) may also occur. Protozoal or parasitic organisms may also result in pneumonia. Pneumonia is very rare in cats but

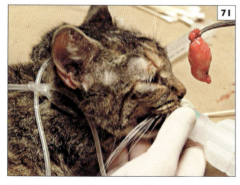

71 A large nasopharyngeal polyp following removal from a cat. The cat, as could be anticipated, had substantial signs of airway obstruction.

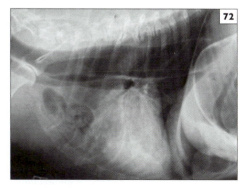

72 Lateral thoracic radiograph of a dog with pneumonia. This dog had a concurrent megaesophagus which predisposed her to aspiration pneumonia and was recovering from surgery to correct a GDV. There is free air in the abdominal cavity.

may develop due to extension of an upper respiratory infection or due to a protozoal infection (e.g. toxoplasmosis).

PATHOPHYSIOLOGY

Infection with bacterial organisms results in a local inflammatory response. Inflammation causes protein-rich edema fluid and neutrophils to fill the airways and pulmonary parenchyma. Gram-negative infections are particularly virulent. Cytokines will magnify the inflammatory response. Severe infection results in systemic signs of sepsis.

CLINICAL PRESENTATION

Dogs with pneumonia will usually show signs of both pulmonary compromise and systemic inflammation/infection. Fever, cough, and nasal discharge are common. Affected dogs may be tachypneic or may have overt respiratory distress. Dogs with megaesophagus may have a history of regurgitation and/or weight loss, and dogs with laryngeal paralysis will often have loud or noisy breathing.

DIFFERENTIAL DIAGNOSES

Pneumonia should be differentiated from other causes of respiratory distress or sepsis/inflammation. Other causes of respiratory distress include CHF, PTE, acute lung injury, allergic pneumonitis, pleural space disease, or trauma. Other causes of sepsis include pyothorax, pancreatitis, septic abdomen, urosepsis, pyometra, or prostatitis.

DIAGNOSIS

Diagnosis of pneumonia is based on documentation of inflammatory pulmonary infiltrates, ideally with a positive culture of the infecting organism. Clinically, thoracic radiographs are very useful for documenting interstitial to alveolar pulmonary infiltrates (**73**). Pneumonic infiltrates are commonly present in the cranioventral lobes, particularly the right middle lobe. Samples for bacterial culture and sensitivity testing and cytological analysis may be collected via a trans-oral tracheal wash or a bronchoalveolar lavage. In some cases, empiric therapy with broad-spectrum antibiotics is initiated without cytology and culture results.

MANAGEMENT / TREATMENT

Treatment of pneumonia should include broad-spectrum antibiotics, intravenous fluids, and physiotherapy. Fluids are beneficial to help hydrate airway secretions and correct any interstitial fluid deficits. Physiotherapy includes nebulization and coupage. Supplemental oxygen therapy is warranted if increased respiratory rate and effort are present or if hypoxemia is documented via an arterial blood gas analysis or pulse oximetry. Lung function may be assessed using a spirometer (**74**) or through arterial blood gas analysis or pulse oximetry. Nasal oxygen is an especially beneficial technique for providing supplemental oxygen. The underlying cause for the pneumonia should be actively sought and corrected if possible.

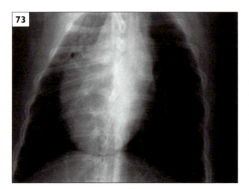

73 Ventrodorsal thoracic radiograph of a dog with aspiration pneumonia. In this case, the alveolar infiltrate is confined to the right cranial lobe. Air bronchograms can be seen. Two views are very helpful in confirming a radiographic diagnosis of pneumonia.

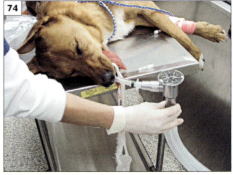

74 A spirometer being used to assess tidal volume and lung function.

Feline asthma

KEY POINTS
- Common signs of asthma include cough and respiratory distress.
- Affected cats usually respond well to glucocorticoids.

DEFINITION / OVERVIEW
Feline asthma is a catch-all term representing lower airway disease in cats. Cats with airway disease may cough frequently or may be normal between bouts of severe respiratory distress.
- Asthma is defined as reversible bronchoconstriction with intermittent bouts of respiratory distress due to airway narrowing.
- Chronic bronchitis is defined as bronchial wall edema with excessive mucus production, resulting in excessive secretions and airway inflammation.

ETIOLOGY AND RISK FACTORS
The cause of feline asthma is unknown. One study has documented an increased incidence in Siamese cats and, anecdotally, cats with severe respiratory infections as kittens or those exposed to high concentrations of allergens seem more commonly affected. Some cats also appear seasonally affected.

PATHOPHYSIOLOGY
Inflammatory or reactive airways develop in response to a stimulus. The bronchial wall may become edematous and goblet cells hypertrophy, resulting in excessive mucus production. Smooth muscle hypertrophy develops. The end result is a narrowing of the airway lumen and subsequent increase in resistance to air flow. Expiratory flow limitation may develop and hyperinflation and prolonged expiratory times may be clinically apparent.

CLINICAL PRESENTATION
Clinical presentation of affected cats is for either severe respiratory distress or cough. Cats with respiratory distress may be very agitated and have prolonged expiratory efforts. Changes in the timing of the respiratory cycle may be difficult to appreciate clinically during marked tachypnea. Cats with cough will appear outwardly normal, although they may have relatively easily induced tracheal cough upon palpation.

DIFFERENTIAL DIAGNOSES
Differential diagnoses include other causes of respiratory distress, such as CHF or pleural effusion. Cats with airway disease are usually normothermic. Cats with respiratory or pulmonary disease may have crackles, representing fluid in the airways. Cats with pleural effusion may have short and shallow respiratory patterns. Cats with occult heartworm infection or lungworm infestation may have similar signs. Pneumonia is very rare in cats.

DIAGNOSIS
Diagnosis is based upon clinical signs, thoracic radiography, and exclusion of other causes. Thoracic radiographs usually document an interstitial to bronchial pattern (75) coupled with evidence of hyperinflation. Screening for parasitic diseases is warranted depending on the part of the world that the cat lives in.

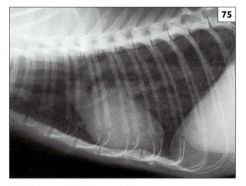

75 Lateral thoracic radiograph from a cat with lower airway disease. There is a profound bronchial pattern. Lungworm was isolated from this cat, who had recently been a stray. Moderate cardiomegaly is also present.

A trans-oral tracheal wash may be performed for collection of a sample of respiratory fluid for cytological evaluation and bacterial culture and sensitivity testing (76). Secondary bacterial infection may complicate a variety of respiratory conditions, although infection was not the initial inciting cause. A tracheal wash is performed by first pre-oxygenating the cat with either flow-by or a face mask with supplemental oxygen. The cat is next briefly anesthetized, usually using propofol (slow intravenous injection to effect). The trachea should be intubated with a sterile endotracheal tube, and aliquots of sterile saline should be infused via a long catheter and then collected for analysis. Usually 3 ml of sterile saline are used and the washing is repeated up to three times. It is often beneficial to allow the excessive fluid to drain into a sterile specimen container, in addition to re-aspiration from the syringe and catheter system. A tracheal wash should *not* be performed in a cat with overt respiratory distress.

MANAGEMENT / TREATMENT

Management and treatment are directed towards removing an underlying cause if possible. Smokers in the household should be discouraged and excessive exposure to allergens limited.

Bronchodilators and anti-inflammatory agents are the mainstay of therapy. Bronchodilators used in cats include theophylline or beta-2 agonists. Beta-2 agonists may be administered either orally or via aerosol. Aerosol medications are gaining popularity in feline practice, due to the proliferation of 'feline-friendly' delivery apparatuses. Anti-inflammatory agents most commonly used include prednisone (prednisolone), either orally or as a reposital injection. Some clinicians advocate the use of human leukotriene antagonists, although objective evidence of their efficacy is currently lacking.

PROGNOSIS

Most cats with feline asthma respond well to therapy, although it is considered a chronic disease requiring life-long treatment.

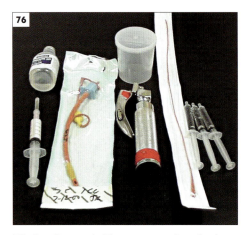

76 Supplies needed for a trans-oral tracheal wash. The procedure is described in the text.

Pulmonary thromboembolism

KEY POINTS
- PTE may result in sudden hypoxemia that is moderately responsive to oxygen supplementation.
- Immune-mediated hemolytic anemia, sepsis, DIC, Cushing's syndrome, heartworm disease, and neoplasia are common predisposing factors in dogs.
- PTE is uncommon in cats.

DEFINITION / OVERVIEW
PTE is characterized by the development of a clot within the pulmonary vasculature. Successful oxygenation of the blood requires both adequate ventilation (V) and adequate blood flow (perfusion: Q). V–Q mismatch may result in hypoxemia.

A small clot may be hemodynamically insignificant while a large clot can result in substantial limitation of perfusion, with subsequent cardiovascular collapse or even death.

PATHOPHYSIOLOGY
PTE results from an alteration in Virchow's triad, which is represented by alterations in blood characteristics (hypercoagulability), endothelial damage, and/or vascular stasis. Common disease processes that have been associated with PTE in dogs include Cushing's syndrome, immune-mediated hemolytic anemia, sepsis, DIC, and heartworm infection. PTE is extremely rare in cats.

CLINICAL PRESENTATION
The clinical signs surrounding PTE are usually peracute with a rapid onset of labored breathing. Occasionally, small showers of PTE may be progressive, with a dog looking simply tachypneic for several hours to days, prior to progressing to overt dyspnea.

DIFFERENTIAL DIAGNOSES
As PTE is usually hospital-acquired, it should be differentiated from other causes of respiratory distress, including pneumonia, volume overload/heart failure, or ARDS.

DIAGNOSIS
Diagnosis of PTE is based upon exclusion of other causes of respiratory distress and upon appropriate imaging results. Thoracic radiographs may be normal, or may document oligemia (reduced blood flow). The gold standard is selective angiography, with injection of iodinated contrast material into the pulmonary artery. V–Q scans may be useful, although they are not widely available. Finally, echocardiography may document right-sided changes consistent with the presence of a pulmonary thrombus. In human medicine the use of CT has proven very useful in documenting PTE noninvasively.

MANAGEMENT / TREATMENT
Treatment and management of PTE include supplemental oxygen and anticoagulants. Additionally, specific treatment directed at the underlying cause is obviously ideal. Anticoagulants used may include aspirin (0.5–3 mg/kg), heparin (200–300 U/kg SC q6hr), low molecular weight heparins (dosage based on type), and coumadin (warfarin sodium). The anticoagulant chosen should reflect the underlying disease. In rare cases, thrombolytic therapies have been attempted, although these have met with mixed success.

PROGNOSIS
The prognosis for PTE is guarded, with severely affected dogs often succumbing to severe respiratory failure. Dogs with mild to moderate PTE may recover with supportive care. Acute fatal PTE has also occasionally been documented on post-mortem examination.

Noncardiogenic pulmonary edema

KEY POINTS
- NCPE reflects the development of increased lung water (pulmonary edema) due to either increased vascular permeability or lowered vascular oncotic pressure.
- Common causes of NCPE in dogs include electrocution, upper airway obstruction, and seizures.
- Pulmonary infiltrates are most commonly dorsocaudal in distribution.

DEFINITION / OVERVIEW
NCPE reflects the presence of high-protein edema fluid in the lung parenchyma. NCPE may be used to describe the presence of any form of pulmonary edema not associated with heart failure, and includes acute lung injury/ARDS or pulmonary contusions. However, in veterinary medicine, NCPE is more commonly used to refer to a specific form of protein-rich pulmonary edema that forms following an insult.

PATHOPHYSIOLOGY
Protein-rich pulmonary edema fluid forms due to changes in capillary permeability, which permit the extravasation of fluid into the alveoli. The underlying mechanism may reflect vasculitis, or a sudden elevation in circulating catecholamine levels, or it may occur via an unknown mechanism.

CLINICAL PRESENTATION
The clinical signs surrounding NCPE are usually acutely progressive over minutes to hours. NCPE is much more common in dogs and is rare to nonexistent in cats. Usually, an antecedent cause is identified, such as a seizure. However, in some cases, no event is recalled other than minor activity, such as restraint for vaccination or a bath. Puppies are more commonly affected than adult dogs. Affected dogs will be tachypneic or have overt respiratory distress. Crackles may be present. Usually, no murmur or gallop is auscultated and the body temperature is normal.

DIFFERENTIAL DIAGNOSES
Differential diagnoses include pneumonia, congenital heart disease, or trauma. Cough is usually absent with NCPE and rectal temperature should be normal. Puppies with severe congenital heart disease will usually have loud murmurs, with the exception of right to left shunts that result in polycythemia. Animals which have suffered trauma severe enough to cause pulmonary infiltrates will commonly have external signs of trauma. Metastatic disease should also be excluded in older dogs.

DIAGNOSIS
Diagnosis of NCPE is typically a diagnosis based on historical and radiographic abnormalities. The radiographic distribution is typically dorso-caudal, although it may be diffuse (77, 78). Peri-hilar or cranioventral distribution should prompt consideration of other differential diagnoses.

MANAGEMENT / TREATMENT
Treatment is strictly supportive, with rest and supplemental oxygen. Any underlying cause should be treated directly. Fluid support should only be provided if clearly indicated, as additional intravenous fluids could result in worsening edema. Mildly to moderately affected animals will usually respond to simple measures quickly. Severe NCPE may be fatal.

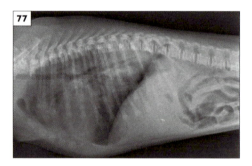

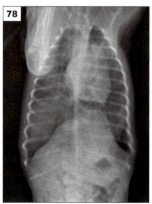

77, 78 Ventrodorsal and lateral thoracic radiographs from a Cocker Spaniel with NCPE. The infiltrates have a diffuse distribution.

Pneumothorax

KEY POINTS
- Pneumothorax should be classified as to its origin.
- Spontaneous pneumothorax should be considered a surgical disease.
- Thoracocentesis or thoracostomy tube placement should be considered in a pet with respiratory compromise and a pneumothorax (**79**).

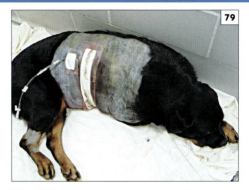

79 A light bandage or occlusive dressing should be placed covering the site of the chest tube.

DEFINITION / OVERVIEW
Pneumothorax is defined as the accumulation of air within the pleural space. Air in the pleural space will prevent adequate expansion of the lungs and may limit ventilation and oxygenation.

A tension pneumothorax represents the most severe form and is defined as a large-volume pneumothorax with supra-atmospheric pleural pressure, with limited or no ability to ventilate, and evidence of cardiovascular collapse.

ETIOLOGY AND RISK FACTORS
Pneumothorax develops due to a communication between the pleural space and the lungs or the chest wall. It most commonly occurs either due to a blunt or penetrating trauma damaging the lung parenchyma or chest wall. Vehicular trauma and thoracic bite wounds are the most frequent causes of traumatic pneumothorax. It may also develop spontaneously due to abnormalities in the lungs, such as bullae/blebs, neoplasia, or infection. One study documented an increased incidence of spontaneous pneumothorax in Huskies and other northern-breed dogs. Finally, pneumothorax may be iatrogenic, subsequent to thoracocentesis or barotrauma. Patients with chronic pleural effusion and pleuritis are at particular risk of iatrogenic pneumothorax.

PATHOPHYSIOLOGY
The normal intrapleural pressure is negative. The addition of air to the pleural space results in a loss of the normal coupling of the visceral and parietal pleura. This causes collapse of lung parenchyma and results in a restrictive breathing pattern, characterized by short, shallow respirations. In cases of a large-volume pneumothorax, the chest cavity will appear larger than normal ('barrel-shaped'). Gas exchange is compromised, due to increasing V–Q abnormalities. Cardiac output may be decreased due to the loss of venous return.

CLINICAL PRESENTATION
In all cases, the severity of the clinical signs of the pneumothorax is related to the relative volume, rather than necessarily the source of the pneumothorax.

Animals with traumatic pneumothorax will most commonly present for stabilization of the initial injury. Animals will be tachypneic and often appear anxious. Breath sounds may be muffled, although if concurrent pulmonary contusion is present, they may sound normal or increased.

Spontaneous pneumothorax will most often have a more insidious onset, with coughing and tachypnea over a period of usually hours to days. Some dogs with spontaneous pneumothorax will present with acute severe respiratory distress and cardiovascular collapse following a period of several days of vague malaise.

Iatrogenic pneumothorax is most commonly appreciated clinically via either the sudden detection of a moderate to large volume of air retrieved during thoracocentesis, the development of respiratory distress in a patient following thoracocentesis, or the desaturation of a patient undergoing mechanical ventilation.

DIFFERENTIAL DIAGNOSES
Traumatic pneumothorax should be differentiated from respiratory distress caused by pulmonary contusion, chest wall instability, or diaphragmatic hernia. Many animals with thoracic trauma will have multiple causes of respiratory distress.

Spontaneous pneumothorax should be differentiated from other causes of respiratory distress, such as pneumonia or CHF. Thoracic radiography is diagnostic.

Iatrogenic pneumothorax should be distinguished from progression of underlying disease, hemorrhage, or mechanical complication, such as endotracheal tube occlusion.

DIAGNOSIS

In animals that are exhibiting severe respiratory embarrassment, needle thoracocentesis will be both diagnostic and therapeutic.

Thoracic radiography is the diagnostic test of choice for confirmation of pneumothorax (80, 81). Radiography is both sensitive and specific for the diagnosis of pneumothorax. The source of the pneumothorax must be determined by integrating the historical and clinical findings. Other imaging modalities, such as CT, may be employed if an underlying cause is not apparent. Ultrasonography is not generally useful in the presence of free air.

MANAGEMENT / TREATMENT

Traumatic pneumothorax is most commonly successfully managed conservatively, with needle thoracocentesis as needed. Animals that require multiple (more than three) thoracocenteses over a 24-hour period for management of a pneumothorax may benefit from the placement of a thoracic tube and the application of continuous suction to ensure re-inflation. Traumatic pneumothorax is rarely surgical, although penetrating bite wounds may damage the lung lobe severely enough to necessitate lobectomy. Resolution of residual pneumothorax will occur over days to weeks, depending upon the volume of the pneumothorax. If desired, supplemental oxygen will hasten the re-absorption of the pneumothorax by creating a nitrogen gradient between the blood and the pneumothorax.

Spontaneous pneumothorax is considered a surgical disease in dogs. Most cases are due to the presence of a bulla or sub-pleural bleb and will not resolve without resection. In a few cases, such as pneumonia, asthma, or dirofilarasis, medical management may be warranted. Careful attention to patient condition and clear communication with the owner are required for successful outcome.

Iatrogenic pneumothorax may be treated conservatively or by surgical intervention. The treatment plan selected should reflect the patient's underlying disease and the severity of the pneumothorax. If the patient has pre-existing pleural space disease/pleuritis and a large-volume pneumothorax, it is unlikely to seal without surgical intervention. However, if a patient has been successfully weaned from mechanical respiration, removal of the barotraumas will commonly result in the success of medical management.

PROGNOSIS

In general, traumatic pneumothorax carries a good prognosis, and spontaneous pneumothorax carries a good prognosis with surgical intervention and a guarded to fair prognosis with medical management. The prognosis for iatrogenic pneumothorax reflects the underlying disease.

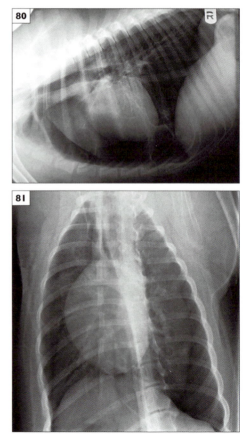

80, 81 Lateral and ventrodorsal thoracic radiographs from a Golden Retriever documenting severe pneumothorax resulting from trauma. There is an apparent 'elevation' of the heart on the lateral projection due to the presence of the pneumothorax.

Pyothorax

KEY POINTS
- Pyothorax is usually a surgical disease in dogs and a medical disease in cats.
- Sepsis may accompany pyothorax and requires aggressive treatment.
- Outdoor cats, cats in multiple-cat households, and hunting dogs are at increased risk of developing pyothorax.

DEFINITION / OVERVIEW
Pyothorax is defined as the accumulation of purulent material (pus) within the pleural space. Pyothorax may result in systemic signs of infection (sepsis) or respiratory distress due to inability to ventilate adequately because of large volumes of pleural effusion.

ETIOLOGY
Pyothorax may develop from a penetrating wound (e.g. bite wound or foreign object) or from rupture of a lung abscess introducing infection into the pleural space. An inhaled plant awn may result in lung abscessation. Lung tissue may abscess in response to severe pneumonia or, rarely, neoplasia.

PATHOPHYSIOLOGY
Pleural effusion from a patient with pyothorax contains a large number of white blood cells (primarily neutrophils) with intra- and extracellular bacteria. The effusion volume may limit respiration, while the infection usually contributes to signs of systemic inflammation, such as fever, tachypnea, and tachycardia.

CLINICAL PRESENTATION
Cats will typically present for lethargy, anorexia, and depression. They may also have labored breathing. Cats may be febrile or hypothermic. Most cats are indoor–outdoor, or live in multi-cat households.

Dogs will usually present for respiratory distress, although occasional dogs will present for signs of sepsis (fever, anorexia, lethargy). Large-breed hunting dogs are more commonly affected than other breeds.

DIFFERENTIAL DIAGNOSES
Pyothorax should be differentiated from other causes of pleural effusion, such as CHF, neoplasia, or hemothorax.

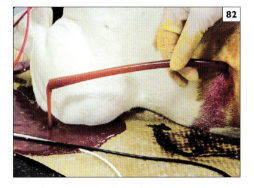

82 A large amount of purulent material flows freely following placement of a thoracostomy tube in this Pointer. There are 'sulfur granules' present in the exudate.

DIAGNOSIS
In animals that are exhibiting severe respiratory embarrassment, needle thoracocentesis will be both diagnostic and therapeutic. Fluid cytology and culture are the methods of choice for documenting pyothorax. In some cases, bacterial culture may be negative, despite visualization of bacteria or severe degenerative change. This may reflect prior antibiotic therapy or delay before a culture swab reaches the laboratory. If an underlying foreign object or abscess is suspected, further imaging, such as thoracic ultrasonography or CT of the chest, may be warranted.

MANAGEMENT / TREATMENT
Appropriate management requires drainage of the infection. In most cases, thoracostomy tubes are placed to permit repeated drainage (**82**). Saline lavage (with the addition of 1000 U/l of unfractionated heparin) may be used at 10–20 ml/kg q6–8 hr. Cats generally respond well to medical management while dogs often require thoracotomy for resolution of the infection.

Broad-spectrum antibiotics should be used until the bacterial culture results are available. Anaerobic coverage should be continued regardless of culture results, due to the frequency of anaerobic infection. Intravenous fluid therapy is warranted. The additional fluid losses into the chest cavity should be replaced by crystalloids.

Pulmonary neoplasia

KEY POINTS
- Thoracic neoplasia may be primary or metastatic.
- The presence of significant volumes of pleural effusion is a negative prognostic indicator.
- Neoplasia will often have an indolent clinical course.

DEFINITION / OVERVIEW
The lungs and pleural space are commonly affected by neoplasia. Lymphoma will affect animals of any age, while carcinoma and sarcoma will more commonly affect older animals.

PATHOPHYSIOLOGY
Neoplasia may result in clinical signs due to diffuse lung involvement resulting in respiratory distress and hypoxemia, due to airway obstruction from a mass, or due to pleural space disease. Pleural space disease may present as large volumes of effusion or a spontaneous pneumothorax. Neoplasia may be primary or metastatic.

CLINICAL PRESENTATION
The clinical signs surrounding pulmonary neoplasia in dogs are usually vague and progressive. Dogs may present with cough, hemoptysis, tachypnea or respiratory distress, or weight loss. Occasionally, dogs may present for 'swollen legs' due to the presence of hypertrophic (pulmonary) osteopathy (83). Cats may have a more rapid appearance of clinical signs, and will often have large volumes of pleural effusion.

DIFFERENTIAL DIAGNOSES
Differential diagnoses of nodular pulmonary disease include abscess or granuloma formation. Tumors may become necrotic and abscessed. Diffuse pulmonary infiltrates may reflect pulmonary fibrosis, allergic lung disease, sepsis, or pneumonia.

DIAGNOSIS
Diagnosis is typically based on historical, radiographic (84), and cytological abnormalities. Radiographic distribution reflects either primary or metastatic disease, but is classically nodular. Lymphoma will exfoliate well into pleural effusions while other cell types exfoliate less well. Other imaging techniques may also be useful.

Biopsy is the gold standard for the diagnosis of tumor type. Fine needle lung aspirate may be diagnostic, although, rarely, patients may develop a pneumothorax following aspiration. Tracheal wash cytology is rarely supportive of neoplasia.

MANAGEMENT / TREATMENT
Isolated masses may respond well to surgical removal, with extended survival times or even cures. However, large masses or those that have spread to regional lymph nodes carry a poor prognosis. Additionally, the presence of pleural effusion, particularly large volumes, is associated with a grave prognosis. Chemotherapy, both local and systemic, has been associated with some improvement in survival. Lymphoma, in particular, is very chemoresponsive.

PROGNOSIS
Overall, the prognosis is very guarded.

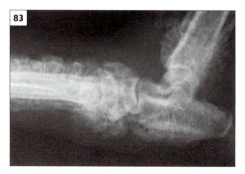

83 Hypertrophic (pulmonary) osteopathy may be observed in animals with thoracic masses. There is marked bony proliferation.

84 Thoracic radiograph documenting a large cranial mediastinal mass.

CHAPTER 4

Hematological emergencies

- **Blood loss anemia**

- **Hemolytic anemia**

- **Nonregenerative anemia**

- **Thrombocytopenia/thrombocytopathia**

- **Acquired coagulopathy**

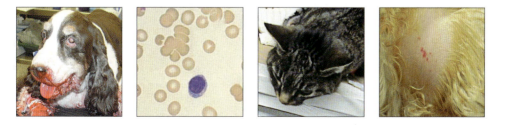

KEY POINTS

- Determine the underlying cause of the anemia (**85**).
- Acute blood loss may not appear regenerative for 48 hours.
- Define coagulopathy as primary (platelet) or secondary (clotting factor) and then as acquired or congenital (**86**).

Blood loss anemia

KEY POINTS

- Blood loss anemia is usually accompanied by a low circulating total protein level.
- Acute blood loss most commonly occurs as a result of trauma, or internal hemorrhage secondary to neoplasia or severe thrombocytopenia.
- Chronic blood loss is most often associated with GI hemorrhage.

85 Flow chart for anemia.

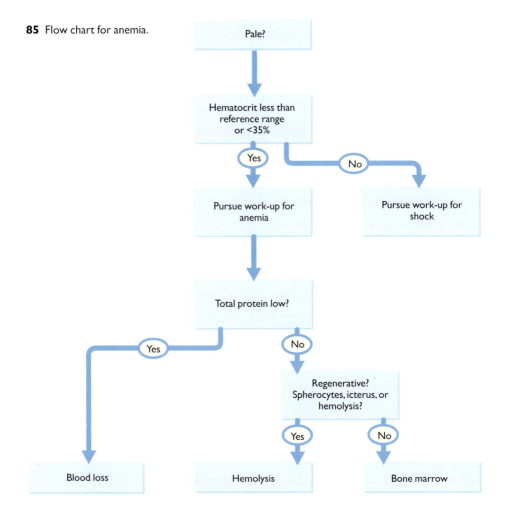

DEFINITION / OVERVIEW

Anemia resulting from blood loss may be caused by acute or chronic hemorrhage. It can further be characterized as internal or external hemorrhage, and as spontaneous or traumatic. Most cases of mild traumatic blood loss do not cause clinical abnormalities in perfusion. If blood loss is severe, hypovolemia will result. Clinical signs depend on the amount of blood lost, period of time during which bleeding occurred, and site of hemorrhage.

86 Flow chart for coagulopathy.

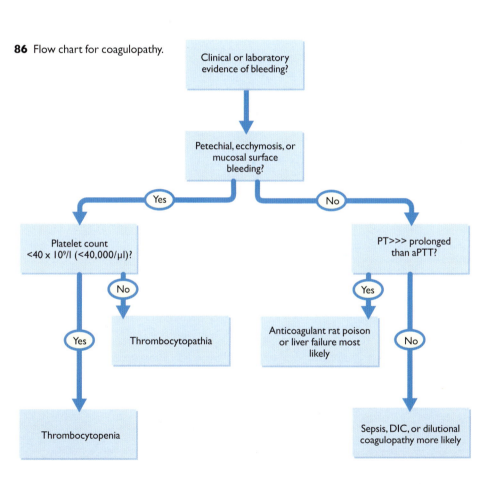

ETIOLOGY

Blood loss commonly results from trauma, including vehicular trauma, bite wounds, or other injuries. External traumatic blood loss is easy to detect. Traumatic injuries may also result in internal hemorrhage, typically into the abdomen from splenic or hepatic injury, but also occasionally into the thorax or retroperitoneal space.

Spontaneous blood loss is usually a consequence of neoplasia (**87**), GI ulceration (**88**), an acquired coagulopathy, such as ACR toxicity, or ITP.

PATHOPHYSIOLOGY

Blood loss results from damage to blood vessels, either from trauma or erosion, or from lack of effective hemostasis at mucosal barriers, such as occurs with thrombocytopenia.

Regeneration

Within hours of blood loss, the marrow begins to increase the production of erythrocytes. It takes the bone marrow approximately 48–96 hours to release enough reticulocytes for detection of circulating reticulocytosis. Therefore, during that time, the blood loss may appear to be nonregenerative. The spleen contracts following blood loss in dogs, which causes delivery of a high hematocrit blood (80%) into the circulation, temporarily increasing the hematocrit. Once the bleeding has been arrested, the anemia typically resolves

within days to weeks. Starting about 2–3 hours after onset of hemorrhage and continuing for about 48–72 hours, the blood volume is restored by the addition of interstitial fluid. Astute clients may detect polydipsia in pets with internal blood loss.

CLINICAL PRESENTATION

Traumatic injuries resulting in blood loss are relatively straightforward to detect (**89, 90**). Animals presenting after vehicular trauma should have their PCV and total solids assessed. Animals with low total solids (i.e. <60 g/l [<6.0 g/dl]) should be assumed to have had blood loss until proven otherwise. Ultrasonography is gaining widespread acceptance as a rapid screening tool for the presence or absence of abdominal effusion (e.g. hemorrhage) (**91**).

Animals with spontaneous hemorrhage may have evidence of external blood loss (e.g. epistaxis or melena), or may be weak or collapsed from internal blood loss. Hypovolemia may be appreciated by tachycardia, pale mucous membranes, and weak pulses.

DIFFERENTIAL DIAGNOSES

Blood loss anemia should be distinguished from hemolytic anemia or nonregenerative anemia. In some cases, the source of anemia may be twofold. For example, a dog may have both hemolytic anemia and thrombocytopenia, resulting in both loss and destruction, or it may have pancytopenia, resulting in loss from thrombocytopenia

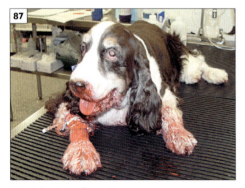

87 A Springer Spaniel with severe epistaxis due to a nasal tumor.

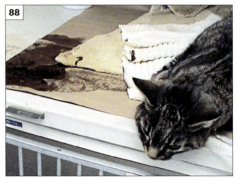

88 Coffee-ground vomitus associated with esophageal and gastric ulceration in a cat on long-term prednisone therapy.

and production failure. Malignant histiocytosis may result in anemia coupled with hypoproteinemia. Thus, if a source of hemorrhage is not identified, it is prudent to consider performing a bone marrow or splenic aspirate, particularly in 'at risk' dogs, such as Bernese Mountain dogs or Flat-Coated Retrievers.

DIAGNOSIS

The diagnosis of blood loss anemia is based upon confirming the presence of anemia and detecting a source of blood loss (either external or internal).

MANAGEMENT / TREATMENT

The underlying cause of the hemorrhage should be determined and corrected if possible. Intravenous fluids should be given to treat hypovolemic shock. A 'shock' dose of crystalloids may be administered, recalling that the end-point of fluid resuscitation is stabilization of vital signs, not the delivery of a specific volume of fluid. If the blood loss is moderate to severe and the patient is showing signs of tachycardia or weakness, a transfusion should be performed. Treatment for other causes of blood loss include: antiparasiticidal therapy; topical treatment for fleas/ticks; vitamin K for suspected rodenticide toxicities; H2 antagonist, sulcrafate or protonpump inhibitors for GI hemorrhage; and doxycycline or tetracycline for possible blood-related infectious agents.

PROGNOSIS

The prognosis is dependent on the underlying cause. Traumatic blood loss usually has a good prognosis. The prognosis for neoplasia is more guarded.

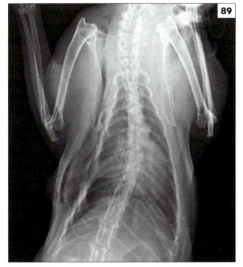

89 Ventrodorsal thoracic radiograph of a cat that was impaled on a stick. Note the pneumothorax, subcutaneous emphysema and large stick. The wood is a soft tissue density.

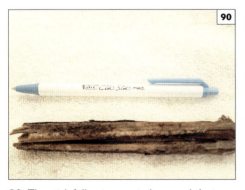

90 The stick following surgical removal. A pic pen is shown for size comparison. The cat made an uneventful recovery although blood transfusions were required to replace blood loss.

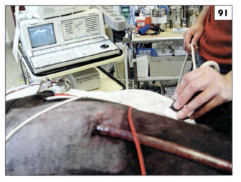

91 Ultrasonography may be used in the emergency room to document free abdominal fluid in patients suffering trauma. Fluid will appear hyperechoic (dark) on ultrasonographic examination.

Hemolytic anemia

KEY POINTS
- Premature destruction of red blood cells may result in anemia.
- Hemolysis may occur intravascularly or extravascularly.
- Most often, hemolytic anemia is idiopathic. However, some toxins or infections may cause hemolysis.

DEFINITION / OVERVIEW
Hemolytic anemia occurs when the rate of erythrocyte destruction is accelerated. Clinical signs become apparent when the rate of red blood cell destruction exceeds the rate of production. Red blood cells may be destroyed extravascularly, by the activities of the reticuloendothelial system, or intravascularly, by the circulating components of the immune system.

ETIOLOGY AND RISK FACTORS
Hemolytic anemias are classified based upon their cause.

Intrinsic (or inherited) hemolytic anemia
These comprise erythrocyte defects, including erythroenzymopathies, erythrocyte membrane-related abnormalities, and hemoglobin disorders. In dogs, phosphofructokinase deficiency is occasionally observed in hunting Springer Spaniels. However, intrinsic hemolytic anemias are rare.

Extrinsic (or acquired) hemolytic anemia
This group includes primary immune-mediated hemolytic anemia, where no underlying cause is identified, and secondary acquired hemolytic anemia, where the anemia results from some identifiable underlying cause. Documented causes of hemolytic anemia include drug reaction (sulfonamides/vaccines), infections (viral, bacterial, and parasitic, such as *Babesia*, *Hemobartonella*, dirofilariasis, ehrlichiosis), neoplasia (lymphoma, hemangiosarcoma), toxicities (zinc, onions/garlic, vitamin K), and hypophosphatemia.

Middle-aged female dogs, particularly Cocker Spaniels, are over-represented.

PATHOPHYSIOLOGY
Immune-mediated hemolytic anemia occurs when an immune response targets the red blood cell directly or indirectly causing its premature destruction. The destruction occurs when IgG antibodies, IgM antibodies, or complement bind to the surface of the red blood cell. Reticuloendothelial cells can phagocytize and destroy the opsonized erythrocytes. Sometimes macrophages remove only a portion of the red blood cell membrane resulting in spherocytes. Spherocytes are subsequently trapped in the spleen and removed from circulation. Non-immune hemolytic anemias may result in the simple destruction of the red blood cell in circulation.

CLINICAL PRESENTATION
Most animals with hemolytic anemia are presented for evaluation of clinical signs reflective of the anemia, including anorexia, lethargy, and collapse. Some dogs are presented for pigmenturia. On examination, dogs will usually appear weak. Fever is common and reflects inflammation, rather than infection. Tachycardia with bounding pulses will be present with moderate to severe anemia. Hepatosplenomegaly, due to extravascular hemolysis, may be pronounced.

DIFFERENTIAL DIAGNOSES
Hemolytic anemia should be distinguished from other causes of anemia. It is important to recall that some anemic pets will have several reasons for anemia.

DIAGNOSIS
Diagnosis of hemolytic anemia is based upon confirming the presence of anemia and detecting evidence of hemolysis. Signs of hemolysis include icterus (pre-hepatic) (**92**), hepatosplenomegaly, evidence of regeneration, auto-agglutination or Coombs positive results, and the presence of spherocytes (**93, 94**).

History or signalment may support an underlying cause. Minimum database includes a CBC, reticulocyte count, evaluation for auto-agglutination or Coombs status, serum chemistry profile, and urinalysis. Many dogs with immune-mediated hemolytic anemia will have a profound leukocytosis with a left shift. This finding alone should not be thought to represent infection in the absence of other clinical signs. A Coombs' test is unnecessary in the presence of auto-agglutination. Coagulation tests, thoracic radiographs, and abdominal ultrasonography, as well as serology for infectious disease, may be warranted. All dogs with evidence of intravascular hemolysis should have abdominal radiography performed to exclude a metallic object.

MANAGEMENT / TREATMENT

Ideally, any underlying cause should be removed, if possible. Treatment is directed at supporting the patient with intravenous fluids and/or blood transfusion to maintain an adequate circulating volume. Immunosuppressive therapy is required in patients with a suspected immune origin for the anemia. Commonly used immunosuppressive drugs include prednisone (prednisolone), azathioprine, cyclosporine (ciclosporin), human IVIG and cyclophosphamide (see Appendix 2 for doses). To date, no controlled trials in large numbers of affected dogs support the benefit of any specific treatment protocol beyond prednisone alone. Other treatments are as clinically indicated. Non-essential medications should be withheld. The patient should be slowly weaned off immunosuppressive therapy over a period of at least 6–12 months following clinical remission. Dogs developing hemolytic anemia after exposure to a specific drug or vaccine should not receive that product in the future.

PROGNOSIS

The prognosis is dependent on the underlying cause and severity of illness. Dogs with severe immune-mediated hemolytic anemia have a very guarded prognosis, with survival commonly <50%. Specific negative prognostic indicators include markedly elevated bilirubin, marked leukocytosis, neurological signs, and failure to respond to therapy. Many critically ill dogs are hospitalized for 7–14 days and may require multiple blood transfusions.

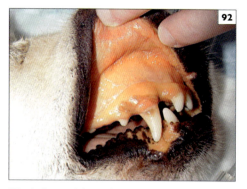

92 A dog with hemolytic anemia may appear clinically very jaundiced.

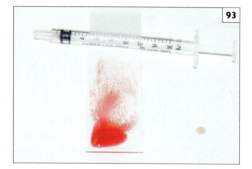

93 Auto-agglutination may be observed in animals affected with immune-mediated hemolytic anemia. Auto-agglutination may be macroscopic, as in this case.

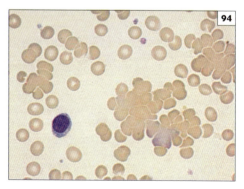

94 Auto-agglutination may only be observed during microscopic analysis of the blood film. Spherocytes can be seen on this microscopic view.

Nonregenerative anemia

KEY POINTS

- Nonregenerative anemia results from failure of adequate erythropoiesis.
- An underlying cause should be sought.
- Extended treatment times are often required to see clinical remission.

DEFINITION / OVERVIEW

Nonregenerative anemia results from a failure of the bone marrow to produce adequate red cells. Nonregenerative anemias tend to develop slowly and thus animals are able to tolerate remarkably low hematocrits. Most frequently, the cause is from within the bone marrow, although other causes are possible.

ETIOLOGY

The causes of nonregenerative anemia may be either within the bone marrow or outside the marrow. Bone marrow causes include a toxic insult, such as occurs with certain drugs or infections (e.g. *Ehrlichia*), deficiencies, such as iron, neoplasia, or immune-mediated disease. Extra-marrow causes most commonly reflect the lack of erythropoietin which accompanies renal failure. A mild nonregenerative anemia may accompany critical illness.

PATHOPHYSIOLOGY

Normal red cell survival is approximately 120 days in dogs and 70 days in cats. Therefore, most often nonregenerative anemia develops slowly as senescent red cells are lost and not replaced. Chronic anemia is much better tolerated by the animal than an abrupt drop in hematocrit. Toxins or viruses (e.g. FeLV) may directly damage the precursor cells in the bone marrow and result in a failure of the production of all cell lines or only selected lines. Iron deficiency will result in nonregenerative anemia due to the obligate requirement of iron in heme synthesis. Immune-mediated destruction of red cell precursors will result in severe anemia, as it is often coupled with destruction of circulating red cells. Finally, infiltration with neoplastic cells may result in the near-extinction of red cell precursors.

CLINICAL PRESENTATION

Most animals with severe nonregenerative anemia will present for signs referable to anemia, such as lethargy, exercise intolerance, and collapse. Cats may be markedly anemic with a hematocrit of <10%. Dogs tend to be symptomatic at a slightly higher hematocrit, in the range of 15%. Both species will often have a flow murmur present on cardiac auscultation and 'boundy' or hyperdynamic pulses with tachycardia as their bodies attempt to compensate for decreased oxygen delivery. Clinical signs will also reflect any other disease processes that are present, such as peripheral lymphadenopathy with neoplasia. Often, animals appear 'pale' but the clinician is surprised at the degree of anemia detected.

DIFFERENTIAL DIAGNOSES

The major differential diagnosis is early blood loss or hemolysis, which will not permit adequate time for effective erythropoiesis. If in doubt, careful evaluation for signs of blood loss or hemolysis, and re-evaluation of the reticulocyte count in 2–3 days' time should help clarify the diagnosis.

DIAGNOSIS

The diagnosis is based upon finding an anemia without evidence of regeneration. Evidence of regeneration includes anisocytosis, macrocytosis, and polychromasia. The presence of circulating nucleated red blood cells is *not* evidence of regeneration. A reticulocyte count should be performed in animals with anemia. The reticulocyte count should be corrected for the degree of anemia, as a higher degree of reticulocytosis should be present with a more severe anemia.

The formula used to correct the reticulocyte count is: Patient's hematocrit/normal dog hemocrit (45%) × percentage of reticulocytes.

This number should be >2. For example, a dog with a hematocrit of 9% and a reticulocyte count of 3% would have a value of 0.6, which is not regenerative, while a dog with a hematocrit of 22% and a reticulocyte count of 5% would have a value of 2.4, which is regenerative.

It is very important to determine if just the red blood cell line is affected, which is termed pure red cell aplasia or if two (bicytopenia) or three (pancytopenia) lines are affected. Thus, the white blood cell count and differential and platelet counts should be scrutinized for abnormalities.

A bone marrow biopsy is recommended to classify the cellular components of the bone marrow. Typically, an aspirate is ineffective and a core biopsy should be performed. Titers for *Ehrlichia canis* are advised in endemic areas.

MANAGEMENT / TREATMENT

Management is directed at replacing red cell mass via a transfusion and searching for the underlying cause. Transfusion is usually in the form of packed red cells, and should be administered slowly as patients are normovolemic. Specific treatment is warranted if a cause is detected. Iron is replaced in packed cell transfusions, but additional therapy may be warranted. If tick-borne disease is suspected, doxycycline should be administered. Neoplasia may respond well to chemotherapy. Immune-mediated destruction will often respond well to immunosuppressive therapy, although a longer course is required to see remission than is common with peripheral destruction.

PROGNOSIS

The prognosis is guarded. Many animals recover, but they commonly require dedicated owners and multiple transfusions. Animals with pancytopenia have a grave prognosis, as sepsis or life-threatening hemorrhage is common.

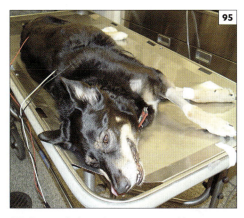

95 Dog with thrombocytopenia and brain hemorrhage.

Thrombocytopenia/ thrombocytopathia

KEY POINTS

- Platelet dysfunction usually results in surface hemorrhage, such as epistaxis or gastrointestinal bleeding.
- Spontaneous hemorrhage is associated with a platelet count of $<40 \times 10^9/l$ ($<40,000/\mu l$).
- Most cases of severe thrombocytopenia in dogs are associated with immune-mediated destruction.

DEFINITION / OVERVIEW

Thrombocytopenia is defined as a platelet count that is below the lower limit of the reference value. The normal reference range for platelets is $200–900 \times 10^9/l$ ($200,000–900,000/\mu l$) for dogs and $300–700 \times 10^9/l$ ($300,000–700,000/\mu l$) for cats. Severe thrombocytopenia can result in spontaneous bleeding, usually from body surfaces. Hemorrhages may be either petechial or ecchymotic. Spontaneous bleeding can occur in the nasal cavity, urinary tract system, respiratory system, cardiovascular system, nervous system, and GI system (**95**).

ETIOLOGY

Platelets are produced by megakaryocytes in the bone marrow by cytoplasmic demarcation. They are released directly into the blood stream and circulate for about 2–10 days. Platelet production is regulated by the hormone thrombopoietin. This hormone is controlled by the circulating platelet mass, not the platelet number. The platelet count remains relatively stable because the amount of platelets produced is equal to the amount of platelets removed from the circulation. The spleen is a reservoir for platelets and can hold up to 20–30% of the platelet pool. Platelets form a hemostatic plug that is sufficient to control bleeding from minute injuries of small vessels. They do this by adhering to exposed sub-endothelial collagen within seconds after injury.

PATHOPHYSIOLOGY

Thrombocytopenia can be the result of one or more of the following abnormalities:
- Decreased platelet production.
- Increased platelet destruction.
- Increased platelet consumption.
- Increased platelet sequestration.

Decreased platelet production

This is relatively rare in dogs, but more common in cats. Cats can develop bone marrow disorders induced by retroviral infections which result in decreased production of platelets. Other causes of decreased platelet production include drug-induced megakaryocytic hypoplasia (estrogens, phenylbutazone, melphalan), myelophthisis, idiopathic bone marrow aplasia, immune-mediated megakaryocytic hypoplasia, and cyclic thrombocytopenia. Late stages of ehrlichiosis and other rickettsial diseases may also decrease production of platelets.

Increased platelet destruction

This is the most common cause of thrombocytopenia in dogs, but it is extremely rare in cats. Platelet destruction may be immune mediated, the direct effect of infectious agents on platelets, or a consequence of a hyperactive macrophage system. ITP can be primary or secondary. Secondary ITP can result from drugs, vaccinations, neoplasia, and infectious agents. Infectious causes include ehrlichiosis, Rocky Mountain spotted fever, distemper, FeLV and FIV. Primary ITP is found more commonly in females than in male animals, and they are usually middle-aged. Common breeds associated with primary ITP include Poodles, Old English Sheepdogs, Cocker Spaniels, and German Shepherd dogs.

Increased platelet consumption

This can be found in animals with DIC, vasculitis, and blood loss.

Increased platelet sequestration

This is found in animals with splenomegaly, splenic torsion, and hepatomegaly.

CLINICAL PRESENTATION

Hemorrhage does not usually develop until the platelet count is $<40 \times 10^9/l$ ($<40,000/\mu l$). An animal may present with petechial (**96**) and ecchymotic hemorrhages in the skin and mucous membranes. They may also present with epistaxis, melena, hematochezia, hematemesis, or hematuria. Animals may have scleral hemorrhages, retinal hemorrhages, and hyphema. If there is significant blood loss caused by the thrombocytopenia, they may have pale mucous membranes, weakness, lethargy, and collapse. They may also present with neurological signs if there is bleeding in the brain or spinal cord.

DIFFERENTIAL DIAGNOSES

Thrombocytopenia and thrombocytopathia should be distinguished from one another. Mechanisms of platelet dysfunction may be from:
• von Willebrand's disease.
• Hereditary platelet function defects, such as Basset Hound thrombopathy and thrombasthenic thrombopathia of Otterhounds, Foxhounds, and Scottish Terriers.
• Acquired platelet function defects, including uremia, DIC, and drug-induced (e.g. by aspirin).
Prolongation of a BMBT is useful to document thrombocytopathy in the face of a normal platelet count (**97, 98**). A BMBT is not warranted with thrombocytopenia.

DIAGNOSIS

Platelet counts can be performed manually or electronically. Electronically determined platelet counts are usually much more precise than manual counts. However, electronic platelet counting methods may give false low numbers of platelets in animals with clumped platelets. Platelet evaluation can be obtained from a blood smear. Generally 1 platelet/hpf is equivalent to a platelet count of $10–15 \times 10^9/l$ ($10,000–15,000/\mu l$). The feathered edge of the blood smear should be evaluated for platelet clumps.

Once platelet numbers are determined to be low, further evaluation should be performed to determine the cause of the thrombocytopenia. A full history, including vaccination history, recent medications, and exposure to infectious agents should be elucidated. A bone marrow aspirate may be performed to evaluate the megakaryocytes, particularly if other cell lines (white or red blood cells) are affected. FeLV/FIV tests should be performed in cats to rule out viral infections. Heartworm antigen tests should be performed to exclude dirofilariasis in endemic areas.

Serum titers may be evaluated if tick-borne diseases are suspected. A coagulation profile may be performed to evaluate for concurrent secondary coagulopathies, including DIC. A Coombs' test may be performed if concurrent immune-mediated hemolytic anemia is suspected. Thoracic radiographs should be evaluated for tumor metastasis and abdominal ultrasonography can also be useful to evaluate for neoplasia, hepatomegaly, splenomegaly, or

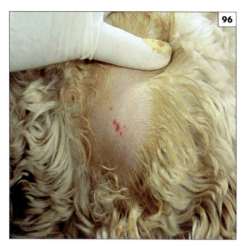

96 Petechiae are evident on the skin of this Cocker Spaniel. The site had been clipped and prepped in preparation for a bone marrow aspirate.

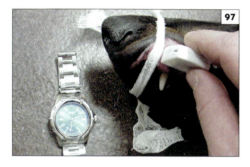

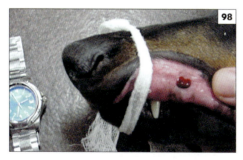

97, 98 A BMBT is performed by making a standardized incision with a commercial device (Simplate II, Organon Tecknika Corp) in the mucous membranes of the patient and then monitoring the length of time for a clot to form. The normal time is <4 min in dogs and <2 min in cats.

internal bleeding. Splenomegaly could indicate splenic sequestration of platelets, or the spleen may be increased in size due to extramedullary hematopoiesis.

MANAGEMENT / TREATMENT
If the animal is severely affected, its activity should be restricted to prevent bleeding. Through-the-needle catheters should not be placed and the jugular vein should be avoided if possible. Cystocentesis should not be performed. Blood transfusions are warranted as needed to support red cell mass. Fresh whole blood or platelet-rich plasma may be used. However, rapid immune-mediated (<15 min) destruction of platelets occurs so, if ITP is the underlying cause, transfusion should be administered only for red cell needs, not for platelet numbers. Synthetic colloids (e.g. etherified starch) should be avoid due to the potential magnification of thrombocytopathia, and medications like aspirin should be discontinued.

Underlying disease should be treated if found. If ITP is suspected treatment with immunosuppressive drugs is warranted. Prednisone (prednisolone) at 2–4 mg/kg/day is the foundation of immunosuppressive therapy. The early addition of vincristine at 0.02 mg/kg IV, once, appears to result in a more rapid platelet rise.

PROGNOSIS
The prognosis for acquired (immune-mediated) thrombocytopenia is fair to good. Platelet rebound generally occurs in 4–7 days. However, life-threatening hemorrhage may ensue prior to the achievement of adequate platelet numbers, so death is possible. Most dogs with von Willebrand's disease may be adequately managed as long as care is given when invasive procedures are undertaken. Neoplastic or septic causes of platelet dysfunction have a grave to guarded prognosis.

Acquired coagulopathy

KEY POINTS

- Acquired coagulopathy may be life-threatening when hemorrhage occurs in specific locations, such as the nervous system, lung, or myocardium.
- Common acquired coagulopathies include DIC, liver failure/dysfunction, and ACR intoxication.

DEFINITION / OVERVIEW

Coagulopathy may be either inherited or acquired. Most commonly, it is acquired, although inherited disease, such as hemophilia A, should be suspected in any young male dog with unexplained hemorrhage. Acquired bleeding tendencies reflect either the failure of primary hemostasis through thrombocytopenia or thrombocytopathy, or failure of secondary hemostasis through factor deficiency. Clinically recognized coagulopathies, such as DIC or ACR intoxication, often have failure of both primary and secondary hemostasis. Untreated, coagulopathy may be fatal.

ETIOLOGY AND RISK FACTORS

The development of an acquired coagulopathy usually occurs due to inadequate clotting factor quantity, although occasionally clotting factor function is inadequate, such as with ACR. Clotting factor quantities may be decreased through failure of production or excessive loss.

Cats are particularly predisposed to the development of hepatic lipidosis with subsequent coagulopathy.

PATHOPHYSIOLOGY

The liver is responsible for the generation of most of the clotting factors. Liver dysfunction may result in inadequate factor generation. Severe systemic inflammation results in the development of DIC. DIC results in rapid depletion of clotting factors through the formation of intravascular fibrin strands and loss into the sites of infection or inflammation. ACR intoxication results in the formation of nonfunctional clotting factors, although their quantities are adequate. Massive fluid resuscitation may result in the development of a dilutional coagulopathy.

CLINICAL PRESENTATION

Dogs with ACR intoxication may present for signs of hemorrhage. However, most other animals affected with acquired coagulopathy will present due to the underlying disease. Thus, they may have signs of sepsis, multiple organ dysfunction, icterus, or polytrauma. Coagulopathy should be suspected in any dog or cat that is critically ill.

DIFFERENTIAL DIAGNOSIS

Isolated thrombocytopenia may result in signs of hemorrhage. Unrecognized trauma may also result in 'appropriate' hemorrhage which may be misinterpreted as a coagulopathy.

DIAGNOSIS

The diagnosis of acquired coagulopathy is based upon identifying prolongation in clotting times. Commonly measured clotting times include the ACT, the PT, and the aPTT. If DIC is present, elevations in the FDP may also be observed. Again, acquired coagulopathy is classically associated with another disease process, thus animals affected with other severe systemic disease should be evaluated for coagulopathy.

MANAGEMENT / TREATMENT

Management is directed at correcting the underlying cause if possible. ACR intoxication will respond rapidly to supplemental vitamin K. If marked prolongations (>25–50% upper limit of normal) exist, transfusion with fresh frozen plasma (5–15 ml/kg) is warranted. In cases of suspected DIC, prior to prolongation of clotting times, heparin therapy is often administered in an attempt to decrease the consumptive aspect of the coagulopathy. The dose is variable, although either 75 U/kg q8hr of unfractionated heparin or 10–25 U/kg/hr by CRI are commonly used.

PROGNOSIS

The prognosis reflects the underlying disease. ACR intoxication carries an excellent prognosis if detected promptly. Other forms of acquired coagulopathy are markers of severe systemic disease and thus carry a grave to poor prognosis.

Toxicological emergencies

- **Overview**

- **Poisonous plants**

- **Ethylene glycol**

- **Anticoagulant rodenticides**

- **Acetaminophen (paracetamol)**

- **Chocolate**

- **Tremorgenic mycotoxicosis**

- **Pyrethrin and pyrethroids**

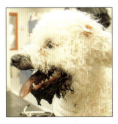 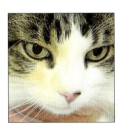 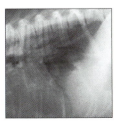 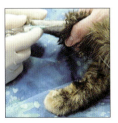

KEY POINTS
- Rapid identification and treatment of life-threatening toxin ingestion is essential for a positive outcome.
- Major body systems (heart, brain, lungs) should be addressed initially.
- Most toxins do not have specific antidotes.
- A 'tox screen' is not widely available for companion animals.

Overview

Management of potential toxicities can be both challenging and rewarding. There are numerous resources available to the veterinarian, including textbooks on toxicology and veterinary poison control hotlines. Since no veterinarian can have adequate knowledge of all possible toxicities these resources should be available when needed.

99 General approach to toxicology.

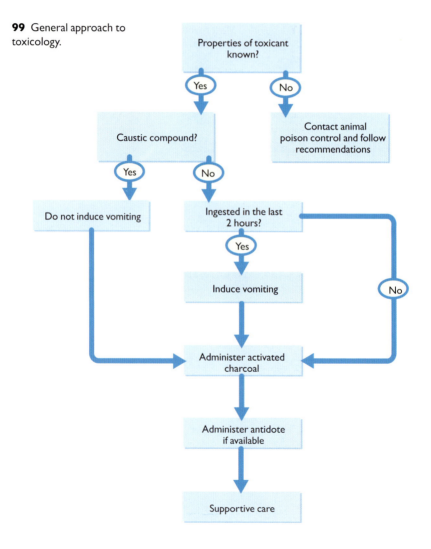

Once a determination of a likely toxicity is made, the following general approach should be taken (**99**):

- Stabilization of major body systems (heart, brain, lungs).
- History and complete physical examination.
- Minimum database.
- Decontamination if indicated.
- Administration of antidote if available.
- Provision of symptomatic and supportive care.
- Monitoring of patient for changes in status.

STABILIZATION OF MAJOR BODY SYSTEMS

Any patient that appears critically ill should be treated with supplemental oxygen. If hypoventilation or severe respiratory distress is present, the patient should be intubated and manually ventilated. Cardiac abnormalities should be addressed with intravenous fluids if hypovolemia or hypotension is present. Arrhythmias are relatively common in toxicological emergencies and may require therapy. Seizure or seizure-like activity should be controlled. Hyperthermia from excessive muscle activity or seizures should be treated to prevent complications associated with heat stroke.

HISTORY AND COMPLETE PHYSICAL EXAMINATION

Once the patient's vital signs are stabilized, the veterinarian should obtain a complete patient history. Important information to be collected includes:

- Suspected toxin.
- Maximum amount of toxin exposure.
- Maximal and minimal possible time elapsed since exposure.
- Patient or environmental clues that toxin exposure occurred (e.g. chewed medication bottle, anxiety, vomiting).

MINIMUM DATABASE

A large amount of important information can be obtained from basic laboratory analysis. A simple minimum database performed in-house should include PCV, serum total protein, urinalysis, serum glucose, and BUN. Samples should be submitted for a CBC and serum biochemical analysis. Blood gas analysis, if available, is very useful in determining acid–base and oxygenation status. Blood may be saved for further analysis, such as serum osmolality for ethylene glycol testing. In addition, any vomitus should be saved for potential toxicological analysis if warranted. Most toxins seen in veterinary medicine represent accidental rather than malicious exposure.

DECONTAMINATION

The goal of decontamination is to prevent further absorption of the toxin. Items to consider when deciding the best route to achieve decontamination include time since ingestion, existence of enterohepatic circulation of the toxin, severity of possible toxicities, and the ability of the patient to protect the airway due to neurological dysfunction.

The time since exposure is important in determining the appropriate steps. Studies have shown that within 1 hour most of the toxin has moved out of the stomach and therefore emesis or gastric lavage may not be effective and may delay the administration of an absorbent, such as activated charcoal. The general recommendation is to induce vomiting if the potential toxin was ingested within the preceding 2 hours.

Toxins that undergo enterohepatic circulation require special treatment. These toxins may require repeated dosing with activated charcoal in order to maximize absorption.

The severity of the potential toxicity should be evaluated. If a toxin will cause only mild signs, extensive decontamination is not indicated. If the potential dose approaches life-threatening toxic levels, a more aggressive decontamination is indicated. Options for decontamination include topical decontamination for cases of dermal exposure, emesis, gastric lavage, and the use of absorbents.

Table 1 Emetic drugs for administration to dogs and cats

Apomorphine (dogs only)

Dose: 0.02–0.04 mg/kg. The tablet is placed in the conjunctival fornix and allowed to dissolve. The conjunctiva should be lavaged after emesis

Onset: 5 min

Adverse effects: respiratory depression, protracted vomiting, undesirable CNS excitation. Excessive emesis may be reversed with metaclopramide

Hydrogen peroxide (3% solution)

Dose: 1–2 ml/kg orally, can be repeated once. Emesis is more likely with a full stomach

Onset: 10 min

Adverse effects: none known

Xylazine (cats only)

Dose: 0.5–1.0 mg/kg IM

Onset: 5–10 min

Adverse effects: bradycardia, depression. Can be reversed with yohimbine

Emesis

Emetics (*Table 1*) should only be used if the animal is cardiovascularly stable and mentally appropriate. Emetics should never be given to patients that are unable to control their airway due to the risk of aspiration.

Gastric lavage

Gastric lavage is a useful tool when gastric decontamination is desired, but emesis is contraindicated. Gastric lavage should only be performed in patients that are endotracheally intubated in order to protect their airway. As a result, anesthesia is required.

A large-bore orogastric tube should be placed into the stomach. A second small-bore tube may be passed to act as an ingress tube if desired. Lavage should be performed with at least 5–10 ml/kg of water and repeated until the egress fluid is clear (**100**). The animal's head should be kept lowered during lavage. Moving the animal on to its back and both sides may aid in gastric emptying.

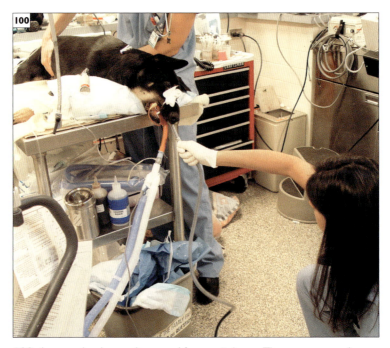

100 A stomach tube may be passed for gastric lavage. The contents may be saved for analysis if clinically indicated.

Absorbents

Activated charcoal is the most effective absorbent available to veterinarians. It is available in combination with sorbitol, which acts as a cathartic. It can be used as the sole decontamination step when emesis and gastric lavage are not performed. Activated charcoal absorbs many common toxins. It should be noted that it does not absorb small charged molecules, such as alcohols and strong acids/alkalis, and metals, such as lead and zinc.

The initial dose of charcoal is 1–2 g/kg of body weight. This can be repeated at a dose of 0.25–0.5 g/kg q6hr for toxins that undergo enterohepatic circulation. Some dogs will readily eat the activated charcoal, however, most animals will require syringe feeding or administration of activated charcoal via a nasogastric or orogastric tube (**101**, **102**).

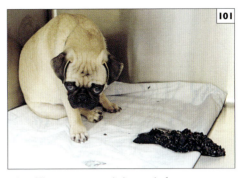

101 This pug vomited charcoal after administration following inadvertent ingestion of anticoagulant rat poison. Rat poisons are often dyed bright blue or green.

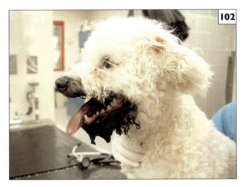

102 A Bichon Frisé after administration of activated charcoal following ingestion of ibuprofen. Charcoal administration may be messy.

Poisonous plants

Some common plants are potentially poisonous to dogs and cats. Ideally, clients should be advised to determine the potential toxicity of any plant prior to bringing it into the house or yard (**103**). A number of sources are available to evaluate the potential toxicity of various plants. It is important to know the particular plants near the practice area, as there are regional variations. Specific highly poisonous plants include lily, oleander (*Nerium oleande*), sago palm (*Cycas revoluta*), yew (*Taxus* spp.) and foxglove (*Digitalis* spp.). Of note, the frequently mentioned poinsettia (*Euphorbia pulcherrima*) is only minimally toxic, even if eaten in large quantities. Most plants will cause only gastrointestinal upset with rapid improvement. A few plants, notably foxglove, yew and oleander, may result in cardiac arrhythmias and even sudden death. For cats, lilies in particular present the greatest poisoning hazard. All parts of the plant are poisonous and only

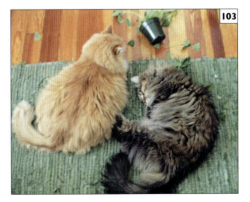

103 Some household plants can be toxic to animals, particularly cats. Owners should be advised to know the common and scientific names of house plants.

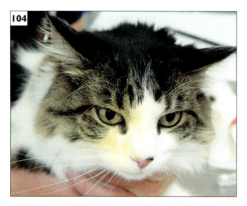

104 This cat's face is covered with pollen from a tiger lily. Lilies are very toxic to cats.

a small amount need be ingested, or even just mouthed, to cause lily toxicity (**104**). Lilies, including day lilies (*Hemerocallis* spp.) and Easter lilies (*Lilium longiflorum*), have been implicated in acute renal failure in cats for over 10 years.

DIAGNOSIS

The diagnosis is based upon the potential for exposure to lilies and appropriate clinical signs, including vomiting and lethargy. As well as being a popular garden plant, lilies are common in many cut-flower arrangements, so even cats that are kept indoors are at risk. Cats will usually vomit after eating even a few bites. However, frequently clients do not recognize the potential risk of the lily and do not pursue treatment. Over the 72 hours following exposure, acute renal failure develops. The renal failure is severe and is commonly associated with hyperkalemia and anuria.

TREATMENT AND PROGNOSIS

Early treatment, after initial ingestion, is associated with trying to remove any remaining leaves by induction of emesis and forced diuresis with 120–180ml/kg/day of intravenous fluids to support renal function. Cats treated early usually recover uneventfully. Conversely, cats who present with severe renal failure have a very guarded prognosis, associated with a high fatality rate. Treatment is similar to any other case of ARF, with intravenous fluid support to promote hydration and, in severe cases, peritoneal or hemodialysis.

Ethylene glycol

DEFINITION / OVERVIEW

Ethylene glycol is commonly used as antifreeze in the cooling systems of cars and trucks. It is a colorless, odorless, sweet-tasting liquid. Many manufacturers add either a bright green or pink color to their product in order to make coolant leaks easily detectable.

PATHOPHYSIOLOGY

Ethylene glycol is rapidly absorbed after ingestion. Metabolism occurs primarily in the liver. The ethylene glycol molecule is metabolized by the enzyme alcohol dehydrogenase to several toxic metabolites, including glycolic acid, glycoxylic acid, and calcium oxalate. An oral dose of 4.4 ml/kg in dogs and 0.9 ml/kg in cats may be lethal.

CLINICAL PRESENTATION

The initial clinical signs associated with toxicity consist of PU/PD that develops within 1–3 hours of ingestion due to hyperosmolality. Animals will frequently act 'drunk' or may have seizures. When untreated, the deposition of calcium oxalate crystals in the renal tubules results in ARF.

DIAGNOSIS

Qualitative assays for ethylene glycol are available. It should be remembered that these assays can be negative as soon as 12 hours after ingestion, since all the parent molecules have been metabolized by that time. A human toxicology lab can perform high-performance liquid chromatography in order to detect glycolic acid, which can remain elevated for up to 60 hours after exposure.

A biochemistry profile may document azotemia, hypocalcemia, and severe metabolic acidosis. Patients with ethylene glycol toxicity will also have increased anion and osmolal gaps. Urine sediment analysis of patients with ethylene glycol toxicity may detect calcium oxalate crystals.

MANAGEMENT / TREATMENT

Early and aggressive treatment of ethylene glycol toxicity is required. Early hemodialysis is the treatment of choice in humans, but it is not widely available to animals. The traditional antidote for ethylene glycol toxicity has been 20% ethanol (40° proof clear alcohol, such as vodka).

- The recommended protocol for dogs is 5.5 ml/kg IV q4hr for five treatments then q6hr for four treatments.
- The protocol for cats is 5 ml/kg q6hr for four treatments then q8hr for three treatments.

The ethanol will competitively inhibit the alcohol dehydrogenase enzyme preventing the formation of toxic metabolites. The major drawback of ethanol therapy is that it produces profound stupor ('drunkenness'), making patient evaluation difficult.

There is an alternative treatment available for use in dogs: 4-methylpyrazole (4-MP, fomepizole). Fomepizole is an inhibitor of alcohol dehydrogenase and does not have the side effects seen with ethanol. Recent studies suggest that high doses (five to six times the dog dose) of fomepizole are effective in cats treated within a few hours of ethylene glycol ingestion. The key to success with both ethanol and fomepizole is to institute treatment early in the course of toxicity before azotemia develops.

The remainder of therapy is directed towards supporting the patient. Therapy with sodium bicarbonate is warranted for severe metabolic acidosis. Intravenous fluid therapy is indicated, although the rate of urine production should be carefully monitored due to the high risk of developing oliguria or anuria and the subsequent potential for volume overload.

PROGNOSIS

The prognosis varies tremendously depending upon when treatment is initiated. If ingestion is witnessed, and early therapy instituted, a complete recovery is possible. On the other hand, patients treated after the onset of azotemia have an extremely poor prognosis.

Anticoagulant rodenticides

DEFINITION / OVERVIEW

Anticoagulant rodenticides (ACRs) are amongst the most frequently encountered rodenticides. They are divided into first, second, and third generations, based upon their ability to kill anticoagulant-resistant rats. They have a duration of action from as few as 2 weeks to as long as 60 days, depending upon the specific rodenticide and total dose consumed. Commonly encountered ACRs include warfarin, bromadialone, and brodifacoum. Owners should be asked to bring the packaging to confirm the exact toxin ingested. Some commercially available rodenticides contain bromethalin rather than ACR.

PATHOPHYSIOLOGY

ACRs are well absorbed orally and are metabolized in the liver. ACRs work by blocking the production of vitamin K-dependent clotting factors II, VII, IX, and X, as well as proteins C and S. Clinical signs appear 72 hours or more after ingestion due to the large reserve of clotting factors normally present.

CLINICAL PRESENTATION

Initial clinical signs may be vague and nonspecific. Often the first sign is anorexia or lethargy. The most common clinical signs are tachypnea and dyspnea. These occur due to hemorrhage into the pleural cavity or the lung parenchyma. Some animals will display large amounts of subcutaneous hemorrhage or hematuria. Less common sites of hemorrhage include joints, the CNS, the spinal cord, the pericardial space, and the nasal sinus (epistaxis). ACR toxicity is quite common in dogs, but very rare in cats.

DIFFERENTIAL DIAGNOSES

Differential diagnoses include congenital factor deficiencies and other acquired coagulopathies, such as DIC or liver failure.

DIAGNOSIS

Animals that have developed clinical signs may have a history of blue/green stool, since many products contain nondigestible dyes. Measurement of the PT, ACT, and aPTT will be markedly elevated. In early cases, the PT will be prolonged due to the shorter half-life of factor VII. By the time clinical bleeding is observed, however, all clotting times (except the TT) will be massively prolonged.

Any young animal with atypical pulmonary infiltrates, pleural effusion, or pericardial effusion should be tested for possible ACR toxicity. Additionally, PIVKA (proteins induced by vitamin K absence or antagonsim) may be measured. The results of this test will be elevated in cases of ACR toxicity as well as any other vitamin K- responsive coagulopathy, so this is not a sensitive test for ACR toxicity. Some laboratories can perform assays for circulating levels of ACR. This testing is usually not necessary, but may be beneficial if the diagnosis is in question.

MANAGEMENT / TREATMENT

In cases of recent exposure to ACR, the treatment should focus on decontamination and monitoring for changes in coagulation times. The previously discussed steps for gastric decontamination should be implemented. After decontamination, there are two options for therapy:

- The patient may be discharged without therapy and instructed to return in 48–72 hours for evaluation of PT. If the PT is then normal, no further therapy is needed. If it is prolonged, even by one second, therapy with 2.5–5 mg/kg/day of vitamin K should be promptly instituted and continued for 30 days, or as guided by the type of toxin ingested. This option avoids unnecessary medication and limits the cost. It does require that clients return for testing, as failure to do so may be life-threatening.
- The patient may directly be started on vitamin K at 2.5–5 mg/kg/day for 30 days. This option has the benefit of not requiring an immediate recheck, but may result in pets being unnecessarily treated.

In all cases, when a dog is prescribed vitamin K, a PT recheck should be performed 2–3 days after completing the course, to ensure no further therapy is required. Vitamin K should be administered with food to maximize absorption.

Patients with clinical signs due to ACR toxicity may require emergency stabilization including intravenous fluids, blood or plasma transfusions, and oxygen therapy. In addition to stabilization of the patient's cardiovascular status, replacement of the vitamin-K-dependent clotting factors should be instituted. Clotting factors can be supplied by transfusion of fresh whole blood, fresh frozen plasma, or frozen plasma. After transfusion, a clotting profile should be rechecked and additional blood products provided as indicated. In addition, a dose of vitamin K should be administered subcutaneously (5 mg/kg) as a loading dose. Oral therapy should then be continued.

A patient with ACR toxicity may present with severe hemothorax (105, 106). These dogs should receive replacement of clotting factors prior to thoracocentesis due to the dangers inherent in performing this procedure on patients with a severe coagulopathy.

PROGNOSIS

The prognosis is generally good to excellent providing that the toxicity is identified early and appropriate therapy initiated.

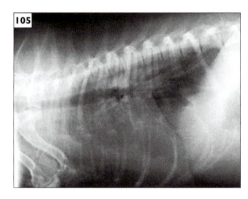

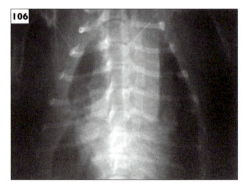

105, 106 Lateral (**105**) and ventrodorsal (**106**) radiographs from a Dachshund with ACR intoxication. The mediastinum is widened and there is pleural effusion. Thoracacocentesis *must not be* performed until the coagulopathy is corrected.

Acetaminophen (paracetamol)

DEFINITION / OVERVIEW
Numerous over-the-counter pain relievers contain acetaminophen alone or in combination with other drugs.

PATHOPHYSIOLOGY
Acetaminophen is rapidly absorbed from the GI tract and metabolized in the liver via sulfation or glucuronidation. It exerts its toxic effects by overwhelming normal conjugation pathways, resulting in the formation of toxic metabolites and depleting glutathione, which normally acts as a scavenger of these metabolites.

CLINICAL PRESENTATION
Cats are far more sensitive than dogs to the effects of acetaminophen. Clinical signs in cats are most often attributable to methemoglobinemia. Cats may have chocolate-colored blood or mucous membranes. The toxic dose in cats is 60 mg/kg, thus one 250 mg tablet will cause toxicity. Cats may present with vague signs, including anorexia or lethargy; however, most cats are collapsed with respiratory distress, a swollen face and paws, and blue mucous membranes (107).

Dogs are more likely to develop hepatic toxicity after acetaminophen exposure. The toxic dose in dogs is approximately 100 mg/kg. Again, clinical signs can be vague, including vomiting, anorexia, lethargy, and depression. Dogs may also exhibit icterus or elevation of liver enzymes. Centrilobular hepatic necrosis is found on biopsy or post-mortem examination. Dogs will exhibit methemoglobinemia and a swollen face less frequently than cats.

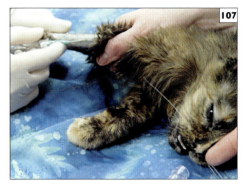

107 A cat who was hit by a car the preceding evening and then administered acetaminophen for analgesia by the well meaning owner. The face is swollen.

MANAGEMENT / TREATMENT
Initial treatment should focus on limiting absorption as previously described. Most toxicologists recommend *against* treatment with activated charcoal due to fear of binding with the antidote. Treatment should then be directed at restoring glutathione stores. Treatment consists of N-acetylcysteine, which serves as a sulfhydryl source that binds toxic metabolites and as a glutathione precursor.

Cats with severe methemoglobinemia may require red cell transfusion or purified bovine hemoglobin transfusion in order to provide additional oxygen-carrying capacity. Additional supportive care should be provided as indicated.

PROGNOSIS
Prognosis depends upon the total dose ingested and the time to treatment. Treatment is generally very successful when initiated before the onset of clinical signs. Cats with severe methemoglobinemia have a more guarded prognosis. Dogs that develop liver failure have a poor prognosis due to the severity of the hepatic insult.

Chocolate

DEFINITION / OVERVIEW
The toxic ingredient in chocolate is theo-bromine. The amount of theobromine varies widely between chocolate products. In general, milk chocolate contains less theobromine than dark chocolate, which contains less than baker's chocolate. Symptoms occur with ingestion of 100 mg/kg of theobromine. Milk chocolate contains 1.6–2.1 mg/g (45–60 mg/oz), semi-sweet or dark chocolate contains 4.6–6.5 mg/g (130–185 mg/oz) and unsweetened (baking) chocolate contains 5.3–21.1 mg/g (150–600 mg/oz). Cocoa powder contains 4.6–6.5 mg/g (130–185 mg/oz).

CLINICAL PRESENTATION
Symptoms of toxicity are consistent with increased levels of circulating catecholamines and may include hyperexcitability, ataxia, seizures, hypertension, tachycardia, and arrhythmia. In addition, vomiting and diarrhea are common when a large quantity of chocolate has been consumed.

TREATMENT
There is no specific antidote. Gastric decontamin-ation may be performed as indicated by the time from exposure and the patient's mental and cardiovascular status. Treatment is mainly supportive and symptomatic. Sedation may be necessary in patients with severe hyperexcitability or seizures. Choices for sedation would include diazepam, pentobarbital, and propofol. Patients with arrhythmia may require treatment with lido-caine, propranolol, or another anti-arrhythmic. Patients with tachycardia severe enough to cause cardiovascular compromise should be treated with beta-blockers, such as propranolol. A urinary catheter should be placed to limit reabsorption of the toxin from the bladder. Theobromine has a long half-life and treatment for as long as 72 hours may be required in severe cases.

PROGNOSIS
Dogs with chocolate toxicity typically have an excellent prognosis and full recovery, however, dogs that ingest extremely large quantities of theobromine or have severe clinical signs have a more guarded prognosis.

Tremorgenic mycotoxicosis

DEFINITION / OVERVIEW
Tremorgenic mycotoxins are fungal metabolites commonly found in moldy foods, which can produce signs of CNS excitation when ingested. To date there are two tremorgenic mycotoxins that have been reported to cause muscle tremors, ataxia convulsions, and death in dogs: penitrem A and roquefortine, which are both produced by *Penicillium* spp.

PATHOPHYSIOLOGY
The exact mechanism of action of tremorgenic mycotoxins is not well understood. Several theo-ries have been proposed, however, it is generally accepted that penitrem A and roquefortine inter-fere with neurotransmitter release at central and peripheral nerve synapses.

CLINICAL PRESENTATION
Signs are related to CNS stimulation and will often progress from mild tremors and ataxia to constant muscle contractions and seizure-like activity. The onset of clinical signs is usually rapid, occurring within 2–3 hours of ingestion of moldy foods or garbage. A history of vomiting is also commonly reported, although it remains unclear if this is a direct result of the mycotoxin ingestion or the result of ingesting other vomitogenic materials in the moldy foods/garbage. Moldy foods confirmed to cause tremorgenic myco-toxicosis include moldy dairy products, moldy walnuts or peanuts, stored grains, moldy bread, moldy blue cheese, and moldy spaghetti; however, a history of possible ingestion of any moldy food should raise a suspicion of myco-toxicosis.

The clinical signs tend to vary depending on the concentration of the mycotoxin present in the food, the amount of toxin ingested, and the species affected. There are several reports of tremorgenic mycotoxicosis occurring in dogs, but to date there are no reports of tremorgenic mycotoxicosis occurring in cats, suggesting that cats may be resistant to the effects of neurogenic mycotoxins or simply that cats are more selec-tive foragers. Although most cases will respond to early recognition and prompt treatment, death has been reported in severe cases with uncontrollable convulsions with or without concurrent aspiration pneumonia. Mycotoxin ingestion should be suspected in previously healthy dogs that present for an acute onset of tremors, particularly if the dog has had access to moldy foods or garbage.

DIFFERENTIAL DIAGNOSES

Other common neurological toxins, such as strychnine, metaldehyde, pyrethroids, organophosphates, carbamates, methylated xanthines (caffeine, theophylline, theobromine), and lead, should be ruled out, as should less common neurological toxins, such as bromethalin rodenticides, hexachloraphene, chlorinated hydrocarbons, and zinc phosphide. Finally, nontoxin-induced causes of tremors and seizures, including cerebellar disorders, tremor syndrome of white dogs, hypomyelination, dysmyelination, metabolic disorders, and infectious diseases, should also be ruled out.

DIAGNOSIS

Tremorgenic mycotoxicosis should be suspected in dogs that present for vomiting and sudden signs of CNS stimulation manifesting as tremors, ataxia, and convulsion, especially if there is a history of garbage ingestion. A definitive diagnosis of tremorgenic mycotoxicosis is made by analysis of stomach or intestinal contents of suspected animals.

MANAGEMENT / TREATMENT

The goals of therapy are to minimize absorption of the mycotoxin from the GI tract, control the tremors and seizures, and provide supportive care. As aspiration pneumonia has been reported in dogs with tremorgenic mycotoxicosis, especially following sedation to control the tremors and seizures, the potential benefit from the administration of activated charcoal and gastric lavage must be carefully considered. Animals with active tremors and seizures should not have these procedures attempted until the CNS excitement can be controlled. If the medication needed to control the CNS excitement causes severe sedation and suppression of the gag reflex, administration of activated charcoal and gastric lavage should be approached with great care due to the risk of development of aspiration pneumonia.

Although diazepam is often the initial treatment given to dogs presenting with seizures, its efficacy in the treatment of tremorgenic seizures has been questioned. Therefore if tremors and seizures fail to respond to diazepam, methocarbamol and pentobarbital sodium in combination should be administered, as they are currently considered the most efficacious medications to control mycotoxin-induced CNS excitement.

Supportive care should be implemented to prevent associated complications, including hyperthermia, exhaustion, dehydration, and acid–base/electrolyte disturbances. Fluids should be administered to combat dehydration and help correct electrolyte and acid–base imbalances. Hyperthermia is common in dogs with tremors and seizures. With the use of sedatives, such as pentobarbital sodium and diazepam, to control CNS excitement, it is not uncommon for animals to experience hypothermic episodes and continual temperature assessment is warranted.

PROGNOSIS

The prognosis varies with the severity of symptoms and promptness of therapy, but overall the prognosis is favorable with most dogs making complete recoveries in 2–3 days if they do not succumb to the initial convulsions or develop aspiration pneumonia.

Pyrethrin and pyrethroids

DEFINITION / OVERVIEW
Pyrethrin and pyrethroid insecticides work by increasing normal nerve membrane sodium ion conduction. They are insecticides used in flea control products and as agricultural products. Typically, they are supplied as shampoos, foams, dips, sprays, and topical applications. Toxicity most commonly occurs when a product labeled for use in dogs is applied to a cat.

CLINICAL PRESENTATION
Clinical signs include ataxia, hyperexcitability, convulsions, tremors, salivation, and whole body tremors.

DIAGNOSIS
In most cases there is a history of pyrethrin/ pyrethroid application. Clinical signs will typically develop between 2 and 48 hours after exposure. Animals will also frequently smell strongly of pest control products.

TREATMENT
In cases of dermal exposure, the dog or cat should be thoroughly bathed with warm soapy water. The remainder of therapy is directed at alleviation of clinical signs and supportive care. Treatment usually consists of a muscle relaxant (methocarbamol) and a sedative (diazepam). Acepromazine and other phenothiazines should be avoided since they can exacerbate clinical signs.

PROGNOSIS
The prognosis for recovery is usually excellent. Some cats exposed to large doses may require therapy for as long as 5–7 days, however, 2–3 days of supportive care is more typical.

CHAPTER 6

Gastrointestinal emergencies

- **Vomiting**

- **Acute diarrhea**

- **Gastrointestinal obstruction**

- **Gastric dilatation–volvulus**

- **Gastrointestinal hemorrhage**

- **Pancreatitis**

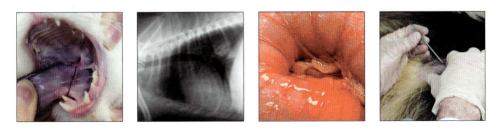

GI disturbances are a common cause of presentation to the emergency clinic. Knowledge of common disease processes, thorough and systematic physical examination, and diagnostic imaging can lead to prompt recognition and successful treatment of diseases of GI origin.

KEY POINTS
- Vomiting may represent GI or non-GI problems.
- The primary question an emergency clinician needs to answer for an animal presented with vomiting is 'Is this problem surgical?'
- GDV should be ruled out with a right lateral abdominal radiograph in any large-breed dog that presents with a history of GI disturbance, as gastric distension may be concealed beneath the ribs and thus not be evident on physical examination.
- Serial physical examination and diagnostic imaging may be required to determine the presence of a small bowel obstruction.

Vomiting

The general approach to vomiting is outlined in (**108**).

KEY POINTS
- Vomiting may be due to an intestinal or an extra-intestinal problem.
- Surgical disease should be excluded.
- Most vomiting is self-limiting in dogs.

DEFINITION / OVERVIEW
Vomiting is defined as the ejection of part or all of the contents of the stomach through the mouth, usually in a series of involuntary spasmodic movements. Persistent vomiting may lead to dehydration, acid–base and electrolyte disturbances, esophagitis, aspiration pneumonia, and bradycardia resulting from stimulation of the vasovagal reflex.

108 General approach to vomiting.

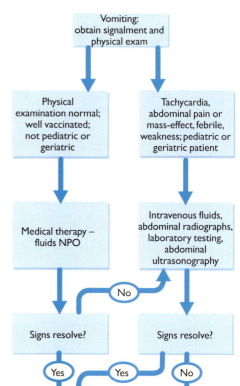

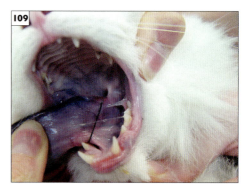

109 A string is noticed under the tongue of this cat. A linear foreign body may result in severe vomiting and is a common cause of intestinal perforation.

ETIOLOGY

Vomiting occurs due to both GI and non-GI diseases. GI diseases which cause vomiting include:

- Obstruction (foreign body (**109, 110, 111**), intussusception, neoplasia, volvulus, mesenteric torsion, constipation).
- Viral infections (parvovirus, distemper, coronavirus).
- Bacterial infections (*Salmonella*, *Campylobacter*).
- Parasitism (*Trichuris, Giardia, Physaloptera, Ollulanus tricuspis*, coccidia, ascarids, salmon poisoning).
- Gastroduodenal ulceration, inflammatory bowel disease, GI perforation, HGE.

Non-GI causes of vomiting include:

- Systemic disease (kidney failure, liver failure, sepsis, acidosis, electrolyte disturbances).
- Endocrinopathies (hypoadrenocorticism, diabetic ketoacidosis, nonketotic hyperosmolar diabetes).
- Neurological disturbances (vestibular syndrome, meningitis, encephalitis, CNS trauma).
- Drugs and toxins.
- Abdominal diseases (pancreatitis, peritonitis, pyometra, pyelonephritis).
- Anaphylaxis.
- Heat stroke, dietary indiscretion, motion sickness.

PATHOPHYSIOLOGY

Vomiting is a reflex act initiated by both humoral (blood-borne) and neural stimulation of the vomiting center in the medulla oblongata. Humoral factors indirectly affect the vomiting center by activating the CRTZ. The CRTZ, located in the area postrema, is on the dorsal surface of the medulla oblongata at the caudal end of the fourth ventricle. It is not completely protected by the blood–brain barrier and can, therefore, detect emetic toxins in both the blood and CSF. Neural stimulation occurs via afferent vagal, sympathetic, vestibular, and cerebrocortical pathways. Stretch receptors, osmoreceptors, and chemoreceptors for these pathways are located throughout the body in the GI tract, other abdominal organs, peritoneum, and pharynx.

CLINICAL PRESENTATION

The severity of clinical signs due to vomiting depends on the duration and severity of vomiting and on the underlying etiology. The animal may present with varying degrees of dehydration (dry mucous membranes, prolonged capillary refill time, reduced skin turgor) or hypovolemia (tachycardia, pale mucous membranes).

Abdominal pain, either diffuse or localized to a specific region of the abdomen, will be present in cases of mesenteric torsion, GDV, GI obstruction, pancreatitis, pyelonephritis, perforated or ulcerated bowel, peritonitis, and HGE. The lack

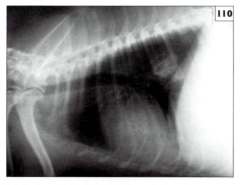

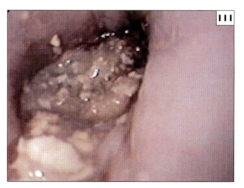

110 A caudal esophageal foreign body (bone) is observed in a West Highland White Terrier which was presented for 'vomiting'. The terrier breeds are predisposed to esophageal foreign bodies.

111 Endoscopic appearance of the bone observed in **110**.

of detectable abdominal pain does not exclude surgical disease. Animals with severe hypovolemia (due to protracted or severe vomiting), or in those that are in shock (i.e. hypoadrenal crisis, GDV, mesenteric torsion, and HGE) may be hypothermic. Fever may be present in cases of neoplasia, infection (sepsis), and inflammation.

Clinical signs due to complications associated with vomiting may also be present. Animals with aspiration pneumonia may have elevated respiratory rate and effort, or abnormal bronchovesicular sounds on auscultation. Animals with severe hypernatremia or hyponatremia often have altered mentation. Hyperkalemic animals may be bradycardic and display neuromuscular weakness, while hypokalemic animals display muscle weakness.

DIFFERENTIAL DIAGNOSES

Vomiting must be differentiated from regurgitation and dysphagia, as the underlying causes and diagnostics required are often significantly different. The act of vomiting can be separated into three components. The first is nausea, which can be characterized by increased salivation, swallowing, lip licking, anxiety, depression, and/or shivering. The second, retching, is characterized by forceful contraction of the abdominal musculature against a closed glottis. During the third phase gastric contents are forcefully expelled from the mouth.

Regurgitation usually indicates esophageal dysfunction. During regurgitation, food or fluid passes retrograde from the esophagus into the oral or nasal cavities. There are no prodromal signs and there is no abdominal effort associated with regurgitation. It should be noted that, although these are two different syndromes, they are not mutually exclusive. Esophagitis from persistent vomiting may lead to regurgitation.

Dysphagia is defined as difficulty or pain associated with swallowing. It can be caused by problems in the oral cavity, pharynx, or proximal esophagus. Clinically, these animals may drop food, gag, have exaggerated swallowing efforts, salivate excessively, appear uncomfortable while swallowing or chewing, or regurgitate shortly after eating. A thorough history and clinical examination will aid in differentiating between vomiting, regurgitation, and dysphagia.

DIAGNOSIS

Because vomiting is a fairly nonspecific clinical sign of disease, there is no one test which can be performed to identify the cause or determine the course of treatment in all cases. The physical examination will provide a significant amount of information. Abdominal palpation may lead to the diagnosis of, or increase the clinician's index of suspicion for, intussusception, GI foreign body, intra-abdominal neoplasia, or GDV.

A basic diagnostic evaluation consisting of CBC, serum chemistry panel, urinalysis, and abdominal radiographs should be obtained of all animals that have signs of systemic or metabolic complications. A venous blood gas is useful to identify acid–base disturbances. The CBC, serum chemistry panel, and urinalysis may be suggestive of or diagnostic for metabolic and electrolyte disturbances, or may document changes that have occurred secondary to the underlying disease.

Radiographic results which warrant surgical intervention include the presence of GDV, free air in the abdomen, an obstructive pattern in the small intestine (112), and fluid-filled uterus in the non-pregnant female. If initial abdominal radiographs are nondiagnostic and illness persists, further imaging with abdominal ultrasonography or a contrast study is warranted.

If there is loss of serosal detail on radiographs or if abdominal effusion is suspected from physical examination findings, abdominocentesis or diagnostic peritoneal lavage should be performed to further evaluate the type of effusion

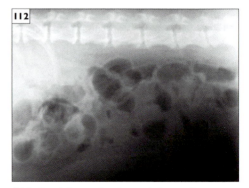

112 An abdominal radiograph from a Bassett Hound with a linear foreign body (carpet). Note the obstructed pattern.

present. If the abdominal fluid analysis documents the presence of intracellular bacteria, or if the abdominal fluid glucose concentration is >1.1 mmol/l (>20 mg/dl) lower than that of peripheral blood, then bacterial peritonitis should be suspected and the abdomen should be explored surgically.

Percussion of the distended abdomen of the GDV may result in the auscultation of a high pitched 'ping' rather than the dull sound auscultated in cases of abdominal effusion or mass. However, the absence of such a finding does not exclude the possibility of GDV.

Additional testing, including tests for the presence of parasites, ACTH stimulation, coagulation profile, fecal occult blood, ethylene glycol assay, lead level, and endoscopy, may need to be performed.

MANAGEMENT / TREATMENT

Treating the underlying cause and ceasing administration of oral feedings and medications will often be sufficient to eliminate continued vomiting. However, if vomiting does persist, antiemetic therapy may be instituted.

- Phenothiazines, such as chlorpromazine (0.5 mg/kg IV, IM, SC q6–8hr) and prochlorperazine (0.13 mg/kg IM q6–8hr), and antihistamines (diphenhydramine at 2–4 mg/kg PO q8hr) can be effective in some situations but often cause drowsiness.
- Metoclopramide (0.1–0.5 mg/kg IM or PO or 1–2 mg/kg/day by slow intravenous infusion) is a dopamine antagonist which acts at the CRTZ and has a prokinetic effect at cholinergic receptors in the GI tract. It is contraindicated in cases of intestinal obstruction.
- Ondansetron (0.11–0.22 mg/kg IV q6–12hr or 0.11–1 mg/kg PO q12–24 hr) and dolasetron (0.6 mg/kg IV or PO q 24hr) are serotonin antagonists which are thought to act either at the CRTZ or at receptors in the periphery or both. They are effective but expensive.

Acute diarrhea

KEY POINTS
- Diarrhea is usually self-limiting.
- In a pet that is not drinking adequately, dehydration may result from excessive fluid losses.
- Differentiating large bowel and small bowel diarrhea can help in determining the cause.

DEFINITION / OVERVIEW
Acute diarrhea is characterized by the abrupt onset of watery or watery–mucoid feces.

ETIOLOGY
Acute diarrhea may result from GI or non-GI disease. GI diseases associated with acute diarrhea include sudden dietary changes, overeating, and food allergies or intolerance.

Causes of GI inflammation which result in acute diarrhea include inflammatory bowel disease, parasitism (*Trichuris vulpis*, *Toxocara canis*, *Toxocara cati*, *Toxascaris leonina*, *Ancylostoma* spp., *Uncinaria* spp., *Diplydium caninum*, *Taenia* spp., and *Strongyloides stercoralis*), salmon poisoning, HGE, *Isospora* spp., *Cryptosporidium parvum*, *Giardia* spp., viral enteritis (feline and canine parvovirus, feline and canine coronavirus, canine distemper virus, and FIV-associated diarrhea), histoplasmosis, prototothecosis, and bacterial enteritis (caused by *Salmonella* spp., *Campylobacter jejuni*, and *Clostridium* spp.).

Several drugs and toxins can cause acute diarrhea (anti-inflammatory medications, antimicrobial drugs, digoxin, chemotherapeutic agents, heavy metals, and organophosphates) as can functional or mechanical ileus.

Extra-intestinal diseases which can cause acute diarrhea include acute pancreatitis, hepatic disease, renal disease, and hypoadrenocorticism.

PATHOPHYSIOLOGY
Diarrhea results from one or a combination of pathophysiological processes:
- *Osmotic diarrhea* occurs when increased unabsorbed solute remains in the intestinal lumen and holds water with it.
- *Secretory diarrhea* results when abnormal amounts of ions and fluid are secreted into the intestinal lumen via activation of intracellular second messenger systems.

The second messengers, such as cAMP and cGMP, stimulate chloride secretion and inhibit sodium absorption. Water then follows along its concentration gradient.

• *Increased intestinal permeability* can cause diarrhea, as mild inflammation alters tight junctions between cells allowing leakage of fluid and ions into the bowel lumen. Severe lesions can cause the loss of macromolecules (albumin, globulin, red blood cells) into the lumen.

• *Altered intestinal motility* can lead to diarrhea by affecting (either decreasing or increasing) transit time.

CLINICAL PRESENTATION

Many animals with acute diarrhea will have no other signs of systemic illness providing that the onset has been recent or the underlying disease is minor. Varying degrees of dehydration may be present as evidenced by the presence of dry mucous membranes, prolonged capillary refill time, and reduced skin turgor. Hypovolemia, whose presence is signaled by tachycardia or pale mucous membranes, may also be present, depending on the quantity of fluid lost and the animal's ability to rehydrate voluntarily. Vomiting may also be present, depending on the underlying cause (e.g. pancreatitis, viral and bacterial enteritis, severe parasitism, HGE, some toxicities, metabolic diseases, hypoadrenocorticism, dietary indiscretion). Abdominal pain may be present in cases of pancreatitis, severe HGE, viral and bacterial enteritis, and hypoadrenocorticism. Animals affected by salmon poisoning, seen primarily in the Pacific northwest, will also have peripheral lymphadenopathy.

DIFFERENTIAL DIAGNOSES

Acute diarrhea, with a duration of <7 days, must be differentiated from chronic diarrhea, as they may have differing underlying etiologies. Small bowel diarrhea, characterized by an increased frequency and volume of diarrhea, must be differentiated from large bowel diarrhea, which is characterized by tenesmus, production of small volumes, and an increased mucus content of the feces.

DIAGNOSIS

The feces should be grossly evaluated for the presence of foreign material, melena, fresh blood, and mucus. The feces should also be evaluated microscopically using the following tests:

• A fecal float to evaluate for ova and parasites.
• A direct smear with saline to check for *Giardia*.
• Fecal cytology to evaluate for sporulated clostridial organisms, the seagull-shaped *Campylobacter*, and white blood cells.
• If *Campylobacter* or *Salmonella* infections are suspected, the feces should be submitted for Gram stain and culture.
• When parvovirus is suspected, a simple in-house test can be performed on a small amount of fresh feces for diagnosis.

In addition to fecal analysis, any animal that is displaying systemic signs of illness should have a CBC, serum chemistry analysis, and urinalysis performed. Abdominal radiographs and ultrasonography may become necessary if pain is noted during the physical examination. Other tests that may be required include a trypsin-like immunoassay for exocrine pancreatic insufficiency, cytology of a lymph node aspirate for salmon poisoning, an ACTH stimulation test for hypoadrenocorticism, and a bile acids test or ammonia level for liver disease.

MANAGEMENT / TREATMENT

The majority of cases of acute diarrhea are mild and self-limiting and do not require any treatment. However in severe cases, anti-diarrheal medications may be administered. Opioids (anhydrous morphine (Paregoric) at 0.25–0.5 mg/kg PO q8hour, diphenoxylate at 0.1–0.2 mg/kg PO q8hour, loperamide at 0.1–0.2 mg/kg PO q8hour) directly increase rhythmic segmentation and decrease propulsive contractions of the intestinal smooth muscle. Some opioids also inhibit intestinal secretion and increase mucosal absorption of fluids, electrolytes, and glucose. They are contraindicated in cats and in animals with bacterial enteritis. Bismuth-subsalicylate, an anti-secretory and gastroprotectant (1 mg/kg PO) may be used in dogs but not in cats due to its salicylate content.

Gastrointestinal obstruction

KEY POINTS
- GI obstruction may be challenging to identify definitively. Mechanical ileus should be distinguished from functional ileus.
- Electrolytes and acid–base disturbances are common.
- Surgical intervention is commonly required to correct the obstruction.

DEFINITION / OVERVIEW
The term GI obstruction refers to a blockage (either partial or complete) of the stomach, or small or large intestine. Obstruction in any of these areas will affect acid–base and electrolyte status, hydration, and GI functions, including peristalsis and secretion or absorption of ions.

ETIOLOGY
The causes of GI obstruction are varied and include foreign bodies (linear and nonlinear), neoplasia (intra- and extraluminal), inflammatory disease, hypertrophy/hyperplasia, strangulation, volvulus, intussusception, and stenosis. GI obstruction is usually a naturally occurring phenomenon, but iatrogenic causes can include post-surgical stenosis, strangulation, or excessive angulation post plication. Any disease leading to a decrease in peristalsis (ileus) can easily be mis-attributed to obstruction.

GI obstruction can be acute or chronic. The degree of obstruction and subsequent duration, timing, and severity of clinical signs are determined by the remaining luminal opening. Partial GI obstruction is more likely to lead to chronic signs.

PATHOPHYSIOLOGY
Obstruction of the GI tract leads to physical impedance of the passage of ingesta, secreted fluids, and gas. With complete obstruction, gas and fluid accumulate proximal to the affected segment causing increasing intraluminal distension (113). Intraluminal distension will interfere with normal peristalsis, absorption, and secretion, disrupt mucosal integrity and vascularity, and allow bacterial growth and translocation. Local capillary bed congestion can occur when intraluminal pressures rise to >40 mmHg, shunting arterial blood away from the affected intestinal segments. Mucosal blood supply and integrity are

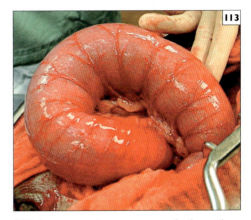

113 Intra-operative appearance of a dog with a colonic obstruction due to colonic torsion. (Photograph courtesy of Dr A. Bentley)

also decreased directly by contact with foreign bodies (large, rough, sharp, linear), local neoplastic infiltration, or extraluminal disease. Mucosal damage can manifest as GI ulceration, mural necrosis, and serosal perforation.

Intraluminal trapping of electrolytes, hydrogen, and bicarbonate will cause the observed acid–base and electrolyte abnormalities. Gastric or proximal SI obstruction may cause a hypochloremic metabolic alkalosis due to intraluminal trapping of hydrochloric acid. Potassium and sodium are often trapped as well. Vomiting of these fluids can lead to severe losses of electrolytes and depletion of body stores. Mid or lower intestinal obstructions may cause metabolic acidosis due to bicarbonate sequestration and loss.

CLINICAL PRESENTATION
The clinical signs of GI obstruction can manifest in many ways depending on the duration, degree, and severity of obstruction, as well as the presence of other related disease (i.e. primary or secondary neoplasia, peritonitis, and pancreatitis). Generally, complete obstructions are usually more acute than partial, proximal SI obstructions are more acute than distal SI, and strangulating obstructions are more severe than simple.

Common clinical signs related to GI obstruction include anorexia, vomiting, diarrhea, dehydration, lethargy, abdominal pain/discomfort, hematemesis, hematochezia, and melena. Further signs of fever, collapse, tachycardia, or tachypnea may be related to secondary sepsis due to peritonitis or bacterial translocation. If obstruction is accompanied by severe ulceration or thrombocytopenia, cardiovascular collapse may be caused by severe blood loss.

DIFFERENTIAL DIAGNOSES

GI obstruction must be differentiated from any disease causing secondary ileus, vomiting, diarrhea, and ulceration. These diseases include hypoadrenocorticism, infection by parasites (*Ancylostoma*, *Trichuris*, etc.), viruses (parvovirus, distemper) or bacteria (*Salmonella*, *Escherichia coli*), inflammatory bowel disease, infiltrative but not obstructive neoplasia, or pancreatitis. Foreign body ingestion should be considered highly likely in any young animal, while neoplasia may be more likely in older animals.

DIAGNOSIS

Baseline diagnostics include a CBC, biochemical profile, and urinalysis to assess hydration, electrolytes, acid–base, and organ function. Thoracic radiographs should also be included in the minimum database if neoplasia is suspected.

Plain radiography may be clearly indicative of an obvious foreign body, abdominal mass, or severe accumulation of air within bowel segments (**114**). When assessing severe intestinal dilation on radiographs, calculating the ratio of the maximal intestinal diameter to the height of the body of the fifth lumbar vertebra at its narrowest point can be helpful. Values >2 indicate a high probability of obstruction. Serial radiographs are also helpful when the first plain radiographs are suggestive of, but not diagnostic for, GI obstruction. Other plain radiographic signs may include parallel intestinal layers connected by hairpin turns ('stacking'), unequal gas–fluid interfaces, plication, 'bunching' of intestinal loops to the right of midline, and decreased abdominal detail.

Ancillary imaging techniques may be needed if plain radiography cannot clearly define the disease entity. These include ultrasonography, contrast radiography, and gastroduodeno- or colonoscopy with or without biopsy. Despite advances in both the operators and technology of these ancillary techniques, exploratory laparotomy with biopsy may still be necessary to identify fully the cause of GI obstruction. Other diagnostic tests that may be necessary include an ACTH stimulation test, parvovirus antigen detection, and fecal examination.

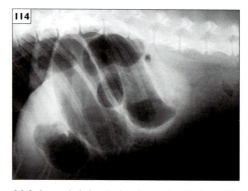

114 Lateral abdominal radiograph of a dog with an intestinal obstruction, showing dilated loops of bowel. (Photograph courtesy of Dr A. Bentley)

MANAGEMENT / TREATMENT

The presentation of animals with GI obstruction is variable and can range from mild (lethargy, anorexia) to severe (shock, sepsis). Paramount in treating GI obstruction successfully is to address any cardiovascular, acid–base, or electrolyte abnormalities in a timely fashion. Restoration of homeostasis will also increase the likelihood of a successful anesthesia and allow proper GI healing.

Fluid therapy with replacement-type crystalloids or colloids is the mainstay of treatment. Normal saline may be indicated in severe cases of hypochloremic metabolic alkalosis. If severe hypokalemia is present, potassium can be supplemented aggressively but should not exceed 0.5 mmol/l/hr (0.5 mEq/l/hr). Blood products, such as packed red blood cells or whole blood, may be necessary in cases accompanied by severe anemia.

Medical management with intravenous fluids may be all that is necessary for some cases of GI foreign body, as they may be small enough to pass through the intestines. Gastric foreign bodies can sometimes be removed endoscopically. If a foreign body has reached the colon, it is likely to pass without intervention. Close monitoring is needed, including serial physical examinations, radiographs, blood work, and visual assessment of fecal material for the foreign body.

Most cases of GI obstruction require surgical intervention. Surgical procedures can include simple enterotomy (single foreign body), multiple enterotomies (linear foreign body), re-section and anastamosis of a portion of the stomach or intestines (neoplasia, foreign body, hypertrophy), or pyloromyotomy. Histopatho-logical analysis of any questionable tissue is advis-able, especially when no gross disease is visualized at the time of surgery.

PROGNOSIS
Post-operative prognosis is generally good and usually depends on intestinal viability at the surgical site and any underlying systemic disease. Poor prognostic indicators for surgical site dehis-cence include the presence of pre-operative peritonitis and hypoalbuminemia. In one study, animals that had a resection and anastomoses performed secondary to the presence of a foreign body dehisced more often than those with neoplasia. That study also found that cats are less likely to dehisce than dogs, but a full assessment has not been performed. Prognosis in animals with intestinal neoplasia varies, depending on the nature of the neoplasm and extent of metastasis at the time of surgery.

Gastric dilatation–volvulus

KEY POINTS
- GDV should be suspected in large-breed dogs that present for abdominal distension and retching.
- Aggressive fluid resuscitation and timely surgical intervention are warranted for successful patient outcome.
- Gastric necrosis increases the risk of peri-operative morbidity and mortality.

DEFINITION / OVERVIEW
GDV occurs most commonly in large and deep-chested dogs, but has also been reported in small dogs, cats, and ferrets. Gastric distension and subsequent rotation of the stomach leads to progressive gastric distension, cardiovascular collapse, and ultimately, if untreated, death. Commonly affected breeds of dog include German Shepherd dogs, Standard Poodles, and Great Danes.

ETIOLOGY
GDV occurs when gas or fluid accumulation develops together with either a functional or mechanical gastric outflow obstruction induced by altered positioning of the pylorus or lower esophageal sphincter. This leads to progressive gastric distension that cannot be relieved by vomiting, eructation, or pyloric gastric emptying. Gastric dilatation can occur alone, or can be followed by volvulus or twisting along the long axis of the stomach. Studies investigating pre-disposing causes of GDV have identified that anxiety or a stressful event may contribute to its development.

PATHOPHYSIOLOGY
Physiological consequences of gastric dilatation include reduced venous return to the heart due to compression of the posterior vena cava and portal vein, leading to reduced cardiac output, hypotension, and signs of shock. Subsequent reduction in tissue perfusion contributes to the development of lactic acidosis, cellular injury, and organ dysfunction.

CLINICAL PRESENTATION
Dogs presenting with GDV typically have an acute history of abdominal distension, nonpro-ductive attempts at vomiting, and/or salivation.

Clinical presentation may range from anxiety and abdominal pain to collapse and signs of shock. Clinical signs of shock include tachycardia, pale (or gray) mucous membranes with prolonged capillary refill time, altered mentation, and weak femoral pulses. Abdominal palpation frequently identifies a firm, distended, and sometimes tympanic abdomen, with a mass effect often palpable in the mid-abdominal region. This effect is due to an engorged displaced spleen. Lack of abdominal distension on palpation does not rule out the presence of GDV, as much of the gastric distension may occur under the ribcage.

DIFFERENTIAL DIAGNOSES

Gastric dilatation without volvulus should be considered. In these cases simple gastric decompression may be all that is required, although gastropexy is a possibility in dogs with multiple episodes of gastric dilatation as they are at high risk for torsion. Mesenteric torsion must also be considered a possibility in the large-breed dog with acute abdominal distension and pain.

Abdominal distension caused by abdominal effusion, such as ascites, should be ruled out, as dogs with a predilection for dilated cardiomyopathy are similar to those that commonly develop GDV. Other diseases that may cause abdominal effusion include pancreatitis and neoplasia causing hemoabdomen.

DIAGNOSIS

Abdominal radiographs should be performed to document GDV. A right lateral abdominal exposure is most beneficial in detecting compartmentalization. This is sometimes referred to as the 'double bubble' appearance of the gastric silhouette (115). Lack of visualization of a displaced pylorus may support the diagnosis of simple gastric dilatation, or may occur with a 360° torsion, and the presence of free air is suggestive of gastric rupture.

Blood samples should be drawn at the time of catheter placement for minimum database (PCV, total solids, glucose, and azostick) along with electrolyte concentrations, venous blood gas, and lactate measurement. Lactate, in particular, has been shown to be helpful in identifying those animals at risk for gastric necrosis, with a lactate concentration >6 mmol/l (>54 mg/dl) associated with a higher incidence of gastric necrosis.

The ability to pass a stomach tube does not exclude the presence of GDV.

MANAGEMENT / TREATMENT

Gastric decompression and fluid resuscitation are the mainstay of stabilization of the GDV patient. A large-bore, short over-the-needle catheter should be placed in each cephalic vein for rapid fluid administration. The hind limbs should be avoided due to the potential for reduced venous return to the heart. A shock dose of crystalloids (90 ml/kg/hr) should be calculated, and administered in increments of about 25% with intermittent re-evaluation until improvements in heart rate, mucous membrane color, and mentation are obtained. Hypertonic saline (7.5%) at a dose of 4–5 ml/kg may be administered for an immediate improvement in intravascular volume status. Once fluid resuscitation has been initiated, a right lateral abdominal radiograph can be taken to confirm the diagnosis of GDV. If the animal is cardiovascularly unstable, immediate decompression may be required.

Gastric decompression
Gastric trocarization

This is the most rapid method of achieving gastric decompression in animals that present with cardiovascular collapse, and rapid trocarization may increase venous return to the heart. The abdomen is palpated, and a tympanic region on the upper right quadrant of the abdomen is identified. That area is shaved, and briefly prepped with chlorhexidine or betadine solution.

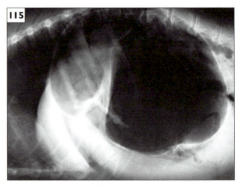

115 Right lateral abdominal radiograph demonstrating a classic 'double bubble' appearance of the stomach caused by dorsal displacement of the pylorus. This finding confirms the presence of GDV.

Trocarization can be performed using any 16 ga or large over-the-needle catheter long enough to reach the stomach (116). The stylette should be removed as soon as the stomach is entered, and the catheter held in place until escaping gas is no longer heard. Alternatively, a 3.8 cm (1.5 inch) 18 ga needle may be used.

Orogastric intubation

While some animals may tolerate orogastric intubation, most require some form of sedation, so gastric trocarization may be preferred if cardiovascular collapse seems imminent. A protocol consisting of anesthetic agents with minimal cardiovascular depressant properties, and, ideally, that are reversible, should be chosen. Appropriate combinations include opioids (hydromorphone 0.1 mg/kg or oxymorphone 0.01 mg/kg) along with diazepam (0.1–0.2 mg/kg), or ketamine (0.3 mg/kg) and diazepam (0.1–0.2 mg/kg) administered intravenously. Endotracheal intubation should be performed to protect the airway during gastric lavage, and to prevent accidental insertion of the orogastric tube into the trachea. The orogastric tube should be premeasured to the level of the last rib, lubricated, and inserted into the esophagus. The correct location of the tube can be confirmed by placing a hand on the ventral aspect of the neck as the tube is directed down the esophagus. Gentle but persistent pressure should be applied when the tube reaches the cardia. If the tube does not pass easily into the stomach, twisting of the tube, shifting the position of the animal, or passage of a smaller tube may be helpful. Once the tube is passed into the stomach, gastric lavage using warm water can be performed and should be continued until clear fluid is obtained.

Fluid therapy

If shock persists despite administration of crystalloids, synthetic colloids (etherified starch, e.g. hetastarch 10–20 ml/kg) can be administered. Laboratory testing, in particular lactate concentration, PCV, and total solids, should be rechecked 15–20 min following initiation of therapy to document improvement in acid–base status and lactate concentration. PCV and total solids should be rechecked following stabilization, as rupture of the short gastric vessels may lead to significant blood loss and necessitate transfusion of packed red blood cells. If cardiovascular instability persists despite decompression and aggressive fluid resuscitation, then an exploratory celiotomy should be performed immediately. Prophylactic antibiotics are warranted in the perioperative period.

Surgery

GDV is a surgical emergency, and an exploratory celiotomy and gastropexy should be performed once hemodynamic stability has been restored. A ventral midline incision should be made, and the stomach should be replaced in its correct location. As the most common rotation is clockwise in direction, proper repositioning of the stomach can be performed by grasping the pylorus with the right hand and pulling it toward the incision while pushing the fundus with the left hand toward the table. Once correct positioning has been restored, all anatomic structures, in particular the stomach and spleen, are assessed for viability before a gastropexy is performed. A splenectomy can be performed if blood flow to the spleen is compromised, if viability is questionable, or if significant avulsion of splenic vessels has occurred. The stomach should be assessed for evidence of gastric necrosis, and necrotic areas should be resected. Devitalized gastric mucosa can be difficult to identify. In general, black, blue-black, or greenish discoloration of the mucosa is consistent with devitalized tissue, while red areas can often be preserved. Questionable areas should be re-evaluated 15–20 min after repositioning of the stomach.

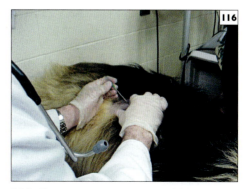

116 Gastric trocarization using a 16 ga over-the-needle catheter for emergency gastric decompression. A small area is clipped and prepped over the site of proposed gastrocentesis.

Several techniques for gastropexy have been described. The most common techniques employed are the incisional gastropexy and belt loop gastropexy. Intra-operatively, fluid therapy should be continued for blood pressure support. Crystalloids (10 ml/kg/hr) should be used, along with colloid support (etherified starch, e.g. hetastarch 10 ml/kg/hr) if hypoproteinemia is documented or if crystalloids alone are insufficient to maintain blood pressure. If hypotension persists despite aggressive fluid therapy, pressor support using dopamine (starting at 5 µg/kg/min and titrating the dose to effect) or norepinephrine (noradrenaline) (0.5–2 µg/kg/min) can be used. Blood products (packed red blood cells, fresh frozen plasma, or fresh whole blood) can be administered as needed in cases of anemia or coagulopathy.

Post-operatively, baseline information consisting of PCV and total solids, acid–base status, electrolyte concentrations, and lactate level should be obtained. Heart rate and rhythm should be monitored continuously, as dogs with GDV have a high incidence of ventricular tachyarrhythmias. In many cases these are mild and resolve within 48 hours of surgery. Lidocaine therapy can be initiated (2–5 mg/kg IV followed by 40–80 µg/kg/min) if the ventricular beats are multiform in nature, if the phenomenon of R on T can be identified, or if reduced cardiac output results in hypotension or altered mentation. Blood pressure should be closely monitored and fluid therapy (either crystalloids or a combination of crystalloids and colloids) should be continued. If pressor support was required during surgery, then it should be continued in the post-operative period until repeated measurements show consistent normalization of arterial blood pressure. Pain management in the peri-operative period should consist of reversible drugs with minimal cardiovascular depression, such as pure opioids (hydromorphone 0.1 mg/kg IV q4–6hr or oxymorphone 0.01 mg/kg IV q4–6hr). Broad-spectrum antibiotics are indicated if gastric resection is required.

PROGNOSIS

The overall survival rate following GDV is approximately 80%. However, severe complications of GDV may occur and in some cases gastric necrosis is too severe to attempt resection and animals must be euthanized.

Gastrointestinal hemorrhage

KEY POINTS

- GI hemorrhage may be associated with local factors, such as ulceration or neoplasia, or systemic coagulopathy, such as severe thrombocytopenia.
- Chronic GI hemorrhage will result in microcytic hypochromic anemia associated with iron deficiency.
- Blood transfusions may be necessary to provide support while treating the underlying cause.

OVERVIEW

GI hemorrhage varies from mild and self-limiting to severe and life-threatening, and may result from a number of different disease processes. Although most cases are easily diagnosed on physical examination, even severe cases may occasionally be missed if signs identifying the GI tract as the source of blood loss are not present, or concurrent diseases obscure the diagnosis.

ETIOLOGY

The causes of GI hemorrhage can be divided into two broad categories: diseases causing ulcers and diseases resulting in coagulopathies. In people, diseases associated with vascular anomalies are common but these are very rare in animals.

Diseases causing GI ulceration occur most frequently and include:
- Drug therapy (NSAIDs and corticosteroids).
- GI ischemic events (GDV, mesenteric volvulus, mesenteric thrombosis).
- Systemic diseases (uremia, liver disease, pancreatitis, sepsis, hypoadrenocorticism, mastocytosis, and gastrinoma).
- Infectious diseases (parasitic, bacterial, viral, fungal, and algal).
- Inflammatory diseases (inflammatory bowel disease).
- Intussusception, foreign bodies, neoplasia, stress, and idiopathic causes.

In the veterinary literature the most common reported diseases causing GI ulcers include drug therapy (NSAIDs and corticosteroids), liver failure, and renal failure.

Coagulation disorders associated with GI hemorrhage include ACR toxicity, DIC, and thrombocytopenia. Thrombocytopenia is by far the most likely coagulopathy to be associated with GI blood loss.

PATHOPHYSIOLOGY

The pathophysiology of GI hemorrhage varies with the inciting cause, however, as ulcers are the most common cause of GI hemorrhage in veterinary patients, a brief discussion of the pathophysiology of ulcers is warranted.

GI ulceration may result from three major causes: increased acid production, decreased mucosal protection, or direct damage to the GI tract. Increased acid production in turn has been associated with elevated gastrin, histamine, and acetylcholine levels, all of which may act synergistically to increase acid secretion. The mucus layer provides resistance to GI ulceration through several mechanisms, which include bicarbonate trapping, which neutralizes back-diffusion of hydrogen ions, a high viscosity and strong adherence to the mucosa, which minimize mechanical injury, and hydrophobic properties, which inhibit the back-diffusion of hydrogen ions. An important factor in the prevention of GI ulcers is also mucosal blood flow, which supplies bicarbonate ions and removes any hydrogen ions that do diffuse across the mucus layer. Finally, for an ulcer to persist, there must also be some abnormality or inhibition of epithelial cell renewal. The usual cause of ulceration is an imbalance between the rate of secretion of gastric fluid and the degree of protection afforded by the gastroduodenal mucosal barrier and the neutralization of the gastric acid by duodenal secretions.

CLINICAL PRESENTATION

A history of hematemesis (the vomiting of 'coffee grounds' or blood), hematochezia (passage of frank blood in the stool), or melena (presence of black tarry stool) is often reported. It should be kept in mind that melena is not usually seen until significant GI hemorrhage has occurred. Administration of bismuth-containing solutions (e.g. Pepto-Bismol®) may also result in a dark-colored stool. There may be a history of using ulcerogenic medications, such as aspirin or steroids, prior to presentation. Signs consistent with anemia, including pale mucous membranes, lethargy, decreased appetite, and weakness, may also be present, depending on the severity and duration of blood loss.

Severely affected patients may present in a state of shock from blood loss, hypovolemia from concurrent vomiting and/or diarrhea, endotoxemia from mucosal barrier breakdown, or sepsis. In these situations the animal may have signs consistent with cardiovascular instability, including tachycardia, diminished or thready arterial pulses, cool extremities, prolonged capillary refill time, and pale mucous membranes.

DIFFERENTIAL DIAGNOSES

GI hemorrhage should be differentiated from other diseases that may result in melena or hematemesis unrelated to active GI bleeding, such as hemoptysis (coughing of blood secondary to airway or pulmonary disease) and epistaxis (hemorrhage from the nasal cavity). If severe, epistaxis and hemoptysis can both result in melena and hematemesis secondary to the swallowing of blood.

DIAGNOSIS

The diagnosis of GI hemorrhage is made when the presence of blood in the GI tract is identified. This can often be determined based on the history (vomiting blood, dark stool, or bloody stool/diarrhea) and physical examination findings (melena, hematemesis). In cases that are less obvious, a fecal occult blood test may prove useful in detecting the presence of blood that is not grossly obvious on examination of the stool, and can rule out significant GI hemorrhage if the result is negative.

Diagnostic tests
Physical examination
A careful evaluation of the abdomen and a rectal examination should be performed on all patients presenting with GI hemorrhage. Abdominal palpation may localize areas of pain (tenderness, voluntary or involuntary guarding), identify masses or foreign objects, or detect the presence of abdominal distention or a fluid wave. As the animal is being resuscitated, careful rectal examination should be performed to detect the presence of frank blood or melena, and to look for possible masses or foreign objects.

Laboratory tests

In cases where GI hemorrhage is not obvious, certain biochemical abnormalities should prompt its consideration as a differential diagnosis. For example, the finding of microcytic, hypochromic anemia (iron deficiency anemia) is associated with chronic blood loss into the GI tract. However, because iron deficiency anemia takes a long time to develop, a large number of patients with more acute GI hemorrhage will have a normocytic normochromic anemia. A fecal occult blood test, although influenced by diet, may prove useful in detecting the presence of blood that is not grossly obvious on examination of the stool, and can rule out significant GI hemorrhage if the result is negative.

The hematocrit can be misleading with acute GI hemorrhage as the initial bleeding will produce loss of whole blood (an equivalent loss of plasma and erythrocytes) with no change in the hematocrit. The fall in hematocrit will not be apparent until fluid has redistributed from the extravascular to the intravascular space, resulting in a dilution of the erythrocyte mass, which can take up to 24–72 hours. With the administration of crystalloids or colloids, the dilution of the hematocrit and the total solids becomes apparent very quickly, necessitating careful monitoring and interpretation of serial hematocrit and total solid measurements.

Other important hematological parameters that should be evaluated include the coagulation profile, platelet count, serum biochemistry panel, and electrolyte concentrations. The coagulation profile may identify ACR intoxication or specific factor deficiencies, or may identify prolonged clotting times that are not the primary cause of hemorrhage but significantly contribute to blood loss. Platelet counts are important as ITP is a common cause of moderate to severe GI hemorrhage, and was found to be the most common cause of GI hemorrhage requiring blood transfusion in one canine study. Given that renal disease is associated with GI ulceration and hemorrhage, BUN, creatinine, and phosphorus values must be evaluated. In addition, a high BUN:creatinine ratio (>20) may be reflective of upper GI hemorrhage. This phenomenon is caused by volume depletion and subsequent re-absorption of BUN in the proximal tubule of the kidney, and intestinal absorption of proteins, including digested blood, into the circulatory system. However, other disease states associated with increased protein catabolism, including fever, burns, infections, starvation, and use of corticosteroids, can also result in an increased BUN and must be ruled out. It should be noted that many dogs with acute GI hemorrhage do not have an elevation of BUN.

Liver disease has been reported as a common cause of GI ulceration and hemorrhage and particular attention should be paid to hematological parameters reflective of liver disease (ALP, ALT, AST, GGT, and bilirubin). As hypoadrenocorticism has been reported as a cause of severe GI hemorrhage in the dog, electrolytes should be evaluated and an ACTH stimulation test performed if another cause for GI hemorrhage cannot be found. Finally, fecal smears may be required to rule out parasitic diseases such as *Ancylostoma* spp. infestation.

Imaging

Although contrast radiographs may identify mucosal defects, they have generally been replaced by ultrasonography and endoscopy. The use of ultrasonography to identify ulcers in dogs has been described and allows evaluation of intestinal wall thickness and wall layering, and can detect the presence of a defect or crater in the gastric wall. When used serially, it has helped monitor response to therapy and has helped determine the need for surgery. Endoscopy, which is considered the most sensitive test to detect upper GI tract hemorrhage and ulcers, allows direct visualization of the mucosa, permits biopsies for histology and culture, and can occasionally be used for therapeutic intervention (i.e. foreign body retrieval). The disadvantages of endoscopy include requirement for anesthesia, potential to exacerbate the GI hemorrhage, and the possibility of iatrogenic ulcer perforation.

Examination of stool/vomitus

Localizing the site of GI hemorrhage to the upper or lower GI tract should be attempted by visual examination of stool and vomitus. The presence of blood or 'coffee-ground' material in the vomit suggests upper GI hemorrhage, as does the presence of melena. However, it is important to remember that it is the amount of time the blood spends in the GI tract that determines the color of the blood in the stool, and not the source of bleeding. The presence of frank blood may be reflective of large intestinal hemorrhage, however, severe acute GI hemorrhage can act as a cathartic, speeding the passage of blood through the GI tract, and can result in the passage of frank blood as well. If the bleeding occurs in the duodenum and there is insufficient reflux of duodenal contents into the stomach, there may be no blood in the vomit.

MANAGEMENT / TREATMENT

The treatment of GI hemorrhage involves specific therapy directed at the underlying cause and nonspecific measures taken to stabilize the CV system, protect the GI tract, and stop ongoing hemorrhage. As underlying causes are variable, specific therapy for these conditions is also variable (e.g. surgery for foreign bodies or tumors, corticosteroids for hypoadrenocorticism, discontinuation of NSAIDs). In considering the underlying cause, it is important to look for diseases that can exacerbate GI bleeding (e.g. uremia in a patient on NSAIDs) and to identify related or unrelated coagulation abnormalities (e.g. liver disease causing GI ulceration as well as clotting deficiencies). Nonspecific therapy is aimed at controlling ongoing hemorrhage, correcting anemia, fluid and acid–base disturbances, treating existing ulcers, and addressing potential bacterial translocation and GI perforation.

Animals with CV instability must be stabilized with aggressive intravenous fluid therapy using crystalloids, colloids, hypertonic saline, and blood products if warranted. An ECG should be performed and the heart and lungs carefully auscultated prior to starting fluid resuscitation.

Following the initiation of fluid therapy, some type of oxygen-carrying support through the use of packed red cells, whole blood, or recombinant bovine purified hemoglobin solution (Oxyglobin®) should be considered. The question of when to transfuse stable patients with GI blood loss is somewhat controversial. Although some clinicians transfuse patients when a specific hematocrit is reached (a transfusion trigger), this value tends to vary between patients and depends on the degree and rate of blood loss, hemodynamic status, initial and subsequent hematocrit levels, presence of concurrent illness, and the presence of clinical signs. If the patient shows signs of CV instability (e.g. tachycardia) and/or the hematocrit continues to fall after initiating therapy, a blood transfusion is indicated. Close observation and serial hematocrit measurements are required to detect ongoing, or recurrence of, GI hemorrhage.

If the hematocrit fails to rise with transfusion of red blood cells, the patient should be re-evaluated for a source of ongoing blood loss through abdominal ultrasonography, endoscopy, or exploratory surgery. If large amounts of blood products are given, it is important to monitor for adverse effects, such as hypocalcemia, hypomagnesemia, hypothermia, hypervolemia, CHF, and pulmonary edema. Patients with cardiac compromise that require a transfusion may need to have the blood administered over a longer period of time. In animals with severe bleeding secondary to thrombocytopenia, vincristine can be administered. Platelet-rich plasma can be prepared and administered in the hope of reducing blood loss until the underlying cause can be addressed, although in ITP, transfused platelets will be destroyed in minutes.

GI ulcers should be considered present until proven otherwise in animals presenting with hematemesis and/or melena, and medications known to cause ulceration, such as NSAIDs, should be discontinued. The role of steroids in causing GI ulceration is controversial. Given the incidence of GI hemorrhage in dogs receiving steroids, corticosteroids should be discontinued unless they are considered essential to therapy (e.g. in hypoadrenocorticism or immune-mediated diseases). Initiating treatment with gastric protectants prior to identifying the underlying cause is recommended, as ulcerative diseases are commonly identified in patients with GI hemorrhage and intraluminal gastric acid neutralization may slow GI hemorrhage by promoting mucosal homeostasis. GI protectants include acid suppressives, such as histamine-2 receptor antagonists (cimetidine, ranitidine, famotidine), proton pump inhibitors (omeprazol [omeprazole]), mucosal binding agents (sucralfate), and synthetic prostaglandins (misoprostol). Although omeprazol (omeprazole) has been shown to suppress acid secretion more effectively than the histamine-2 antagonists, the higher cost and the need for oral administration may limit its application, as the absorption of enterally administered medications in critically ill patients has been questioned.

Due to the risk of bacterial translocation from a compromised mucosal barrier, broad-spectrum antibiotics (e.g. a penicillin and an aminoglycoside or fluoroquinolone, or a combination of a cephalosporin, metronidazole and an aminoglycoside or fluoroquinolone) are warranted in patients with significant GI hemorrhage. Collection of urine and blood samples for culture and sensitivity is ideally performed prior to starting antibiotic therapy.

Most cases of GI hemorrhage can be managed medically, thus avoiding the need for anesthesia and surgery. However, surgery is indicated in the presence of a pre-existing surgical disease (foreign body or tumor), in patients at risk of exsanguination or perforation (based on endoscopy or serial sonographic evaluation), in the presence of septic peritonitis, or if the patient fails to respond to medical therapy.

PROGNOSIS

The prognosis in dogs with moderate to severe GI hemorrhage varies with the inciting cause; however, in general, a guarded prognosis should be given if a blood transfusion is required to control hemorrhage, as the mortality rate in these cases is 29–45%.

Pancreatitis

KEY POINTS

- Pancreatitis may range in severity from mild to life-threatening.
- Diagnostic testing that helps support the identification of pancreatitis includes laboratory testing, radiography, and ultrasonography.
- Supportive care, including intravenous fluids, anti-emetics, and analgesics if warranted, is the primary method of treatment.

DEFINITION / OVERVIEW

Pancreatitis is defined as an inflammatory process involving the exocrine portion of the pancreas, resulting in autolysis of pancreatic tissue by digestive enzymes. In dogs, acute pancreatitis is a common cause of vomiting, fever, and abdominal pain, and two forms are commonly recognized:
- Mild acute pancreatitis is associated with pancreatic edema and mild inflammation, and typically responds rapidly to treatment.
- Severe acute pancreatitis can be associated with multiple organ failure and/or local complications, such as pancreatic necrosis, abscessation, or cyst formation, and tends to carry a more guarded prognosis.

Pancreatitis in cats tends to be a more insidious disease and thus may be difficult to identify. A number of different types have been recognized, including:
- Acute necrotizing pancreatitis, characterized by acinar and peripancreatic fat necrosis similar to that seen in dogs.
- Acute suppurative pancreatitis, with extensive suppurative inflammation but minimal necrosis.
- Chronic pancreatitis, a relapsing form of the disease with variable degrees of associated pancreatic inflammation and fibrosis.

ETIOLOGY

The inciting cause of pancreatitis in dogs and cats frequently remains undetermined, but a number of risk factors have been suggested. High-fat diets or treats, obesity, and hyperlipidemia are among the more commonly cited factors, though the exact mechanism by which these may trigger pancreatitis is poorly understood. Endocrinopathies, such as diabetes mellitus, hypothyroidism, and hyperadrenocorticism, have also been associated with acute, fatal pancreatitis. Numerous drugs and toxins have been associated with the development of pancreatitis, including corticosteroids, anticonvulsants (phenobarbital, potassium bromide), chlorpromazine, azathioprine, l-asparaginase, thiazide diuretics, sulfa drugs, tetracyclines, and organophosphates. Hypercalcemia, immune-mediated disease, hereditary disease, pancreatic trauma, and pancreatic duct obstruction, secondary to a mass or duodenal foreign body, are other etiologies that have been identified.

PATHOPHYSIOLOGY

The initial event in the development of pancreatitis is intracellular activation of trypsinogen to trypsin, leading to autodigestion of pancreatic cells. The process is perpetuated as trypsin activates other digestive enzymes, such as phospholipase A_2, elastase, lipase, chymotrypsin, and kallikrein, causing further injury to the pancreas and surrounding tissues. As serum protease inhibitors (proteins that regulate the activation of zymogens) are consumed, systemic inflammation and DIC may develop as a result of activation of kinin, kallikrein, coagulation, fibrinolytic, and complement cascades.

CLINICAL PRESENTATION
Dogs
Vomiting is the most common clinical sign reported in dogs with pancreatitis. Abdominal pain frequently develops as a result of inflammation of the pancreas and surrounding structures. Other clinical signs may include fever, dehydration, anorexia, diarrhea, and melena. Clinical signs may range from mild and self-limiting to life-threatening. With severe acute pancreatitis, signs of shock, including tachycardia, decreased pulse quality, and prolonged capillary refill time, may be noted. Some patients may develop icterus as a result of bile duct obstruction.

Cats
Clinical signs of pancreatitis tend to be more variable in cats. Anorexia may initially be the only clinical sign noted. Vomiting, diarrhea, and abdominal pain may also be present, but are recognized less frequently than in dogs. Other symptoms may include weight loss, dehydration, fever, and icterus. Symptoms of shock (hypothermia, tachycardia, bradycardia, tachypnea, and weak pulses) may develop in cats with acute necrotizing pancreatitis. Pancreatitis in cats may also occur in conjunction with cholangiohepatitis, hepatic lipidosis, or inflammatory bowel disease, and symptoms related to these disorders may predominate.

DIAGNOSIS
Laboratory tests
The diagnosis of pancreatitis may be challenging because the commonly used laboratory markers tend to be inconsistent. Although elevations in amylase and lipase are often considered to be diagnostic of pancreatitis, this is not necessarily the case. Amylase and lipase may be elevated as a result of liver disease, primary GI disease, renal disease, or the use of drugs, such as etherified starches (e.g. hetastarch) or corticosteroids. Amylase and lipase may also be normal in cases of acute pancreatitis if inflammation leads to the depletion of stored enzymes. Amylase and lipase have no clinical utility in the diagnosis of pancreatitis in cats, as these enzymes are frequently elevated as a result of nonpancreatic causes and they may be decreased in cats with pancreatitis. Serum TLI, a pancreas-specific marker, is frequently used in cats as an indicator of acute pancreatitis. However, this test has also been shown to become elevated with nonpancreatic

illness, such as azotemia, inflammatory bowel disease, and GI lymphoma, and may be normal in cats with various forms of pancreatitis. For this reason, TLI is best interpreted in conjunction with other diagnostic testing.

Other laboratory abnormalities may include leukocytosis, hemoconcentration or anemia, prerenal azotemia, and elevations in ALT, AST, ALP, and total bilirubin. Hyperglycemia may be present due to release of stress hormones or as a result of concurrent diabetes mellitus. Hypoglycemia may also be seen, particularly in cats, as a result of systemic inflammation. Hypocalcemia may develop from saponification of intraabdominal fat. Thrombocytopenia, hypofibrinogenemia, prolongations of PT and aPTT, and the presence of FDPs or D-dimers may indicate the development of DIC.

Imaging
Abdominal radiographs should be performed to rule out intestinal obstruction. Radiographic changes associated with pancreatitis include ileus, widening of the angle between pylorus and duodenum, thickening of the duodenum, and focal loss of detail or 'ground glass' appearance to the right cranial abdomen. Unfortunately, these changes are nonspecific and are rarely useful in confirming a diagnosis of pancreatitis.

Abdominal ultrasonography (117) is currently one of the most useful tools for diagnosing pancreatitis. Ultrasonographic changes consistent

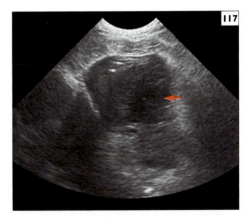

117 Ultrasound image of a dog (Welsh Terrier) with a pancreatitic abscess (arrow) and severe pancreatitis.

with pancreatitis include pancreatic enlargement, hypoechogenicity, and increased echogenicity of the peripancreatic fat. Pancreatic cysts, abscesses, and masses may also be visualized. Disadvantages of ultrasonography include poor sensitivity and the need for a high degree of operator skill.

CT is considered very useful in the identification of pancreatitis in people. Small case series have suggested a similar benefit in dealing with dogs and cats.

MANAGEMENT / TREATMENT

Treatment of pancreatitis in dogs consists largely of intravenous fluid and electrolyte supplementation, pain management, and nothing by mouth. In dogs, food and water should typically be withheld until 24 hours have elapsed with no further vomiting. A low-fat, highly digestible diet may then be reintroduced. Balanced crystalloids should be provided at a rate calculated to replace fluid deficit, provide maintenance needs, and meet ongoing losses. Potassium chloride should be supplemented, based on serial electrolyte monitoring. Anti-emetics are frequently needed to control vomiting, and metoclopramide may be added to intravenous fluids to provide a dose of 1–2 mg/kg/day by CRI. If this is not successful in controlling vomiting, ondansetron (0.1–0.2 mg/kg IV q8hr) or dolasetron (0.6–1 mg/kg SC q24hr) may be added. Appropriate analgesia should also be provided for patients suspected to have abdominal pain. Many clinicians advocate buprenorphine (0.01–0.015 mg/kg q6h) over pure agonist opioids, such as morphine, in patients with pancreatitis, as morphine may induce constriction of the pancreatic duct. Whether this theoretical concern is of clinical significance has not been proven in veterinary patients.

Nutritional support should be instituted in patients with protracted vomiting. TPN is generally preferred in patients unable to tolerate enteral feeding because of its ability to bypass the gut and to avoid stimulating pancreatic secretions. Disadvantages include the potential for catheter-related sepsis, electrolyte disturbances, and hyperglycemia. Additionally, failure to provide enteral nutrition is associated with an increased risk of bacterial translocation due to villous atrophy and increased gut permeability. As an alternative to parenteral nutrition, jejunostomy tubes may be placed surgically or endoscopically to provide enteral nutrition for patients with pancreatitis. Advantages to jejunostomy tubes include the ability to provide enteral nutrition without contributing to ongoing vomiting or increased pancreatic secretions. Disadvantages include the need for invasive surgery (if not otherwise needed) and the equipment and technical skills to place the tube endoscopically. In cats with chronic pancreatitis, there is no evidence to suggest that enteral feeding is associated with worsening of the disease and esophagostomy or gastrostomy (PEG) tubes are frequently placed for long-term nutritional support.

Plasma transfusion has been recommended in the treatment of animals with severe pancreatitis in order to replace α-macroglobulins and other serum protease inhibitors. While there are currently no studies in veterinary species to support this practice, studies in human patients have not documented increased survival with plasma replacement. As such, its use should be limited to those patients with evidence of coagulopathy. Antibiotics are also frequently employed by veterinary practitioners in the treatment of pancreatitis. In contrast to what is described in the human literature, pancreatic infection is rarely documented in dogs and cats with acute pancreatitis, and prophylactic antibiotic therapy is therefore not routinely recommended.

Surgical intervention is occasionally performed in patients with severe necrotizing pancreatitis, particularly in those with focal areas of necrosis, pancreatic masses, or pancreatic abscesses. As sterile abscesses or inflammatory masses may also be successfully managed medically, indications for surgery are currently unclear and are frequently based on the documentation of infection or biliary obstruction, or failure to respond to medical management. Additional benefits to surgical intervention include the ability to obtain a definitive diagnosis, to place jejunostomy tubes for nutritional support, and to place abdominal drains for relief of severe inflammatory effusions.

PROGNOSIS

The overall prognosis for dogs affected with pancreatitis is fair to good with supportive care and time. However, some animals, particularly cats, with necrotizing pancreatitis succumb to multiple organ failure.

CHAPTER 7

Renal emergencies

- **Acute renal failure**

- **Dialysis**

- **Chronic renal failure**

- **Urethral obstruction**

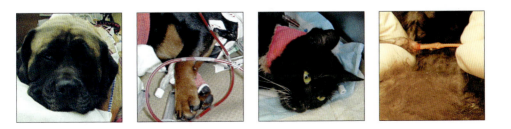

Injury to the renal system is a common cause for presentation to the emergency clinician. The general approach to azotemia is illustrated in 118. Clinical signs are often vague and include depression, lethargy, anorexia, or vomiting. Because the kidneys are integral to electrolyte homeostasis, and maintenance of volume and systemic blood pressure, any alteration in renal function can result in life-threatening disease. Signalment, history, physical examination, and analysis of a minimum database, including serum renal values and electrolytes, are all essential diagnostic components. For example, cats commonly present with urinary obstruction. A roaming dog may be hit by a car and suffer traumatic bladder rupture. A well-supervised, indoor cat may chew on an Easter lily plant and develop ARF. The following section provides a review of ARF, CRF, and urinary obstruction. As veterinary medicine becomes more specialized, more sophisticated treatment options are available. A review of dialysis is thus also presented. Essentially, however, despite the increasing availability of aggressive management options for severe renal disease, the role of the emergency clinician is still vital, recognizing and providing stabilization of the critical animal.

KEY POINTS
- The kidneys are integral to maintaining fluid balance and electrolyte homeostasis.
- Sophisticated treatments for renal failure are available (119).
- Survival of animals with renal disease often depends on the intervention of the emergency clinician.

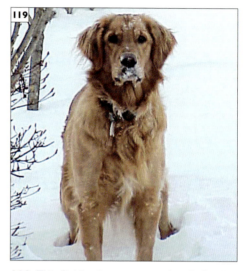

119 This Golden Retriever was identified with congenital renal dysplasia as a puppy. A vascular access device was placed in the jugular vein for home administration of intravenous fluids, which permitted an extended survival with a high quality of life.

118 Flow chart for azotemia.

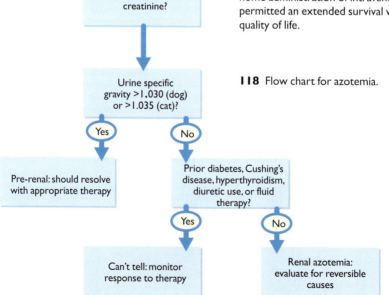

Elevated BUN or creatinine?

↓

Urine specific gravity >1.030 (dog) or >1.035 (cat)?

Yes → Pre-renal: should resolve with appropriate therapy

No → Prior diabetes, Cushing's disease, hyperthyroidism, diuretic use, or fluid therapy?

Yes → Can't tell: monitor response to therapy

No → Renal azotemia: evaluate for reversible causes

Acute renal failure

KEY POINTS
- ARF is classified by pre-renal, renal, and post-renal causes.
- Goals of treatment include correction of volume deficits, dehydration, and electrolyte derangements.
- Prognosis often relies on identification and reversal of an inciting cause.
- Improved prognosis is associated with early intervention and rapid response to therapy.

DEFINITION
ARF is a syndrome characterized by a rapidly progressive (over hours to days) impairment of the kidney's ability to maintain electrolyte homeostasis and excrete nitrogenous wastes. In humans, ARF is determined within the context of an increase of serum creatinine 44.2 µmol/l (0.5 mg/dl) over baseline. ARF is divided into three broad categories based on the origin of the renal impairment: pre-renal, renal, and post-renal. Two or more causes may co-exist simultaneously. Without timely intervention, pre-renal failure may easily and rapidly progress to intrinsic ARF.

ETIOLOGY
Pre-renal ARF
Any condition that causes decreased effective circulating volume can result in decreased GFR and cause pre-renal ARF. Common causes include hypovolemia, dehydration, or decreased cardiac output (*Table 2*). Severe vomiting or diarrhea can result in profound fluid losses. PU/PD in animals with diabetes mellitus, Cushing's syndrome, or CRF results in a high risk of pre-renal azotemia if water intake is limited, as with water restriction or anorexia. Decreased cardiac output due to CHF or cardiovascular collapse (shock) will result in decreased renal perfusion and pre-renal ARF. Hypoadrenocorticism (adrenal insufficiency, Addison's disease) commonly results in azotemia due to pre-renal failure from inability to maintain normal mean arterial blood pressure and effective circulating volume.

Renal ARF
Intrinsic renal tissue damage causes ARF and is categorized by location of injury: tubule, interstitium, glomerulus, or vessels. Common causes of acute tubular necrosis include ischemia, nephrotoxicity, and infection (*Table 3*). Immune-mediated injury can result in glomerular disease, and allergic reaction can cause interstitial nephritis. Additionally, renal injury can result secondary to systemic disease. Sepsis-associated ARF is related to a series of events governed by the production of inflammatory mediators, resulting in systemic hypotension but renal vasoconstriction. With circulatory collapse, the kidneys suffer severe injury due to decreased renal perfusion and local deleterious effects of inflammatory mediators. Without extraordinary critical management, including dialysis, prognosis for survival for severe sepsis with ARF is extremely poor.

Table 2 Causes of pre-renal acute renal failure

Hypovolemia or severe dehydration (vomiting, diarrhea, prolonged anorexia)

Decreased cardiac output (CHF)

Hypotension (hypoadrenocorticism)

Table 3 Common causes of acute intrinsic renal injury

Toxins and drugs
Ethylene glycol (antifreeze)
Toxic plants (lily toxicity in cats)
NSAIDs (salycilates, ibuprofen, ketoprofen)
Aminoglycoside antibiotics (amikacin, gentamicin)
Chemotherapeutic agents (cisplatin)

Infectious agents
Leptospirosis
Rocky Mountain spotted fever
Ehrlichiosis
Pyelonephritis (bacterial)

Other
Immune-mediated (lupus, glomerulonephritis)
Thrombosis or renal infarction
Heat stroke
Sepsis

Table 4 Common causes of post-renal acute renal failure

Urethral or bilateral ureteral obstruction

Uroabdomen

Post-renal ARF

Post-renal ARF occurs when urine outflow is obstructed, or with leakage of urine into the peritoneal cavity (uroabdomen) (*Table 4*). Urinary obstruction is usually the result of urine imped-ance in the urethra or ureters. Calculi, tumors, inflammatory lesions, or blood clots are common causes. In cats with FLUTD, spasms of the urethral sphincters commonly disrupt urine flow. For azotemia to be apparent, obstructive nephropathy has to occur. Obstructive nephro-pathy is caused by increased pressure on the tubules of the kidney imposed by both existing trapped urine and the continued production of urine. Although azotemia commonly occurs with UO, it should not result with obstruction of a single ureter provided the contralateral kidney and ureter are healthy and capable of producing and propagating the flow of urine. In fact, because of continued normal function of the opposite kidney and ureter, it is not uncommon for a kidney and ureter to have been unknowingly obstructed in the past with no clinical signs.

Uroabdomen is caused by any injury that allows urine leakage from the kidney, ureter, bladder, or urethra. The most common cause of uroabdomen in dogs and cats is traumatic rupture of the urinary bladder. Other causes include trauma to the urethra from avulsion of the urinary bladder, or iatrogenic injury incurred during passage of urinary catheters. Trauma to a ureter can result from traumatic avulsion from its attachments to the kidney or urinary bladder, or secondary to inadvertent ligation or resec-tion during OHE (**120**). Bladder rupture is a common injury with blunt or crushing abdom-inal trauma, and should be considered in any animal with pelvic fractures. Ligation or transec-tion of the ureters should be considered in any animal with recent OHE. Perforation of the bladder is an uncommon result of severe bladder inflammation, but should be considered with chronic, long-term cystitis or emphysematous bladder, a complication of diabetes mellitus.

Neoplasia of any region of the urinary tract can be a cause of post-renal ARF by either obstruc-tion or uroabdomen via perforation.

PATHOGENESIS

In ARF, injury to the renal tubule, regardless of its inciting cause, limits the kidney's ability to maintain electrolyte homeostasis and to excrete nitrogenous wastes and other substances that act as uremic toxins. Failure of the tubular cells to reabsorb glucose and protein increases their loss in the urine. As glucosuria and proteinuria continue, osmotic diuresis occurs, exacerbating water loss. Uremia increases, causing gastritis, nausea, and anorexia. Vomiting, diarrhea, and anorexia prevent correction of volume losses, further decreasing effective circulating volume, GFR, and renal perfusion. As diminished renal perfusion progresses, renal oxygen delivery drops, and a devastating spiral of renal injury continues. Eventually, the kidneys' ability to produce urine is diminished, and the animal becomes oliguric. Unless aggressive intervention is provided to restore effective circulating volume and to treat the underlying cause of the ARF, progression to anuria will occur rapidly.

Prognosis often depends on early recognition of disease, prompt intervention, and response of the animal to treatment. In severe cases, dialysis (hemodialysis (**121**) or peritoneal dialysis) may be required to stabilize electrolyte derangements and

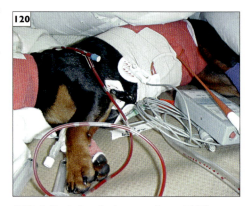

120 A Dachshund who experienced ARF following bilateral ureteral ligation during routine OHE. Peritoneal dialysis and removal of the ligatures permitted return of normal renal function.

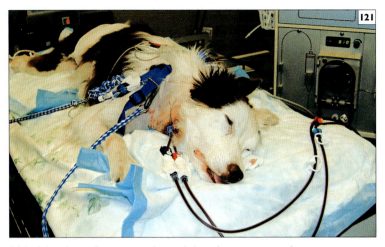

121 A border collie receiving hemodialysis for treatment of acute renal failure.

allow for continued fluid administration during the anuric phase. Fluid overload during anuric renal failure necessitates judicious fluid administration, and management commonly may require both dialysis and mechanical ventilation.

CLINICAL PRESENTATION

Uremia, electrolyte derangements, and the underlying cause for the disease all account for the clinical signs of ARF (*Table 5*).

Uremia causes gastritis, encephalopathy, pneumonitis, and platelet dysfunction. Lethargy, weakness, mental dullness, vomiting, anorexia, respiratory distress, and coagulopathy are common clinical signs. Recent or acute onset of PU/PD is also typical; however, by the time of presentation, anorexia and vomiting may have resulted in severe dehydration and the animal may be unwilling to drink, and oliguria or anuria may have already occurred.

Animals presenting with pre-renal causes will commonly be profoundly weak or even collapsed. Azotemia secondary to hypoadrenocorticism is likely to be accompanied by hypotension, hyponatremia, and hyperkalemia. Oliguria or anuria accompanying a hypoadrenal crisis is often due to profound hypovolemia. The clinical scenario typical of hypoadrenocorticism is similar to that of post-renal ARF.

Hyperkalemia is a major finding with conditions causing urinary obstruction or uroabdomen, and without aggressive intervention will progress to life-threatening cardiac instability resulting in bradycardia, atrial standstill, and, eventually, cardiac arrest. Clinical suspicion of hypoadrenocorticism, in addition to an ability to assess quickly for urinary obstruction and peritonitis, are essential in providing emergency care for animals with signs of ARF.

Respiratory distress may be present as a result of uremic pneumonitis, pulmonary edema associated with concurrent pulmonary contusions (trauma), fluid overload with anuria, or attempts to compensate for accompanying metabolic acidosis. The abdomen may be painful with peritonitis from urine contamination, or from renal swelling caused by obstruction or infection. If renal failure is intrinsic and associated with other underlying disease, such as leptospirosis or lymphosarcoma, additional systemic signs may be apparent, such as icterus or petechiae.

Table 5 Common clinical signs of acute renal failure
Lethargy
Anorexia
Nausea
Dehydration
Hypovolemia

Table 6 Diagnostic tests for acute renal failure

Minimum database (CBC, serum chemistry analysis, urinalysis)

Urine culture and sensitivity

Diagnostic imaging (survey radiography, ultrasonography, IVP, contrast cystourethrogram)

Serology

ACTH stimulation

Ethylene glycol level in blood

DIAGNOSTIC TESTS

All animals with azotemia should have minimum database including CBC, serum chemistry analysis, and urinalysis (*Table 6*). A diagnosis of ARF may be made with as little of an increase in serum creatinine as 44.2 µmol/l (0.5 mg/dl) over baseline. Often, however, baseline values are unknown, and serum values for both BUN and creatinine are already out of the normal range. A loss in the ability to concentrate urine is the hallmark of primary renal parenchymal disease, while a urine specific gravity >1.030 is usually associated with pre-renal ARF. One should remember that pre-renal and renal azotemia may co-exist. Urine aerobic culture with sensitivity should be obtained, unless a clear history of drug or toxin exposure, trauma, or recent surgery is known.

Initial test results that may assist in the rapid determination of the cause of azotemia include arterial blood pressure, urine specific gravity, serum electrolytes, and emergency imaging with survey radiography and ultrasonography. IVP and contrast cystourethrogram are useful for determining obstruction or trauma. Serology may be carried out for infectious and immune-mediated diseases. Azotemia should resolve with fluid resuscitation if the cause were pre-renal. In the absence of an explanation for such dehydration to result in pre-renal ARF, ACTH stimulation should be performed to rule out hypoadrenocorticism. Once pre- and post-renal causes of azotemia have been eliminated, primary or intrinsic ARF should be considered.

The presence of glucosuria in the absence of hyperglycemia is suggestive of proximal tubular dysfunction. A high level of urinary protein, in the absence of bacteria or white blood cells, is likely due to glomerular disease (glomerulonephritis). Urine protein:creatinine ratio should be obtained with the presence of proteinuria and hypoalbuminemia. Because moderate to severe azotemia frequently results in the development of hypertension, and pharmacological control of hypertension is associated with a better outcome, blood pressure monitoring is warranted.

Elevations in the white blood cell count can be associated with pyelonephritis or a systemic infectious disease. Lack of a stress leukogram is suspicious for hypoadrenocorticism. Concurrent thrombocytopenia or polyarthritis may indicate infectious or immune-mediated disease.

Ethylene glycol toxicity should be suspected in any animal that roams unsupervised or has known exposure. Classic signs include mental alteration, ataxia, and seizures. Animals with ethylene glycol toxicity may have metabolic acidosis, hypocalcemia, and increased anion gap prior to the onset of azotemia. Early recognition of this potential intoxication is essential in achieving a positive outcome. Blood tests for ethylene glycol levels are available, and are recommended with any suspicion of potential exposure.

Ingestion of lilies is a common cause of intrinsic ARF in cats during the Easter holiday (**122**), and, like ethylene glycol toxicity, should be suspected in any cat with ARF with potential exposure. Calcium oxalate crystalluria is often present in ARF caused by ethylene glycol and lily toxicities. See also Chapter 5.

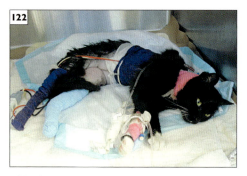

122 Cat receiving peritoneal dialysis for ARF due to Easter lily ingestion. There is severe swelling in the inguinal region. Fluid balance may be very challenging in a patient with anuria or oliguria.

Table 7 Goals of treatment for acute renal failure

Correct fluid deficits

Correct electrolyte imbalances

Correct underlying disease

Improve urine production

MANAGEMENT / TREATMENT

Treatment and management of ARF are aimed at stabilization of electrolyte derangements, correction of fluid deficits, and provision of diuresis to maximize recovery from renal injury (*Table 7*). Outcome often relies on identification and elimination of any underlying, inciting cause.

In most cases, with prompt intervention, pre- and post-renal ARF are associated with an excellent prognosis. This usually involves aggressive intravenous fluid resuscitation, return of normal electrolyte status, and correction of the causative disease. Hyperkalemia is the most common life-threatening electrolyte imbalance encountered in ARF. If hyperkalemia is severe (>7.5 mmol/l [>7.5 mEq/l]), emergency treatment includes intravenous administration of fluid therapy (0.9% NaCl) and 10% calcium gluconate (0.5–1.5 ml/kg IV over 10–15 min) to stabilize bradycardia and atrial standstill. Administration of regular insulin (0.1–0.25 U/kg IV, IM, or SC), and then 50% dextrose (0.5 g/kg bolus IV followed by 2.5% dextrose infusion) may be additionally used for hyperkalemia. Administration of sodium bicarbonate (1–2 mmol/kg [1–2 mEq/kg of body weight] IV over 20 min) requires pH monitoring and is recommended with metabolic acidosis and hyperkalemia due to ethylene glycol toxicity.

Trauma or post-surgical complication usually requires surgical intervention. UO requires urinary catheter placement to relieve the obstruction. Maintenance of the indwelling urinary catheter is beneficial to provide intravenous fluid therapy during post-obstructive polyuria. Bilateral ureteral obstruction and uroabdomen causing peritonitis almost invariably require surgical intervention following diagnostic imaging to identify the cause.

Rapid resolution of azotemia and electrolyte abnormalities with intravenous fluids should prompt suspicion for hypoadrenocorticism. These animals should be administered dexamethasone sodium phosphate, and have an ACTH stimulation test performed.

Animals with ARF of intrinsic renal cause require aggressive management, often in a referral hospital with 24 hours care. Central venous intravenous access allows for monitoring of CVP in addition to administration of fluid therapy. Hypovolemia should be corrected rapidly. Fluid choice should rely on the needs and electrolyte imbalances of the animal. Generally, correction of hypovolemia is best achieved with any isotonic replacement fluid (e.g. lactated Ringer's solution or 0.9% NaCl). Moderate (6.6–7.5 mmol/l [6.6–7.5 mEq/l]) to severe (>7.5 mmol/l [>7.5 mEq/l]) hyperkalemia is usually preferentially treated with fluid containing no potassium (0.9% NaCl). However, hyperkalemia is often the result of decreased GFR due to decreased effective circulating volume, and fluid resuscitation with any isotonic replacement fluid is of paramount importance in providing life-saving emergency treatment. Hypovolemia and fluid needs can be evaluated on the basis of CVP and urine production. Because oliguria and anuria are difficult to assess with hypovolemia and dehydration, a fluid therapy plan designed to maintain CVP between 4 and 7 cmH_2O, and achieve urine production at a rate of >0.25 ml/kg/hr, is optimal.

To attempt to improve diuresis, administration of mannitol to animals not severely overloaded has been advocated. Mannitol (0.25–1.0 g/kg IV over 30 min) is thought to improve fluid movement through the renal tubules, by drawing water from edematous tubular cells and pushing cellular debris (casts) along through the tubules. Furosemide (2 mg/kg bolus IV, followed by CRI at 0.25–1 mg/kg/hr) may also improve diuresis, although its use with ARF due to aminoglycoside toxicity is contraindicated. The use of dopamine in ARF remains controversial, but may be tried at a low dosage (0.5–2.5 µg/kg/min).

Animals with oliguria or anuria despite adequate fluid administration will demonstrate signs of fluid overload, such as tachypnea, subcutaneous fluid accumulation, chemosis, and weight gain. In these cases, CVP will be elevated to >7 cmH$_2$0, and further measures to treat ARF, including dialysis, may be necessary because intolerance of continued diuresis dictates cessation of intravenous fluid therapy.

Hypertension, a common finding in ARF, should be treated with the oral administration of calcium channel blockers (amlodipine) and ACE inhibitors (e.g. enalapril, benazepril). The use of amlodipine as a mono-therapy agent is contra-indicated in hypertensive patients. Intravenous therapies including hydralazine or sodium nitro-prusside should be considered if vomiting precludes the use of oral medications.

Although metabolic acidosis is common in ARF, it is seldom severe enough to require treatment. If, however, metabolic acidosis is severe and life-threatening (pH <7.1), as in ethylene glycol toxicity, calculation of the bicarbonate deficit yields an amount that can be supplemented over 24 hours: Bicarbonate deficit = 20 minus measured HCO$_3$ (mmol/l [mEq/l]) × body weight (kg) × 0.3. (Measured bicarbonate is obtained from blood gas analysis; mmol/l and mEq/l are equivalent to each other, there is no need for conversion.)

The administration of gastric protectants is always advised, in addition to anti-emetics if vomiting is present. Antibiotics should be administered on the basis of culture results, or presumptive diagnosis of underlying infection.

PROGNOSIS

Prognosis depends on the severity of renal failure and the underlying cause. Pre- and post-renal ARF respond well to restoration of volume status, correction of electrolyte derangements, and reversal of the inciting cause. Intrinsic ARF may respond to aggressive supportive management, but increased severity may require critical care including dialysis, and survival is less probable.

Dialysis

KEY POINTS
- Dialysis performs vital functions of fluid management and electrolyte stabilization during anuric or oliguric renal failure.
- Dialysis can remove certain compounds when serum levels become toxic.
- Dialysis cannot treat or reverse renal disease. It can only provide time to allow injury to heal.

DEFINITION

Dialysis removes uremic waste products, corrects electrolyte imbalances, and adjusts fluid volume by mechanical means. Two different technologies are employed: *intermittent dialysis* and *continuous renal replacement therapy* (CRRT). Intermittent dialysis is used to achieve large corrections over a short period of time. It is the most commonly employed method in human medicine in North America. CRRT is utilized to make small, gradual changes in a patient's condition over longer periods of time, and is normally performed in the intensive care setting. While each technology has its theoretical advantages, neither has been proven superior in randomized clinical trials.

Table 8 Indications for dialysis

Anuric or oliguric renal failure not responding to appropriate intravenous fluid therapy

Severe azotemia despite adequate urine production

Toxicities

Table 9 Common substances removable by dialysis

Acetaminophen (paracetamol)

Salicylates

Ethylene glycol

Aminoglycosides

Metaldehyde

Alcohols

Phenobarbital

Theophylline

Tricyclic antidepressants

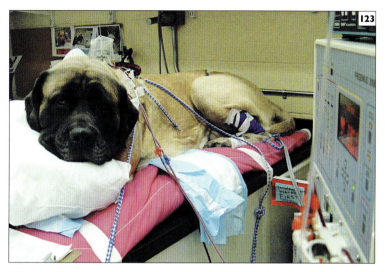

123 Mastiff receiving dialysis for treatment of ARF due to leptospirosis.

INDICATIONS

Indications for dialysis include ARF (**123**) or CRF that has failed to respond to intravenous fluid management (*Table 8*). Anuria or oliguria, electrolyte derangements, and signs of fluid overload (tachypnea, subcutaneous fluid accumulation, chemosis, and weight gain) are common indications for consideration of dialysis. Other indications include severe azotemia (serum BUN >36 mmol/l [>100 mg/dl] or creatinine >884 µmol/l [>10 mg/dl]) despite adequate urine production, and toxic levels of certain medications or other substances. Dialysis in CRF patients may be best utilized for stabilizing patients prior to renal transplantation.

MECHANISM OF ACTION

The removal of a substance with hemodialysis is dependent on specific characteristics: protein binding affinity, molecular size, water solubility, and its volume of distribution. Dialysis is increasingly used in the intensive care setting to treat animals with severe renal failure. Dialysis can perform many life-saving functions, in particular the removal of nitrogenous wastes and excess serum potassium. Dialysis is also employed as treatment for some toxicities, including ethylene glycol, phenobarbital, and ethanol (*Table 9*).

It is important to remember, however, that organ damage that may have occurred prior to removing the offending substance will not necessarily be reversed with dialysis. The Nephrology Pharmacy Associates' website maintains information regarding the ability of dialysis to remove many drugs and illicit substances. This information, which is provided as a service to the medical community, is currently available at: www. nephrologypharmacy.com/pub_dialysis.html.

PROGNOSIS

The time required for return of adequate renal function is variable and cannot be predicted. Not all patients will recover adequate renal function. With the exception of an acute toxicity, dialysis is unlikely to repair a problem, and, in an unstable animal, it is not a risk-free therapy. Dialysis may, however, be a life-saving treatment, supporting the animal while providing the kidneys with time to heal. Prognosis, therefore, depends on the cause and severity of renal failure, and financial resources of the owner. If an owner wishes to explore treatment of renal failure with dialysis, the animal should be transferred to a dialysis center (see Appendices) as soon as possible. The chance of successful treatment increases with earlier intervention.

Chronic renal failure

KEY POINTS
- CRF results from congenital or acquired renal abnormalities.
- Treatment is focused on ensuring hydration and decreasing the signs of uremia.
- CRF is almost invariably progressive, although good quality of life may be maintained for years.

DEFINITION
CRF is defined as a progressive impairment in the kidney's ability to concentrate urine, excrete nitrogenous waste, and maintain electrolyte homeostasis. This deterioration in renal function is due to gradual, irreversible nephron loss, and is the most common kidney disease in companion animals. CRF is divided into two categories based on the underlying cause: congenital and acquired.

ETIOLOGY
Congenital renal disease
This occurs as a result of a lesion present at birth that either causes failure, or will lead to renal failure in the future. Mostly, these lesions are hereditary, and the condition becomes apparent early in life and is progressive. Common congenital renal diseases include:
- Renal dysplasia (Lhasa Apso, Shih Tzu, Poodle, Soft-Coated Wheaten Terrier, Golden Retriever, Chow Chow).
- Glomerulopathy (Samoyed, English Cocker Spaniel, Rottweiler, Newfoundland, Doberman Pinscher, Soft-Coated Wheaten Terrier).
- Amyloidosis (Abyssinian cats, Shar Pei).
- Fanconi syndrome (Basenji).
- Polycystic kidney disease (Persian cats, Cairn Terrier).

Acquired chronic renal disease
This is the result of an insult to the renal parenchyma that results in nephron loss and precipitates a gradual decline in renal function. In some cases, an underlying cause can be determined, such as pyelonephritis. In most instances, however, the inciting cause is never identified. Regardless of the etiology, most cases of CRF have a similar clinical presentation, course, and treatment.

CLINICAL PRESENTATION
Clinical features of CRF are nonspecific, and depend on the severity of the azotemia and presence of concurrent illness. Common clinical signs include dehydration, PU/PD, weight loss, lethargy, anorexia, vomiting, and oral ulcers.

DIAGNOSIS
Initial tests include minimum database of CBC, serum chemistry analysis, urinalysis, and urine aerobic culture with sensitivity. Determination of arterial blood pressure should be carried out in all animals with CRF.

Abnormalities typically identified by urinalysis include isosthenuria (specific gravity 1.007–1.015), glucosuria in the absence of hyperglycemia, proteinuria in the absence of bacteria, white blood cells, or blood. A urine protein: creatinine ratio is indicated when glomerulonephritis is suspected or with proteinuria and hypoalbuminemia.

Azotemia, hyperphosphatemia, and mild hypercalcemia are typical findings on serum chemistry analysis. Nonregenerative anemia is the most consistent hematological finding. Although the white cell count is usually unremarkable, elevations may be present with chronic pyelonephritis or a systemic infection.

Survey abdominal radiography is useful for determination of kidney size, and presence of radio-opaque urinary calculi or mineralization. Abdominal ultrasonography is preferred for examining renal architecture and presence of calculi. Renal biopsies are of questionable benefit when test results and history are overwhelmingly supportive of CRF. Injury to the kidney with biopsy may further decompensate an animal's condition.

MANAGEMENT / TREATMENT
With the exception of dehydration, many of the problems accompanying CRF are part of a chronic process. The key to therapy for the dog or cat with CRF is to separate cause of the acute decompensation from the manifestations of the chronic process. Dehydration can occur quickly in an animal with PU/PD. An animal with PU/PD spends a significant amount of time consuming water, compensating for an inability to concentrate urine. Any problem that may decrease water consumption, such as weakness or lethargy, anorexia or vomiting, may result in rapid

onset of dehydration. It is not uncommon for a cat that prefers to drink from the faucet to develop severe dehydration if weakness prevents it from approaching the sink. Increasing azotemia exerts pressure to pull water osmotically from the interstitium and cellular space, further worsening dehydration. Although urine culture may be negative, intravenous antibiotics should be considered in all patients with chronic renal failure that have undergone a sudden deterioration.

A rapid intravenous bolus of fluid will prove ineffective at correcting dehydration. Therefore, dehydration should be estimated as a percentage, and then replacement calculated according to the following equation: Replacement fluids (ml) = % dehydration × body weight in kg × 1000.

Replacement should then be administered over 24–36 hours. Maintenance fluid requirements should be calculated at a rate of 40–50 ml/kg/day in the cat, and 60–66 ml/kg/day in the dog. Maintenance requirements are administered in addition to replacement resuscitation. The status of the animal should be periodically evaluated to avoid over- or under-hydration. Once dehydration is corrected, fluid therapy should be reassessed. Ideally, a maintenance fluid should be administered if the animal is still inappetent, and unwilling to drink water. It is easy to underestimate the animal's requirement for free water, and it is not uncommon to see hypernatremia occur as a result of continuing administration of replacement fluids in preference to a fluid choice that would deliver more free water.

Other treatments for the management of the animal with CRF include medications to control hypertension, including calcium channel blocking agents (amlodipine) and ACE inhibitors (enalapril and benazepril). The goal of antihypertensive agents is to maintain systemic blood pressure at <160 mmHg. Hypokalemia is a common finding in cats with CRF and should be treated with intravenous supplementation. Hyperphosphatemia is also a common finding, but attempts to correct it in the emergency setting are not recommended. If the patient is symptomatic for anemia, transfusion of packed red blood cells should be administered. To help counter signs of uremic gastritis, gastric protectants should always be given. Chronic pyelonephritis is a common complicating cause of decompensation of CRF. Although urine culture is usually negative, intravenous antibiotics should be considered.

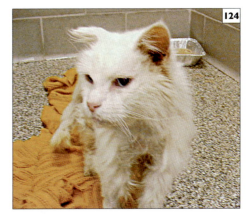

124 Elderly cats are commonly affected with CRF. Committed clients and a good relationship with the family veterinarian may permit many years of added survival with a good quality of life. The cat shown in this photograph was 17 years of age, and had both chronic renal failure and diabetes mellitus.

PROGNOSIS

With management, many animals with CRF survive for years with good quality of life. For this reason, it is essential to consider the dog or cat presenting with acute decompensation of CRF within this context. Infection or other underlying problems that cause inappetence may result in decreased water intake and dehydration. Identification and correction of a cause of acute decompensation may allow the animal with CRF to recover and return home (**124**). End-stage CRF, on the other hand, is unrewarding to treat, and survival to discharge is unlikely. Unfortunately, there is no definitive measure to differentiate end-stage CRF from acute decompensation of chronic disease upon entry to the emergency room. Prognosis depends on severity of disease.

Urethral obstruction

KEY POINTS
- UO is a common cause of post-renal ARF and may be life-threatening.
- Dogs are more commonly affected with uroliths and neoplasia, while cats are more frequently obstructed with plugs of mucus and debris.
- Radiolucent uroliths in a young dog should prompt consideration of a portocaval shunt.

DEFINITION
UO is a common cause for presentation of cats and dogs to the emergency room. Cats are affected more frequently than dogs. In cats, UO usually results from the presence of mucus plugs, grit, or urethral sphincter spasms associated with FLUTD. Tumors and calculi occur more frequently in dogs. Whatever the cause of obstruction, mounting pressure of urine within the urinary bladder eventually results in obstructive nephropathy and ARF. Inability to excrete nitrogenous wastes and potassium will result in azotemia and hyperkalemia. Severe hyperkalemia can cause bradycardia and atrial standstill. If allowed to progress, untreated UO will result in death.

ETIOLOGY
Due to anatomical differences, UO occurs more frequently in males. Urinary calculi affect dogs more commonly than cats. Calculus formation depends on a number of factors, including hereditary predisposition, metabolic disease, or underlying urinary tract infection. Certain breeds of both dogs and cats have hereditary predispositions to formation of various calculi. Dalmatians, for example, are predisposed to the formation of urate calculi. Struvite calculi may precipitate in alkaline urine, which is often associated with urinary tract infections. Ammonium biurate calculi may result from conditions that produce hyperammonemia, such as portocaval shunting, or other liver disease.

Although not entirely understood, FLUTD is a syndrome in cats that is associated with cystitis, spasm of the urethral proximal and distal sphincters, and plugging of the urethra with casts, calculi, mucoproteins, or crystals. Other, less common causes of urethral obstruction in both dogs and cats include neoplasia, trauma, and stricture formation. Regardless of the cause, however, UO almost invariably will progress to post-renal ARF, resulting in the inability to eliminate nitrogenous wastes and potassium.

PATHOGENESIS
An inability to expel urine causes an accumulation of urine within the urinary bladder resulting in increasing intravesicular pressure, mucosal sloughing, and hemorrhage. If this increase in pressure is allowed to continue, intraureteral and intrarenal pressures will eventually increase as well, resulting in ARF.

CLINICAL PRESENTATION
Clinical signs vary based on the severity and duration of obstruction, and differ for dogs and cats.

The dog with UO is often accompanied by a helpful history of stranguria, pollakiuria, or hematuria. Certain types of calculi are common in specific breeds of dogs; such as urates in Dalmatians and calcium oxalates for Bichon Frisé). Any female, middle-aged to older dog should be suspected of neoplasia of the urethra or bladder.

Urinary patterns in the cat are less obvious to the owner. A cat may often not be determined to have UO until found collapsed or moribund. Sometimes the cat will demonstrate anxiety, crying, or howling, or be observed to make frequent trips to the litter box. Outdoor cats with signs of UO may go entirely unnoticed. Less often the owner may report pollakiuria, stranguria, or hematuria.

In both species, as azotemia develops, lethargy, vomiting, and anorexia occur. By the time the animal is presented to the emergency clinician, significant dehydration may have developed. Rarely, however, will the dog present moribund. Almost invariably, animals with UO will have relatively large, hard bladders on palpation. However, animals with large, flaccid bladders secondary to prior neurological disease may also have signs suggestive of UO. Pain may be elicited with physical examination. Dehydration may account for faint pulses. If moderate to severe hyperkalemia (>7.5 mmol/l [>7.5 mEq/l]) is present, sinus bradycardia or atrial standstill should indicate a critical state necessitating emergency intervention.

DIAGNOSIS

Diagnosis is usually easily made based on signalment, history, and identification of a large, hard bladder that is inexpressible. Dogs should have minimum database including CBC, serum chemistry analysis, and urinalysis with urine culture. Because of the likelihood of FLUTD, the minimum database for cats includes serum renal values and electrolytes, and urinalysis. Bacterial urinary infection is not a typical finding in cats, so urine culture is not indicated.

Common abnormal findings include azotemia and hyperkalemia. The urine should be assessed for pH, signs of infection, and presence of crystalluria. All animals with UO should be monitored with electrocardiography, with close attention for bradyarrhythmias, tall T waves, and flattened (undetectable) P waves. The flattening of P waves may falsely be suggestive of a ventricular rhythm, but the clinician must be cognizant of the animal's hyperkalemic condition, and resist treating the animal with anti-arrhythmic medications that may result in death. A sinoventricular rhythm is not a ventricular arrhythmia but a sinus bradyarrhythmia associated with hyperkalemia. Additionally, it is not uncommon in some regions for cats to have concurrent lower urinary tract disease and hypertrophic cardiomyopathy. Therefore, as complete a physical examination as possible should be performed prior to sedation or anesthesia.

Following stabilization only, survey abdominal radiographs should be obtained for assessment of presence of radio-opaque urethral calculi.

MANAGEMENT / TREATMENT

The animal with UO should be considered a medical emergency and receive prompt attention. Intravenous access should be obtained via catheter placement. If possible, electrolytes should be analyzed immediately. Continuous ECG should be monitored. Relief of the obstruction should be achieved as soon as measures to stabilize the animal are accomplished. If dehydrated or hypovolemic, the animal should receive intravenous fluids. It is more beneficial to achieve fluid resuscitation than it is to deprive an unstable animal of fluids on the basis of inability to pass urine.

Sinus bradycardia, sinoventricular rhythm, or atrial standstill should be treated with intravenous calcium supplementation at 50–150 mg/kg IV slowly over 10–15 minutes, to counteract the effect of the hyperkalemia on heart rate and function. Moribund animals with severe bradycardia may, in addition, be administered atropine (0.1 ml/kg IV). Other therapies to treat hyperkalemia include regular insulin (0.1–0.25 U/kg IV, IM, or SC) and 50% dextrose (0.5 g/kg bolus followed by 2.5% CRI), and sodium bicarbonate (0.5 ml/kg IV of a 1 mmol/l [1 mEq/l] solution over 10 min). Calcium supplementation, however, will counter the hyperpolarizing effect of hyperkalemia, and should be administered prior to and above all others.

Attempts to stabilize the animal should be aggressive and timely. Once stabilization has been achieved, the animal should be sedated or anesthetized for passing of a urinary catheter to relieve the obstruction (125). The anesthetic plan will depend on the stability of the animal. Sedative combinations of an opioid/benzodiazepine are commonly used. Ketamine with diazepam may be used in cats without signs of concurrent heart disease. Intravenous propofol with or without intubation and gaseous anesthesia may be used in dogs and cats that are relatively stable.

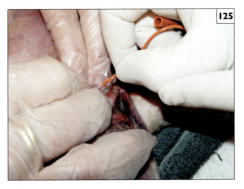

125 A cat affected with UO is sedated in order for the obstruction to be relieved. Sedation is required in all but moribund animals. Hyperkalemia is life-threatening and prompt recognition and treatment are required.

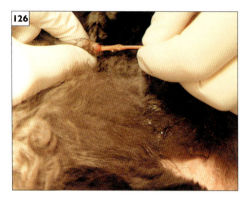

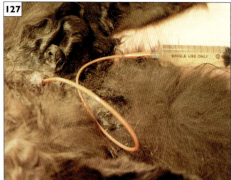

126 To relieve a urethral obstruction in a tom cat, the penis should be extruded and a tom cat catheter used with gentle but firm flushing. The stiff tom cat catheter may then be replaced by a softer red rubber catheter.

127 The catheter should be advanced until urine is freely flowing. The external end of the catheter is typically about 3/4 the length of the tail in cats with average length tails.

UO is relieved by passage of a lubricated urinary catheter (**126**, **127**). Retrohydropropulsion is often required to dislodge the obstruction, flushing it back into the bladder. Rarely, attempts to pass the urinary catheter are not successful, and cystocentesis has been advocated but is considered controversial. Due to the risk of contamination of the abdomen, cystocentesis is contraindicated if the bladder could have infection or neoplasia. Once successful passage of the urinary catheter has been accomplished, the bladder is emptied and a closed collection system is attached for urine output quantification. Many clinics that do not have 24- hour care will often disconnect urinary collection systems during nonsupervised hours allowing free passage of urine. In so doing, the risk of obstruction by twisting of lines is minimized. Post-obstructive diuresis can be significant, requiring large volumes of intravenous fluid to compensate for dehydration and to 'keep up' with ongoing loss. Crystalloids, including lactated Ringer's solution and 0.9% NaCl, are good choices. Once the obstruction has been relieved, and volume deficits have been corrected, potassium loss in the urine can be profound. Hence, it is often not necessary to limit intravenous fluid choices to those containing little or no potassium. If, however, volume deficits have not been met, hyperkalemia may persist until effective circulating volume is corrected enough to improve GFR. The obvious recommendation is to ensure volume deficits are met with appropriate intravenous fluid rates. Urine production in the post-obstructed animal should be high, and if the animal is not demonstrating polyuria, it is unlikely that volume deficits have been met.

Rarely, hemorrhagic cystitis may be severe enough to require transfusion of packed red blood cells. However, despite the bloody appearance of the urine, blood loss is seldom significant enough to result in clinical anemia. Unless pre-existing infection is known to exist, antibiotics are not routinely given. Medications designed to relax urethral sphincters and bladder spasms may be administered, but their use is not universally advocated. Further medical, dietary, or surgical therapy may be indicated on a per patient basis.

PROGNOSIS

Long-term survival for the animal with UO that receives appropriate follow-up therapy is excellent. Unless moribund upon presentation, prognosis for reversal of ARF due to UO is also good.

CHAPTER 8

Neurological emergencies

- **Seizures**

- **Traumatic brain injury**

- **Paralysis and paresis**

- **Vestibular syndrome**

- **Mental alteration**

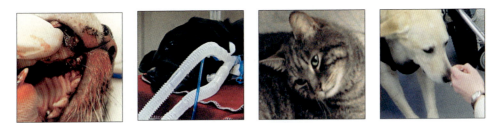

Neurological emergencies are common in small animal practice. As with other body systems, infections, neoplasms, trauma, inflammatory processes, and congenital and hereditary diseases all affect the central and peripheral nervous systems. Advanced forms of imaging provided by CT and MRI in veterinary medicine are allowing improved diagnostic plans and management options. The assessment, stabilization, and treatment of the neurological emergency, however, still rely on the ability of the emergency clinician to consider a complete history, perform a complete physical examination, and analyze readily available emergency test results. The following section provides an overview of common neurological emergencies: changes in mental alteration, seizures, paresis and paralysis, vestibular syndrome, and traumatic brain injury. Basic knowledge of neurological disease processes in animals allows the emergency clinician to consider a variety of differential diagnoses quickly and efficiently. Conditions such as hypovolemia, anemia, and those causing hypoxia, including pulmonary disease, airway obstruction or pleural space disease, can be manifest as mental alteration. Metabolic disorders, such as hypoglycemia or

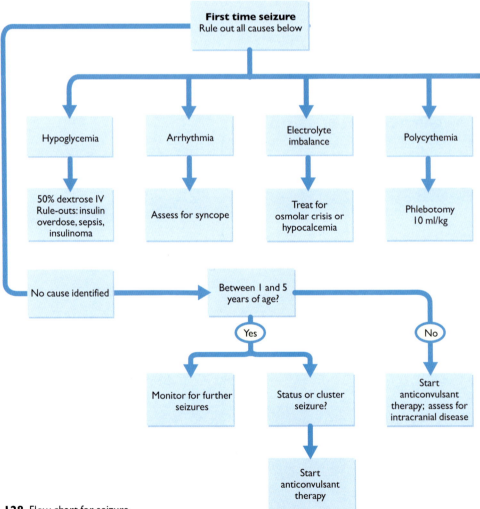

128 Flow chart for seizure.

electrolyte derangements, can cause seizures. Cardiovascular and metabolic instability must be recognized and corrected prior to neurological evaluation. Once satisfied that other underlying causes of central nervous signs have been ruled out, the clinician can consider a primary neurological disorder.

KEY POINTS
- Neurological abnormalities should be localized to help identify the underlying cause.
- Recent advances in diagnostic imaging have dramatically advanced veterinary neurology.
- Many neurological conditions respond well to therapy.

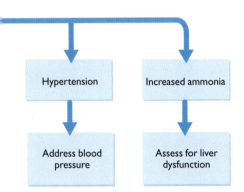

Seizures

KEY POINTS
- Signalment and history provide important information during the emergency presentation.
- Analysis of blood glucose, serum electrolytes, and hematocrit will identify a number of metabolic causes of seizures (**128**).
- Seizures are classified as generalized or partial.
- Seizures in animals <1 year or >5 years of age dictate further testing.
- Most seizures require long-term therapy.

DEFINITION / OVERVIEW
Seizures are the physical manifestation of an abnormal balance between excitatory and inhibitory tone in the central nervous system (CNS). Seizures are categorized as either generalized or partial (*Table 10*). Generalized seizures include those that have traditionally been described as convulsions or *grand mal* seizures. Partial seizures describe atypical behaviors, and are classified as simple partial or complex partial seizures. Generalized and partial seizures commonly require treatment, as both may represent potentially life-threatening conditions.

ETIOLOGY
The CNS relies on a balance of excitatory tone and inhibitory tone. Generally, excitatory tone is mediated by the neurotransmitter glutamate, and inhibitory tone is mediated by GABA. Depolarization of the cell membrane results with binding of glutamate to its receptors. Hyperpolarization of

---

Table 10 Categories of seizures

Generalized
Loss of consciousness
Tonic, clonic, or myoclonic activity

Partial
Unilateral, stereotypical, or bizarre behavior
- Simple partial: no loss of consciousness
- Complex partial: altered mentation or loss of consciousness

the cell membrane occurs when GABA binds to its receptors. Uncontrolled, perpetuated neuronal activity may derail normal mechanisms that act to prevent random excitation, resulting in seizures.

PATHOPHYSIOLOGY

Seizures may occur with a wide variety of conditions. These conditions are grouped according to those with intracranial causes, or *structural epileptic seizures* (SES), those with extracranial causes, or *reactive epileptic seizures* (RES), and idiopathic epilepsy, or *primary epileptic seizures* (PES) (*Table 11*). Although each of these categories should be considered in animals presenting with acute or recent onset of seizures, the age of the animal may suggest one group over another. Animals <1 year or >5 years of age are more commonly represented in the SES group. Recurrent SESs typically occur within 2–4 weeks of the acute onset (first seizure). Dogs aged 1–5 years are more likely to have PESs, and recurrent seizures may not recur for another 4–6 weeks or longer. Cats develop PESs uncommonly, and when they do so usually have a prior inciting cause, such as trauma or inflammation.

CLINICAL PRESENTATION

Generalized or *grand mal* seizures are characterized by loss of consciousness and bilateral muscle activity. Generalized seizures may have increased tone (tonic) and/or muscle flexation (clonic). Loss of autonomic tone is common, so the animal may vomit, urinate, or defecate. The generalized seizure is the most commonly *recognized* seizure in small animals.

Partial seizures are clinically manifest by unilateral, bizarre behavior and are commonly referred to as *focal* seizures. Animals with simple partial seizures remain alert and responsive, while those with complex seizures may have some loss or alteration in consciousness. The stereotypical behavior of the partial seizure is referable to the seizure's origin in a specific region of the brain, often the temporal or frontal lobe. Commonly recognized partial seizures include biting at imaginary flies, tail chasing, circling, ear or whisker twitching, head turning, or pupil dilation or constriction.

The seizure or ictal state can be followed by a post-ictal phase, during which the animal may seem confused, tired, pant, pace, and have visual impairment. A pre-ictal phase, if recognized, is commonly referred to as the aura. During the pre-ictal phase, the animal may seem confused or seek the attention of the owner. A partial seizure that progresses to a generalized seizure is also referred to as an aura.

A cluster of seizures is a series of isolated seizures lasting over minutes to days. Status epilepticus is a prolonged single seizure lasting >3 minutes without recovery. Status epilepticus can be life-threatening, resulting in brain anoxia and residual brain impairment or death.

Table 11 Seizure classification

Structural epileptic seizures (SES)

Common causes:
- Congenital: hydrocephalus
- Hereditary: lysosomal storage disease
- Neoplasia: primary or metastatic
- Infectious: viral (dog: rabies, canine distemper virus; cat: rabies, FIP), bacterial, tick-borne, fungal, protozoal, parasitic
- Inflammatory: Pug dog encephalitis, granulomatous meningoencephalitis, necrotizing encephalitis of Maltese and Yorkshire Terriers
- Trauma
- Vascular or thromboembolic

Reactive epileptic seizures (RES)

Common causes:
- Hypoglycemia
- Hyperammonemia
- Toxin
- Electrolyte derangement (hypernatremia, hyponatremia, hypocalcemia)
- Hypertension
- Polycythemia
- Coagulopathy

Primary epileptic seizures (PES)

(No known cause)
- Common age: >1 year but <5 years of age
- Common breeds: Poodle, Beagle, German Shepherd dog, Retrievers

DIFFERENTIAL DIAGNOSES

Syncope from AV block or sick sinus syndrome may mimic a seizure. Electrocardiogram (ECG) analysis is warranted in any patient with a slow heart rate or with signs that develop on exertion or with excitement.

DIAGNOSIS

Diagnosis of seizures is usually made on the basis of physical examination and historical description of the event. The history that commonly accompanies seizure is a period of abnormal behavior that was preceded and then followed by normal behavior. A major differential to consider is syncope, and a definitive diagnosis can be determined on the basis of the ECG. If the ECG is unremarkable, and the history and physical examination are consistent with seizure, treatment can be administered based on index of suspicion.

The diagnostic plan for seizures is summarized in *Table 12*. Signalment and history are major components of diagnosis. All animals with acute onset or recurrent seizures should have minimum database including CBC, serum chemistry analysis, and urinalysis. Animals <1 year of age with acute or recurrent seizures should be considered for congenital and hereditary diseases. Animals >5 years of age should be considered for neoplasia. Brain imaging with MRI or CT is indicated for animals <1 year or >5 years of age. Cerebrospinal fluid (CSF) analysis may be required to rule out inflammatory, infectious or neoplastic conditions. Due to the increased risk of brain herniation with elevations in intracranial pressure, obtaining CSF should ideally be performed following imaging.

Animals of all ages can be affected by inflammatory diseases, including infections due to viral, bacterial, tick-borne disease, protozoal, fungal, and parasitic diseases. Sterile inflammations are more common in specific breeds, including Pug dog encephalitis, necrotizing encephalitis of Maltese and Yorkshire Terriers, or granulomatous meningoencephalitis, but any breed and any age can be affected. Rabies should be considered in any animal with uncertain vaccination status, or a wound of unknown origin.

Table 12 Diagnostic plan for seizures

1 Minimum database: CBC, serum chemistry analysis, urinalysis
2 Blood pressure measurement
3 Diagnostic imaging: brain MRI or CT, thoracic and abdominal radiography
4 CSF: analysis, culture, titers
5 Serum: titers

Animals of all ages should also be considered for extracranial causes of seizure, including hypoglycemia, hyperammonemia, coagulopathy, toxin, hyperosmolality, electrolyte derangements, or polycythemia. Hyperviscosity, due to profound leukocytosis, polycythemia or hyperglobulinemia, can cause seizure. Young animals suspected for portocaval shunts should be assessed for blood ammonia and bile acids. Animals with portocaval shunts may present with urinary obstruction with ammonium biurate calculi. The presence of petechiae or ecchymoses should prompt assessment of platelets. Retinal examination should always be performed. Assessment of blood pressure should be carried out in all animals with recent onset of seizures. Assessment of the thorax and abdomen with survey radiography or ultrasonography for neoplasms should be performed in older animals. A common cause of seizures in cats is hypoglycemia from insulin overdose. However, any older cat (>10 years of age) should be suspected of primary brain neoplasia, such as meningioma. Outdoor cats in summer and fall may suffer ischemic events from aberrantly migrating larvae. Toxicities such as pyrethrins in cats, mycotoxin (compost or garbage) in dogs, and ethylene glycol in all animals are commonly associated with seizures. Hypocalcemic tetany should be considered in nursing animals.

MANAGEMENT / TREATMENT

Stabilization and emergency treatment typically involve the use of anti-epileptic medications but successful seizure control may depend on the underlying cause of the seizure. Rapid assessment of the clinical signs, history, signalment, and available test results, including blood glucose, hematocrit, electrolytes, and blood pressure, is essential. Intravenous access should be established and maintained for continued anti-epileptic medication administration. Animals with PES and occasional isolated seizures once every 4–6 months may be left untreated, but any animal presenting with ongoing seizure, seizure clusters, or status epilepticus should be treated and managed with long-term anti-epileptic therapy. *Table 13* summarizes the treatment of seizures.

Intravenous anti-epileptic medications that quickly cross the blood–brain barrier are the foundation of emergency seizure control. These include the benzodiazepines, such as diazepam (Valium) at 0.2 mg/kg as an intravenous bolus. This dose can be repeated up to four times. Pentobarbital is a fast-acting barbiturate that causes anesthesia, although its anti-epileptic control is controversial. Phenobarbital is the standard anti-epileptic treatment, and can be administered according to a loading dose protocol. Phenobarbital is not as quick-acting as diazepam or pentobarbital, however, and should be used in place of these options for the emergency control of ongoing seizure only when diazepam is unavailable. Propofol has been used as both an intravenous bolus or administered as a CRI. An additional advantage of the short-acting medications propofol and pentobarbital is their rapid clearance, allowing for a quicker recovery from sedative effects.

Anti-epileptic management producing profound sedation should be accompanied by close monitoring, including continuous ECG and pulse oximetry. Particularly when the cause of seizure has not yet been determined, the sedated neurological patient should be managed with adequate intravenous fluid therapy and maintenance of a patent airway, sometimes requiring intubation and manual ventilation. Efforts to limit aspiration during anesthesia as a means to control seizures should be paramount.

Identified causes of seizures should be addressed:

- Animals with suspected intracranial lesions should be administered mannitol (0.25–2 g/kg IV slowly over 20 min, and this can be repeated once if signs progress). Animals should be assessed to be cardiovascularly stable prior to mannitol administration.
- If a brain tumor or hydrocephalus is considered likely, rapidly acting corticosteroid therapy should also be given (prednisolone sodium succinate (Soludelta Cortef) 20 mg/kg IV slowly over 20 min).
- Hypoglycemia should be treated with dextrose infusions.
- Hypocalcemia should be treated with calcium supplementation.
- Polycythemia should be treated with phlebotomy.

Table 13 Treatment of seizures

For control of repeated seizure or status epilepticus:

Obtain venous access

Diazepam (0.2 mg/kg bolus IV up to four doses)

Propofol (4 mg/kg bolus IV or CRI)

Supportive management (intravenous fluids, supplemental oxygen)

Identify and treat any underlying cause:

Hypoglycemia

Electrolyte disorders

Toxin

Polycythemia

Encephalopathy

Hypertension

For presumptive intracranial mass lesion:

Mannitol (0.5–2 g/kg bolus IV)

Corticosteroids

Long-term anti-epileptic treatment:

Phenobarbital (2.2 mg/kg q12hr)

Potassium bromide (25–50 mg/kg q24hr)

- Hepatic encephalopathy should be cautiously treated with oral medications to reduce blood ammonia only if the animal is awake and appropriate to prevent aspiration. Rapidly progressive encephalopathy due to hyperammonemia should be treated with intravenous mannitol and enemas with lactulose or betadine.
- Traumatic brain injury should be treated with supportive therapies, including fluid resuscitation, with the treatment objective being maintenance of systemic mean arterial blood pressure and adequate oxygenation. Rarely, an animal may require surgical intervention for brain injury that results from depressed skull fractures or subdural hematoma.
- Hypertension at levels >200 mmHg systolic pressure should be treated with oral antihypertensive agents, such as amlodipine, enalapril, or prasozin, or intravenous agents, including hydralazine or sodium nitroprusside.
- Cats with pyrethrin exposure usually respond to intravenous boluses of methocarbamol, diazepam, or propofol.
- Dogs with mycotoxin ingestion usually respond to intravenous therapies, including fluids and diazepam, but may require gastric evacuation and lavage in extreme cases.
- Ethylene glycol toxicity is best treated with dialysis to remove toxin and metabolites of the toxin. Administration of fomepazole or ethanol and aggressive intravenous diuresis may help prevent progression to ARF. However, once ARF occurs, prognosis for recovery is poor.
- Animals with undetermined vaccination status should be considered for rabies, and appropriate measures observed to prevent unvaccinated personnel from potential exposure.

PROGNOSIS

Prognosis depends on the underlying cause for the seizure. Animals with PES typically have excellent long-term prognosis with seizure control. Animals with RES usually have good prognosis for seizure control once the underlying cause has been identified and corrected. Animals with SES have a fair to guarded prognosis, depending on whether the underlying brain disease can be treated.

Traumatic brain injury

KEY POINTS
- The animal with traumatic brain injury should be considered a critical emergency.
- In addition to the consequences of the primary brain injury, the animal can continue to suffer further brain injury if interventions to maintain systemic mean arterial blood pressure and oxygenation are not initiated.
- Prognosis can be estimated by assessment of clinical signs according to the modified Glasgow Coma Scale.
- Outcome relies on appropriate medical and surgical interventions, and provision of nursing care.

DEFINITION / OVERVIEW

Animals can suffer brain injury as a result of traumatic head injury (129) when they are kicked, stepped on, struck by moving automobiles, shot, or attacked by other animals. Primary brain injury describes the initial insult to the brain, and usually includes an area of hemorrhage or edema resulting in cellular hypoxia. Secondary brain injury occurs after the initial event and affects an area surrounding or adjacent to the area of primary injury. The goal of management of traumatic brain injury is to provide measures that will prevent progression of primary brain injury to secondary brain injury.

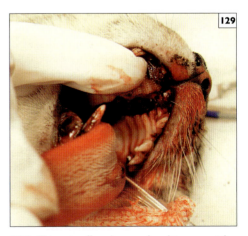

129 This cat suffered severe head trauma, with a split hard palate. Brain injury is always a possible complication of skull fracture.

ETIOLOGY

Primary brain injury involves direct parenchymal brain damage that has been inflicted by blunt forces resulting in contusion, or lacerations resulting from shearing skull fractures. Intracranial hemorrhage producing subdural or epidural hematoma can result in increased intracranial pressure. Subdural or epidural hematomas may increase intracranial pressure as a mass lesion, with adjacent vasogenic edema resulting in cerebral edema. Without surgical decompression, the animal will continue to deteriorate neurologically. Intraparenchymal brain injury, on the other hand, resulting from hemorrhage or edema, results in an area of cellular hypoxia and neuronal death. As hemorrhage, swelling and hypoxia extend from this initial area of injury, increased numbers of neurons are affected. The initial, or primary, injury occurs quickly. The extension of injury, or secondary injury, follows the initial injury and may continue to spread without prompt medical intervention.

PATHOPHYSIOLOGY

Secondary brain injury occurs as a result of the initial primary process and extends into tissue surrounding the damaged area. Hypoxia is the driving force of continued injury within this adjacent brain tissue described as the penumbra, resulting in depletion of cellular ATP. The depletion of ATP leads to membrane pump dysfunction, and increased intracellular sodium and potassium concentrations. Glutamate is the predominant excitatory neurotransmitter in the CNS. Due to limited energy supplies, clearance of extracellular glutamate decreases and glutamate concentration rises dramatically. Binding of glutamate leads to activation of specific cellular receptors, which results in continued cellular calcium and sodium influx. This massive ionic influx causes depolarization of neurons, and, combined with activation of the second messenger system, produces increased intracellular calcium accumulation. The inability of the nerve cells to maintain electrolyte homeostasis results in cytotoxic brain edema. Cytokines and mediators of inflammation initiate further cellular interactions that continue inflammation and derangement of coagulation. As intracranial pressure increases, cerebral perfusion decreases, preventing adequate oxygenation to brain cells within the penumbra. Elevations of $PaCO_2$ cause local vasodilation, which further exacerbates increases in intracranial pressure. Physiological response to these events results in signals to increase systemic arterial blood pressure. The hypertension is quickly recognized, and produces a parasympathetic response to slow the heart rate (Cushing's reflex). This so-called 'inappropriate' bradycardia is a sign of progressive and life-threatening increased intracranial pressure. Without prompt intervention, cerebral edema will progress and result in coma and death.

CLINICAL PRESENTATION

Clinical features (Table 14) will vary depending on the location of injury. Abnormalities may include changes in mental awareness, such as dullness, obtundation, or coma. Generalized or partial seizures may be transient or may result in residual epilepsy. Injury to the brainstem may result in dullness, cranial nerve deficits, and vestibular or cerebellar signs.

Visual impairment may be permanent or transient. Injury to the pituitary gland, due to skull fractures, can result in a variety of neuroendocrine disorders and diabetes insipidus. Progressive, untreated, increased intracranial pressure eventually leads to brain herniation. Signs of increased intracranial pressure and impending brain herniation include:

- Apnea, cranial nerve deficits, and miotic pupils with brainstem herniation.
- Dilated and unresponsive pupils with midbrain herniation.

Inappropriate bradycardia signifies progressive increased intracranial pressure.

Table 14 Common signs of traumatic brain injury

Mental alteration: dullness, obtundation, coma

Paresis

Seizures: generalized or partial

Vestibular signs: head tilt, torticollis, strabismus, nystagmus

Cerebellar signs: intention tremors

Miosis or mydriasis

Apnea

Bradycardia

DIAGNOSIS

Animals with traumatic brain injury should be considered as critical, and tests should be obtained and performed to ensure proper care is provided (*Table 15*). Minimum database includes CBC, serum chemistry analysis, and urinalysis. Serial monitoring of hematocrit, electrolytes, and coagulation parameters is essential. Imaging of the head and brain with CT may be indicated in extreme cases or with progression of CNS signs. A complete assessment of the animal should be undertaken, identifying concurrent thoracic, abdominal, spinal, or skeletal trauma, and serial neurological examinations performed.

MANAGEMENT / TREATMENT

The foundation of management for animals suffering brain injury secondary to head trauma includes maintenance of adequate systemic arterial blood pressure, oxygenation, and nursing care (*Table 16*). Without signs of increasing intracranial pressure, administration of intravenous fluids, pain management, nutrition, comfortable bedding, and physical therapy are probably sufficient to meet the needs of the animal. Seizures should be treated with anti-epileptic therapy, but anti-epileptic prophylactic administration in the absence of seizures is not recommended. Severe brain injury not resulting in increased intracranial pressure may require 7–15 days of hospitalization, and then months of nursing care at home for recovery.

Animals with signs of increased intracranial pressure should undergo imaging of the brain and head. Depressed skull fractures and subdural or epidural hematomas are emergencies that require surgical decompression. Measures to manage increased intracranial pressure include mannitol (0.25–2 g/kg IV over 20 min, repeated twice if no response), and intubation and mechanical ventilation to maintain $PaCO_2$ between 30 mmHg and 35 mmHg. Caution is advised with therapies that may potentially increase venous pressure, such as jugular intravenous catheters and elective intubation.

Intravenous fluid therapy should be based on the needs of the animal to maintain normal systemic arterial blood pressure. Hematocrit, serum electrolytes, and coagulation parameters should be monitored as needed to provide interventions to maintain a stable animal. Limiting fluid administration as a means of decreasing cerebral edema is not effective and is not advised.

Table 15 Tests for cases of traumatic brain injury

Minimum database: CBC, serum chemistry analysis, and urinalysis

CT or MRI of head and brain

Table 16 Management of traumatic brain injury

Maintenance of systemic arterial blood pressure

Maintenance of oxygenation

Seizure control

Nursing care

Nutrition

If indicated, surgical decompression of depressed skull fractures, and subdural and epidural hematomas

If signs of increased intracranial pressure, intravenous mannitol and mechanical ventilation

Supplemental oxygen should be provided to maintain adequate oxygen saturation. Antibiotics should be administered in the presence of wounds or with evidence of aspiration pneumonia. Parenteral nutrition may be necessary if the animal has skull fractures limiting food intake, or persistent mental alteration causing inappetence.

The administration of glucocorticoids for traumatic brain injury has been shown to have no proven efficacy, and use in humans has been associated with worsened outcome. The use of glucocorticoids is not advised for animals with traumatic brain injury. Thus, caution is advised in their use for facial swelling associated with trauma with concurrent CNS signs.

PROGNOSIS

Emergency clinicians are encouraged to evaluate the animal with traumatic head injury and document the findings according to the criteria of the modified Glasgow Coma Scale (*Table 17*). Prognosis relies on severity of signs at the time of trauma, and would be further influenced by deterioration in condition.

Table 17 Modified Glasgow Coma Scale	
Motor activity	
Normal gait, normal spinal reflexes	6
Hemiparesis, tetraparesis, or decerebrate activity	5
Recumbent, intermittent extensor rigidity	4
Recumbent, constant extensor rigidity	3
Recumbent, constant extensor rigidity with opisthotonus	2
Recumbent, hypotonia of muscles, depressed or absent spinal reflexes	1
Brain stem reflexes	
Normal pupillary light reflexes and oculocephalic reflexes	6
Slow pupillary light reflexes and normal to reduced oculocephalic reflexes	5
Bilateral unresponsive miosis with normal to reduced oculocephalic reflexes	4
Pinpoint pupils with reduced to absent oculocephalic reflexes	3
Unilateral unresponsive mydrisasis with reduced to absent oculocephalic reflexes	2
Bilateral unresponsive mydriasis with reduced to absent oculocephalic reflexes	1
Level of consciousness	
Occasional periods of alertness, responsive to environment	6
Depression or delirium, capable of responding to environment but response may be inappropriate	5
Stupor, responsive to visual stimuli	4
Stupor, responsive to auditory stimuli	3
Stupor, responsive only to repeated noxious stimuli	2
Coma, unresponsive to repeated noxious stimuli	1
	Total
Assessment	
Good prognosis	15–18
Guarded prognosis	9–14
Grave prognosis	3–8

Paralysis and paresis

KEY POINTS

- Diagnosis and prognosis for paresis and paralysis rely on history, signalment, lesion localization, severity of signs, and response to therapy.
- Dogs with suspected intervertebral disk disease with decreased or absent voluntary motor function should be referred *urgently* to a facility with diagnostic imaging (e.g. myelography, CT, MRI) and emergency surgical capabilities.
- Other causes for severe weakness such as collapse, including shock, anemia, sepsis, heart failure, and toxicities, should be ruled out prior to diagnosis of paralysis or paresis.

DEFINITION / OVERVIEW

Paralysis denotes a loss of voluntary motor function due to spinal cord or peripheral nerve disease. Paresis represents retention of voluntary motor function despite measurable conscious proprioceptive deficits. Paresis, like paralysis, is caused by defects in the spinal cord, or in the motor nerves as they exit the spinal cord. Plegia describes the loss of voluntary motor function in a single limb. Plegia and paresis are diagnoses based on findings from a complete physical examination. Weakness, lethargy, and lameness should be ruled out, and a neurological examination should be performed prior to the diagnosis of paralysis or paresis.

ETIOLOGY

The common causes of paresis and paralysis are summarized in *Table 18*. Injury to the spinal cord can arise as the result of an external force causing compression and subsequent edema, or from an intradural, parenchymal lesion. Intervertebral disk disease can occur chronically or acutely, and is a common cause of extradural spinal cord compression. Tumors and inflammatory lesions are less common causes, as are traumatic fractures or luxations. Tumors can occur in the intradural, extramedullary, or intramedullary space. Other intraparenchymal lesions include inflammatory lesions, embolism, and vascular accidents.

Peripheral nerve disease or neuromuscular disease can result from inflammatory or neoplastic lesions, or trauma. A common cause of a traumatic neuropathy is the brachial plexus avulsion injury. Generalized lower motor neuron

Table 18 Common causes of paralysis or paresis in small animals

Intervertebral disk disease

Neoplasia

Vascular or embolic events (FCE)

Inflammatory or infectious

Trauma

Peripheral neuropathy (myelinopathy, axonopathy, radiculoneuritis)

Neuromuscular disease

disease should be considered with diffuse loss of tone and spinal reflexes. Electromyography (EMG) is used to identify and classify neuromuscular dysfunction (**130**). Common clinical signs of neuromuscular disease include gas distension of the esophagus, bark change, loss of cranial nerve reflexes, and laryngeal/pharyngeal weakness. Some common neuromuscular disorders include myasthenia gravis, polyradiculoneuritis ('coonhound paralysis'), botulism, organophosphate toxicity, thyroid dysfunction, and adrenocortical deficiency.

CLINICAL PRESENTATION

A neurological examination will provide important information for localization of a lesion.

Animals with altered mentation, tendencies to pace or circle, cranial nerve deficits, or recent onset of seizures may have paresis. Unless comatose or severely obtunded, paralysis would be an unlikely finding in an animal with intracranial disease. Extensor tone and ability to withdraw should be assessed for each limb. A high cervical (C1–C5) lesion should produce convincing, increased tone and reflexia to all limbs. A low cervical–high thoracic (C6–T2) lesion should result in weak withdrawal (flaccid) of the thoracic limbs, but strong withdrawal of the pelvic limbs. A thoracolumbar (T3–L3) lesion will result in increased tone and reflexia of the pelvic limbs, and unaffected thoracic limbs (**131**). With Schiff–Sherington signs, however, the thoracic limbs will demonstrate excessive extensor tone. Lower lumbar (L4–L6) lesions will produce weak extensor tone and reflexia of the pelvic limbs. Lumbosacral disease may produce weak tail and anal tone. Bladder tone may be increased with pelvic limb paralysis or tetraplegia. Weak bladder tone is common with flaccid paralysis. A lack of tone diffusely in all limbs suggests peripheral nerve (lower motor neuron) disease, or neuromuscular disease. Urine leakage is suggestive of bladder atony or flaccid paralysis, but may be present with upper motor neuron disease and an overflow phenomenon. Despite the presence of urine production, the bladder with upper motor neuron disease is inexpressible, and anal and tail tone are likely to be normal.

DIAGNOSIS

Orthopedic injury due to trauma should be considered in animals with acute onset of signs. Arterial thrombosis should be considered in the absence of palpable pulses to the affected limbs, especially with concurrent cold distal extremities

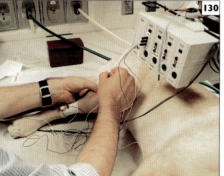

130 EMG may be used to better highlight neuromuscular dysfunction.

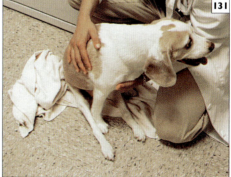

131 This beagle is sitting with the characteristic posture of a dog with a T3–L3 lesion. This dog had a spinal tumor.

and nail base cyanosis. Prior to performing a neurological examination, the animal should be stabilized, with normal or improved cardiovascular and respiratory status.

A neurological examination should assess mentation and cranial nerve and spinal reflexes. Ideally, the examination should be performed prior to the administration of sedation or anesthesia. Localization of the lesion based on examination is essential for continued diagnostic testing, and may help in determination of a prognosis.

History, in addition to examination, is essential in establishing differential diagnoses. A chronic, progressive history is more suggestive of a compressive lesion. Compressive lesions are more likely to cause bilateral signs, such as pelvic limb paraparesis or paralysis. Acute onset of signs can also be caused by a compressive lesion, however embolic or vascular accident, and trauma should be considered as well.

Signalment should be considered. Chondrodystrophic breeds, for example, may more commonly present with intervertebral disk disease. Young dogs should be considered for congenital problems, including occipital-atlanto or atlanto-axial instabilities and defects of the dens. Young Great Danes or middle-aged Doberman Pinschers should be suspected of cervical vertebral instability ('wobbler' disease).

Spinal cord disease is uncommon in cats so pelvic trauma or aortic thromboembolism should be considered. Less commonly, the cat can be affected by spinal cord tumors, including lymphosarcoma, spinal trauma, and infectious disease (FIP, fungal disease, toxoplasmosis).

Rabies should be considered in any animal with unkown vaccination status, and particularly if a wound of unknown origin is identified.

Intradural causes of spinal cord disease or injury should be suspected in animals with acute onset of signs and lack of discomfort. Vascular accidents should be considered in any young animal. Inherited or acquired coagulopathy can present with acute spinal cord hemorrhage. Spontaneous hemorrhage can also occur with severe thrombocytopenias, or neoplastic metastases. Embolism of disk material, known as fibrocartlilagenous embolism, is a common cause of acute plegia or paresis. In rare cases, the embolism may cause concurrent vascular injury and leakage of blood into the extradural space, resulting in compression. Acute traumatic disk extrusions can occur with trauma, such as road traffic accidents.

Accurate diagnosis of paralysis or paresis relies on history and physical examination. Minimum database including CBC, serum chemistry, and urinalysis may provide important information suggesting the presence of underlying diseases, such as infection or neoplasia. Evaluation of clotting by assessing platelet count, prothrombin time (PT), activated partial thromboplastin time (aPTT), and buccal mucosal bleeding time (BMBT) may identify clotting factor deficiency or bleeding disorders.

Survey spinal radiography should be obtained in any animal with known or likely trauma. Survey thoracic radiography, in addition to spinal radiographs, should be assessed for lytic or metastatic lesions. Imaging of the spinal cord with contrast myelography, CT, or MRI is the standard for diagnosis of spinal cord disease. Contrast myelography is useful in providing definitive localization of compressive lesions. Some intradural lesions can be identified as well. CT and MRI may provide improved imaging of both intraparenchymal and extraparenchymal lesions.

Further information may be gained with analysis of CSF. Injection of contrast for imaging should be performed only following fluid inspection in cases with suspected infection.

Assessment with EMG, nerve conduction testing, and evaluation for thyroid disease and hypoadrenocorticism should be considered in animals with nontraumatic peripheral neuromuscular disease. If myasthenia gravis is suspected, an edrophonium response test should be performed, in addition to thoracic imaging with survey radiography or CT to exclude thymoma. Histopathology of peripheral nerve and muscle may be required for definitive diagnosis of neuromuscular disease.

MANAGEMENT / TREATMENT

Cardiovascular and pulmonary compromise should be stabilized prior to assessment of, or therapies for, paralysis or paresis. Animals with high cervical lesions and lower motor neuron diseases may be hypoventilatory and require immediate intubation and manual ventilation (132). Once stabilized, treatment should be aimed at the most highly suspected cause for the animal's signs.

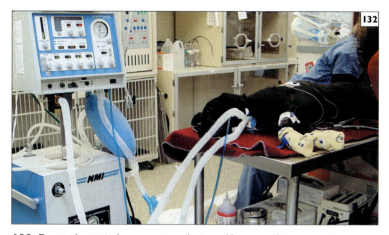

132 Dog with cervical trauma, tetraplegia, and hypoventilation requiring mechanical ventilation.

A surgeon should be consulted for animals suspected of spinal trauma or compressive spinal cord lesions. Prognosis for return of function relies in part on the ability of the animal to display deep pain of the affected limbs, and in part on the length of time the animal has been affected. A course of physiotherapy may be required (**133**). Generally, paralysis due to spinal cord compression is best treated with surgical decompression. The use of nonsteroidal and corticosteroid medications has been widely accepted, although their usefulness remains controversial. Protocols for the use of intravenous high-dose methylprednisolone sodium succinate (Solumedrol, 30 mg/kg over 20 min at time 0, followed by 15 mg/kg over 10 min at 2 and 4 hours) and prednisolone sodium succinate (Soludelta Cortef, 20 mg/kg over 10–20 min) are well described, and have been indicated for the perioperative period. Caution is advised with the use of dexamethasone, which may cause colonic ulceration and perforation.

Animals diagnosed with lower motor neuron disease may need long-term care, including intravenous fluid therapies and mechanical ventilation. If thymoma is present, thymectomy is recommended following stabilization of the animal.

If megaesophagus is present, vigilant measures to prevent aspiration pneumonia are advised. Clotting factor deficiencies should be corrected with blood product transfusions and vitamin K_1 if applicable. Animals with severe thrombocytopenia should be assessed for immune-mediated disease and treated with immunosuppressive therapies, including corticosteroids and azathioprine. The emergency clinician should work closely with the neurologist and surgeon for continued management and diagnostic plans.

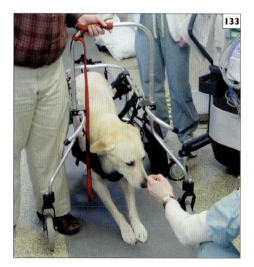

133 A Labrador Retriever undergoing physical therapy during recovery from a traumatic back fracture.

Vestibular syndrome

KEY POINTS

- Vestibular syndrome is a common cause of neurological emergency presentations.
- Vestibular signs should be localized to the peripheral nervous system or CNS.
- Peripheral vestibular syndrome commonly resolves over 15 days.
- Central vestibular syndrome is sometimes static, but usually progresses.
- Animals with vestibular syndrome require supportive therapy and nursing care for optimal recovery.

DEFINITION / OVERVIEW

Vestibular syndrome is manifested principally as a loss of balance and an inability of the animal to correct its orientation. Mildly affected animals may demonstrate head tilt, abnormal eye position, irregular eye movement, and ataxia. Severely affected animals may develop debilitating disease due to an inability to stand or regain orientation, or take adequate nutrition and maintain hydration.

134 Cat with central vestibular syndrome secondary to cerebellar infarction.

ETIOLOGY

Vestibular syndrome results from disease affecting either the peripheral nervous system (PVD) or central nervous system (CVD) (see *Table 19*). PVD involves the vestibular portion of the eighth cranial nerve or the vestibular receptor located within the petrous temporal bone. CVD (**134**) involves the vestibular nuclei, located on the floor of the fourth ventricle, the brainstem on either side of the medulla oblongata, or the cerebellum. PVD is typically less severe than CVD and signs often spontaneously resolve, while CVD is typically progressive and carries a poorer prognosis.

Lesions affecting the vestibular system peripherally include inflammatory conditions, such as infections of the ear or bulla, neoplastic diseases that either arise from the nervous system, such as nerve sheath tumors, or that are locally invasive, such as carcinomas or lymphosarcoma.

Viral or noninfectious inflammatory diseases are commonly suspected of causing self-limiting PVD. Similar processes are likely to affect the brain, causing CVD. Some inflammatory or infectious causes respond to immunosuppressive and antibiotic therapies. Examples are granulomatous meningoencephalitis, tick-borne diseases, including rickettsial, ehrlichial, and anaplasma infections, or protozoal infection, including *Toxoplasma* and *Neospora*. Feline infectious peritonitis is a common cause of CVD in cats and is often progressive and fatal. Rabies should be considered in any animal with uncertain vaccination status or the presence of a wound of unknown origin.

Table 19 Common causes of vestibular syndrome

Peripheral vestibular disease (PVD)

Otitis media–interna

Head trauma

Geriatric vestibular syndrome (dog)

Idiopathic feline vestibular syndrome

Drug toxicity (metronidazole, aminoglycosides)

Mass lesions (neoplasia, inflammatory polyps in cats)

Central vestibular disease (CVD)

Neoplasia

Vascular accident (hypertension, coagulopathy)

Head trauma

Infection (viral, bacterial, fungal, protozoal, tick-borne, parasitic)

Inflammatory (granulomatous meningoencephalitis)

Primary or metastatic neoplastic lesions produce progressive central vestibular signs, whereas vascular or thromboembolic lesions will not progress and may even improve. Aberrant migration of the larva of the *Cuterebra* fly may cause acute onset of vestibular signs in the cat during the late summer and early fall. Occasionally, brain abscess can be caused by infection extending from the ear, or via bacterial embolism with bacteremia. Signs of both PVD and CVD have been reported with toxicities of various drugs, such as metronidazole. Traumatic head injury may cause hemorrhage or swelling in the area of the brainstem and cause signs which may resolve or remain residual. Inflammatory polyps may invade the auditory canal in cats, and ought to be considered as a leading differential diagnosis in any young cat or kitten with peripheral vestibular signs.

CLINICAL PRESENTATION

A primary goal in assessing clinical signs in the vestibular animal is to localize the cause to either the peripheral nervous system or CNS (*Table 20*). Animals with PVD often recover, with signs resolving over 15 days, whereas the prognosis for animals with CVD is poor, often with signs progressing to the point where the animal cannot function without nursing care.

Most animals with vestibular syndrome will demonstrate head tilt and ipsilateral falling or inability to regain balance. More severe cases may roll or circle tightly to that side. Extensor tone of the contralateral limbs and decreased tone in the ipsilateral limbs are usually present. Acutely, abnormal eye movements (nystagmus) are apparent, and normal physiological nystagmus may be depressed or absent. Ventrolateral deviation of the ipsilateral eye can be accentuated with extension of the head. Generally, vertical, rotary, or horizontal nystagmus can be present with CVD, but vertical nystagmus is exceedingly rare with PVD. Typically, PVD is characterized by horizontal nystagmus with the fast phase directed away from the direction of the head tilt. Thus, determination of head tilt and direction of horizontal nystagmus distinguishes the diagnosis of PVD, and additionally localizes the lesion to the side of the head tilt. Rarely, head tilt and horizontal nystagmus are opposite to that which would be expected with PVD. This finding is typical of parodoxical vestibular syndrome, and is highly suggestive of a lesion in the cerebellar

peduncle (CVD). PVD that is associated with otitis media–interna is often associated with Horner's syndrome and facial nerve paralysis. Decreased or absent sensation of the cornea represents trigeminal nerve involvement and is suggestive of CVD, along with changes in mentation, cerebellar signs, including intention tremors or spasticity, and ipsilateral paresis. Animals with vestibular signs and deficits involving the trigeminal and facial nerves invariably have CVD caused by a lesion in the cerebellomedullary pontine angle. Hence, assessment of the complete neurological examination is essential to the diagnosis of vestibular syndrome.

Vomiting is common with onset of vestibular signs. Inappetence or anorexia may be difficult to distinguish from inability to take food and water. Inflammatory lesions due to infections may be accompanied by fever or hypothermia. Septic embolism to the brain, resulting in vestibular syndromes, has been seen in animals with bacterial endocarditis, liver disease and portocaval shunting.

Table 20 Clinical signs of vestibular syndrome

Clinical sign	PVD	CVD
Head tilt	Yes	Yes
Loss of balance	Yes	Yes
Cranial nerve deficits	Possibly VII	Possibly V, VI, and VII
Ventrolateral strabismus	Yes	Yes
Horner's syndrome	Possible	No
Positional nystagmus	No	Yes
Spontaneous nystagmus	Horizontal or rotary	Vertical, horizontal, or rotary
Conscious proprioceptive deficits (ipsilateral)	No	Yes
Abnormal postural reactions	No	Yes
Cerebellar signs	No	Possible
Mental depression	No	Possible

DIAGNOSIS

A minimum database including CBC, serum chemistry analysis, and urinalysis should be obtained in all animals (*Table 21*). A complete physical examination in addition to the neurological examination should include retinal and otoscopic examinations. Blood pressure should be assessed in all animals with neurological signs. Culture of fluid from abnormal ears should be submitted.

Imaging of the brain and skull should be considered in all animals with vestibular signs unless the diagnosis of drug-induced or middle ear infection is obvious and the animal is responding to treatment (removal of the drug or administration of appropriate antibiotic therapy). Survey radiographs of the skull may confirm fluid density in the bullae. Advanced imaging of the brain and skull with CT or MRI will assist diagnosis in identifying neoplastic, traumatic, or inflammatory lesions and should be obtained if these tests are available to the clinician.

A retinal examination may identify signs of hypertension, hemorrhage, anemia, neoplasia, or infectious disease. CSF should be obtained if indicated for analysis, culture, or titers. If indicated, titers should be obtained from serum, whole blood, or aqueous fluid. Myringotomy or bulla osteotomy should be considered if inner/middle ear infection is suspected, and signs are not responding to broad-spectrum antibiotic therapy. Survey thoracic radiographs should be evaluated for signs of infectious and neoplastic disease.

TREATMENT

Although mild cases of PVD in both dogs and cats are self-limiting and will resolve, many animals will require hospitalization for supportive care. Severe cases should be hospitalized for intravenous fluids and nursing care. Commonly, animals will be vomiting or unable to take enough food or water to maintain adequate nutrition and hydration. Animals with difficulty standing will need assistance for urination and defecation, and some larger dogs may benefit from the placement of an indwelling urinary catheter. Bedding should be soft and comfortable, providing protection from trauma caused by uncontrolled spinning and reducing development of pressure wounds.

Table 21 Diagnostic testing for vestibular syndrome

Minimum database: CBC, serum chemistry analysis, urinalysis

CT, MRI, skull radiographs

CSF analysis

Serology and culture of CSF and blood

Survey thoracic radiographs

Animals with concurrent cranial nerve deficits causing an inability to blink or feel the cornea should have topical ophthalmic management to prevent development of corneal ulceration. Development of corneal ulceration can progress rapidly to perforation, requiring surgical treatment or even enucleation.

Anxiety associated with the animal's inability to maintain balance may respond to intravenous boluses of diazepam, and nausea may respond to antihistamines such as diphenhydramine. Maintaining ability to assess changing mental status in the neurological animal is essential, and caution in using therapies that cause sedation is advised. Intravenous antibiotic therapy based on culture and/or titer results, or pending test results but based on index of suspicion is recommended. Some aseptic inflammatory processes will respond to anti-inflammatory doses of immunosuppressive therapies, including corticosteroids. Most peripheral vestibular syndromes due to idiopathic or geriatric disease will resolve over 15 days given appropriate supportive care. Consultation with an oncology specialist is recommended for animals with a neoplastic cause for vestibular signs. While typically inoperable, some lesions may respond to chemotherapy or radiation therapies.

PROGNOSIS

Prognosis is highly dependent upon the underlying cause.

Mental alteration

KEY POINTS
- Mental alteration results from brain hypoxemia, metabolic disease, primary CNS disease, trauma, and toxins.
- Systemically ill animals may appear weak or dull.
- Outcome relies on rapid assessment and treatment, and response to therapy.
- Prognosis depends on the cause of the signs.

DEFINITION / OVERVIEW
Changes in mental status are typically manifest as obtundation, stupor, or coma.

Determination of whether an animal is mentally appropriate is essential in distinguishing altered mentation from lethargy or weakness. Lethary or weakness can result from acute or chronic illness, dehydration, neuromuscular disease, or metabolic disease. Mental alteration, alternatively, requires an assessment that an animal responds in a truly inappropriate manner.

ETIOLOGY
Diagnosis of mental alteration includes consideration of causes of five general categories (*Table 22*).

Brain hypoxia
Decreased tissue perfusion secondary to cardiovascular compromise results in hypoxemia and brain ischemia. As well as cardiogenic and hypovolemic shock, systemic responses to infection induce circulation of inflammatory mediators leading to circulatory collapse. Severe hypoxia can result from primary lung disease, such as pneumonia, pulmonary edema, and pulmonary contusions, or acute anemias caused by hemorrhage or hemolysis. Methemoglobinemia can cause cyanosis in the cat as a result of acetaminophen toxicity. Encephalopathies secondary to hypoxemia can result from hypoventilation, such as with anesthetic accidents, prolonged seizures, or smoke inhalation and carbon monoxide toxicity.

Central nervous system disease
Altered mental status is a common manifestation of primary brain disease. Causes to consider in the animal <1 year of age include congenital diseases, such as hydrocephalus, and hereditary diseases, such as lysosomal storage diseases. In animals >5 years of age, primary or metastatic neoplasia should be considered. Inflammatory diseases can affect all animals, and include viral, bacterial, fungal, rickettsial, protozoal, and parasitic infections. Rabies should be considered in any animal with uncertain vaccination status, particularly with a wound of unknown origin. Although some inflammatory diseases tend to affect particular breeds (Pug dog encephalitis, necrotizing encephalitis of Yorkshire and Maltese Terriers), any breed can be affected by inflammatory diseases categorized as granulomatous encephalitis. Vascular accidents can result from coagulopathies including acquired causes such as thrombocytopenia (see Chapter 4), clotting factor deficiency (e.g. warfarin-induced), or hereditary diseases, such as von Willebrand disease or hemophilias. Cerebrovascular accidents resulting from thrombi or embolisms can occur with infections or conditions which reduce fibrinolysis, such as decreased antithrombin (protein-losing diseases), or cause increased thrombus formation, such as hyperviscosity (severe leukocytosis, polycythemia, or hyperglobulinemia). Traumatic brain injury can result from depressed skull fractures, subdural hematomas, or intraparenchymal hemorrhage and edema. Mentation can also be temporarily altered during seizures – particularly complex partial seizures – or in the post-ictal period.

Toxin
Many toxins and drugs can induce changes in mental status, and intoxication should be considered in any animal with acute inappropriate behavior. Outdoor or unsupervised animals may have exposure to a number of toxins, including ethylene glycol, metaldehyde ('slug bait'), mycotoxins (garbage, compost), strychnine, and wild mushrooms. Potential exposure to 'recreational' drugs such as marijuana, phencyclidines, and alcohol should be considered, in addition to household medications, such as antihypertensive agents, antidepressants, and barbiturates.

Table 22 Causes of altered mental status

Hypoxia or hypoxemia

Infection

CNS disease

Toxin

Metabolic

Metabolic

A metabolic cause for animals of any age should be considered. Encephalopathies can result from hyperammonemia, hypoglycemia, uremia, and electrolyte disturbances such as hypernatremia and hyponatremia (135). Encephalopathy caused by hyperammonemia is typically more common in young animals with congenital portocaval shunting, but can also occur in older animals with acquired shunts secondary to portal hypertension and liver failure. Systemic infection (sepsis) may also affect mentation (136). Uremic encephalopathy can occur with renal failure. Hypoglycemia secondary to insulin overdose can result in irreversible encephalopathy. Any condition resulting in hyperosmolality is likely to cause mentally inappropriate behavior. These include hypernatremia and severe hyperglycemia.

CLINICAL FEATURES

Physical examination and history are essential in determining a cause for mental alteration. Animals with hypoxia will demonstrate dyspnea or respiratory distress, and possibly cyanosis. Cardiovascular collapse will be evident with signs of shock. Tachycardia, bounding pulses, hyperemia, and rapid capillary refill time indicate compensatory shock. Decompensated shock will be apparent, with pale to muddy mucous membrane color, weak pulses, and slow capillary refill time. Animals with anemia will be pale, and icterus may accompany acute hemolysis. The history will likely indicate a recent or acute onset of signs.

Animals with infection may have fever or be hypothermic. A focus of infection may not be readily apparent, and history may suggest either a chronic or acute onset of signs. Toxin involvement should be suspected with an unknown history, or known exposure to certain substances. Central nervous disease should be suspected if the animal appears cardiovascularly stable, and has no signs of respiratory compromise or anemia. Other abnormalities with the neurological examination may or may not be present. Metabolic disease should be considered in any animal with mental alteration.

DIAGNOSIS

Physical and neurological examination should be performed prior to administration of sedation, analgesia, or anti-epileptics. Should the animal's condition warrant emergency anti-epileptic therapy, neurological examination should be performed, but be repeated when the animal is more awake. Any animal presenting with mental alteration should have a minimum database, including CBC, serum chemistry, and urinalysis. Emergency clinicians should have the capability of performing serum electrolytes, blood glucose, and survey radiographs. Other initial tests and monitoring include arterial blood gas analysis, pulse oximetry, and blood pressure monitoring. If the signs are due to cardiovascular compromise or hypoxia, the animal should improve once stabilized. Tests to measure a variety of toxins, such as ethylene glycol and mycotoxins, are available. Coagulopathy should be assessed with

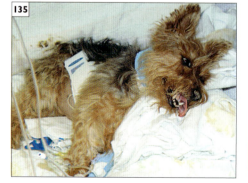

135 An Australian Terrier with altered mentation due to electrolyte disturbances.

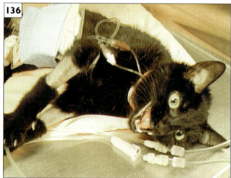

136 A cat with altered mentation associated with a septic abdominal process.

evaluation of platelets, PT, aPTT, and BMBT. Hereditary or acquired coagulopathies should be suspected in any young animal with unexplained bleeding or bruising. Brain imaging with MRI or CT may be necessary to look for other causes of CNS disease, along with obtaining CSF for analysis, titers, and culture. *Table 23* summarizes the diagnostic testing to be carried out for cases of mental alteration.

MANAGEMENT / TREATMENT

Initial therapy goals should provide cardiovascular support and correction of shock (*Table 24*). If dyspnea fails to respond to supplemental oxygen, the animal should be intubated and manually ventilated. Following stabilization, a more complete assessment can be obtained.

If infection is suspected, cultures should be obtained and antibiotics started. Metabolic disorders can largely be determined from analysis of electrolytes, blood glucose, and renal values, and treatment can be directed toward cautious correction of these derangements. Transfusion of fresh frozen plasma can provide life-saving clotting factors quickly, followed by administration of vitamin K_1 if anticoagulant rodenticide (ACR) toxicity is considered likely.

Following assessment of the animal, if no clear underlying cause can be determined for altered mental status, a presumptive diagnosis of primary CNS disease should be considered. If the signs are rapidly progressive, increased intracranial pressure should be suspected and treated with agents effective at treating that, including intravenous dosing of mannitol (0.25–2 g/kg slowly over 20 min, and repeated once if signs progress) or corticosteroids (prednisolone sodium succinate (Soludelta Cortef) 20 mg/kg slowly over 20 min). The animal should be intubated and manually ventilated if hypoventilation is apparent.

Imaging of the brain should precede performing cerebrospinal tap, as brainstem herniation can occur with relief of intracranial pressure due to the presence of an intracranial mass or severe hydrocephalus. Further treatment options for primary CNS disease will be based on the results of imaging and CSF analysis.

Table 23 Diagnostic testing for cases of mental alteration

Minimum database, including CBC, serum chemistry, and urinalysis

Arterial blood gas, arterial blood pressure

Thoracic and abdominal survey radiographs

Coagulation profile, including PT, aPTT, and platelet count

Brain imaging

CSF analysis

Cultures of CSF, blood, urine

Titers for infectious diseases

Table 24 Treatment for cases of mental alteration

1 Obtain intravenous access for administration of fluids, anti-epileptic medications, antibiotics, sedatives
   - Correct shock and fluid balance
   - Provide blood products if anemia present

2 Obtain control of adequate oxygenation. May require intubation and manual ventilation

3 Correct serum electrolytes and glucose derangements, polycythemia, hyperammonemia

4 Correct coagulopathies with clotting factors, vitamin K_1

5 Give intravenous mannitol or corticosteroids for suspected increased intracranial pressure

6 Use poison-control sources for guides on treating intoxications

CHAPTER 9

Metabolic emergencies

- **Diabetic ketoacidosis**

- **Hypoglycemia**

- **Hypoadrenocorticism (Addison's disease)**

- **Disorders of calcium**

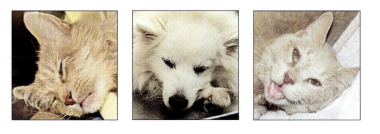

Metabolic disorders encompass a broad group of pathophysiological changes in otherwise normal body systems. As with many diseases, the spectrum of severity of metabolic disorders ranges from mild changes to devastating, life-threatening complications. An in-depth discussion of pathophysiology is beyond the scope of this section. However, a basic understanding of a handful of common metabolic disorders is essential for the practice of emergency medicine.

This chapter includes descriptions of common metabolic emergencies: diabetic ketoacidosis, hypoglycemia, hypoadrenocorticism, and disorders of calcium. Weakness, lethargy, inappetence, PU/PD, and vomiting are signs that are common to each of these disorders. The spectrum of severity of these signs, however, is large. A proper triage may assess the animal as stable. Alternatively, the animal may present collapsed, requiring immediate resuscitation. Interestingly, each of these disorders can be identified with evaluation of a minimum database available in most emergency clinics: CBC, serum chemistry analysis, and urinalysis. Each of these disorders demands medical interventions. Ideally, the emergency clinician must be respectful of the potential of any metabolic disorder to derail and progress rapidly into a spiral of deterioration that may result in the death of the animal (137). Knowledge and experience will enable the emergency clinician to recognize the metabolic disorder before it becomes a metabolic crisis.

KEY POINTS
- Metabolic disorders may progress rapidly into crisis.
- Fluid therapy in a patient with pre-existing PU/PD is very challenging. Patient hydration status and urine production should be carefully monitored.
- Hospitalization following initial diagnosis may be lengthy.

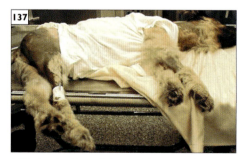

137 A mixed breed dog with long-standing Cushing's disease which developed sepsis from a small wound on the hind leg.

Diabetic ketoacidosis

KEY POINTS
- Patients with DKA require careful monitoring.
- Patients succumb from a lack of fluids and acid–base disturbances, rather than an insulin deficiency *per se*.
- The production of ketones strongly suggests a co-morbid condition, such as pancreatitis, Cushing's syndrome, or infection.

Table 25 Characteristics of the patient with diabetic ketoacidosis. Most patients have all four metabolic changes contributing to the development of DKA

Insulin deficiency (absolute and relative)

Activity of counter-regulatory hormones (catecholamines, glucagon, cortisol, growth hormone)

Unchecked lipolysis and free supply of FFAs for conversion to ketoacids

Concurrent illness (infection, pancreatitis, liver disease)

DEFINITION / OVERVIEW
DKA is a life-threatening complication of diabetes mellitus. The previously undiagnosed diabetic is most at risk, although the poorly regulated diabetic may also develop DKA. The critical nature of the disease requires aggressive treatment and, almost invariably, long-term hospitalization. The most severely affected animals should be referred to specialists capable of providing 24-hour care. Once recovered, animals will likely require lifelong insulin management for diabetes mellitus.

ETIOLOGY
The metabolic changes which contribute to the development of DKA are summarized in *Table 25*. Insulin deficiency (and relative insulin deficiency) causes failure of cellular uptake of glucose, setting in motion a series of actions resulting in a deleterious and potentially life-threatening pathophysiological response. Hyperglycemia persists and actually increases as the result of a combination of the effects of insulin deficiency and the counter-regulatory hormones (catecholamines, glucagon, cortisol, and growth hormone). The counter-regulatory hormones serve to maintain blood glucose at >3.33 mmol/l (>60 mg/dl) under normal conditions. During stress, or concurrent illness, these hormones, particularly glucagon and epinephrine, continue to drive hyperglycemia. Simultaneously, the liver takes up FFAs, released during lipolysis of triglycerides, for conversion to ketone bodies. Ketone bodies can be used as a potential energy source by most cells in the body. Ketogenesis, or oxidation of FFAs, is also driven in the presence of glucagon, a hormone of stress and one of the counter-regulatory hormones. These strong acids, namely β-hydroxybutyric acid and acetoacetic acid, are strong acids and dissociate at physiological pH. Hydrogen ions titrate bicarbonate, which results in the metabolic acidosis of DKA. The decreased bicarbonate is replaced with β-hydroxybutyric acid and acetoacetic acid, and this accounts for the increase in anion gap.

Concurrent illness is almost invariably associated with the onset of DKA, providing the source of stress which promotes secretion of glucagon. Infection, pancreatitis, renal disease, and liver disease are examples of concurrent disease processes. As the levels of glucose and ketone bodies increase in the blood, the kidney's ability to reabsorb them is diminished and severe osmotic diuresis results. Consequently, dehydration occurs, and as effective circulating volume decreases, so does the GFR. This further limits the kidney's ability to eliminate ketoacids, which are continuing to be produced via the unchecked supply of FFAs. The result is continued diuresis, worsening hypovolemia, and increasing serum osmolality from hyperglycemia. As serum osmolality increases, more water is drawn from cells, worsening cellular dehydration. In the brain, glial cells produce osmols that function to control this water loss and prevent brain dehydration. Until insulin is administered, fluid and electrolyte balance is restored, and concurrent illness is identified and treated, this severe metabolic disorder cannot be corrected.

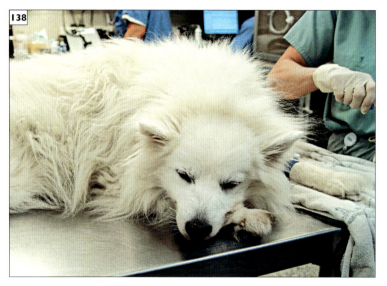

138 A Samoyed affected with diabetic ketoacidosis.

CLINICAL PRESENTATION

Lethargy, weakness, and collapse are common clinical signs (**138**) (*Table 26*). Profound dehydration is usually evident. Metabolic acidosis may cause rapid, deep, and labored respirations (Kussmaul breathing). Because a diagnosis of diabetes mellitus is rarely made prior to the onset of DKA, nonspecific signs of anorexia or vomiting provide little assistance. In fact, clinical signs of other concurrent diseases may be more apparent, such as fever or hypothermia, and icterus. Hyperadrenocorticism may cause insulin resistance, and should be considered in dogs and cats with appropriate signs. History is essential, alerting the clinician to signs which should warrant consideration of diabetes, including recent onset of polydipsia, polyuria, and weight loss despite increased appetite. Vomiting may be associated with concurrent pancreatitis.

DIAGNOSIS

Animals presenting with signs of DKA should have a minimum database that includes CBC, serum chemistry analysis, and urinalysis (*Table 27*). A diagnosis of DKA is typically easily made with these results: hyperglycemia and ketonuria. Diagnosis of metabolic acidosis can be made from a venous blood gas. Once the diagnosis of DKA has been determined, a vigilant search should be performed for a coinciding disease process. Culture of the urine or other appropriate samples should be obtained. Survey radiographs of the thorax and abdomen should be assessed for infection or masses. Ultrasonography of the abdomen should be performed to evaluate for pancreatitis, and liver or other abdominal disease. Prostatitis or pyometra should be considered in any intact animal.

MANAGEMENT / TREATMENT

To correct DKA, the primary goals are to restore effective circulating volume, stabilize electrolyte imbalances, administer insulin, and to treat coinciding illness (*Table 28*). Intravenous fluids with isotonic crystalloid solutions should be aggressively administered until volume is restored and hydration status improved. Fluids can be administered subcutaneously only if venous access cannot be obtained due to profound dehydration and vascular collapse. Venous access should be attempted promptly, however, because subcutaneous fluid administration is largely ineffective in correcting the fluid losses of DKA.

Antibiotic therapy should be instituted from the outset, as underlying infection is a common inciting cause of glucagon secretion. General anesthesia or sedation for surgical interventions should be untaken judiciously, as the animal with newly diagnosed DKA is rarely able to undergo such procedures safely.

Cautious stabilization of electrolyte derangements should be made. Serum sodium is often decreased, which likely represents profound free water excess, but may additionally mask total body sodium depletion. Estimation of serum osmolality should be made from the calculation:
$2(Na^+ + K^+) + glucose + BUN = $ serum osmolality (mmol/l).

If sodium, potassium, glucose and BUN have been determined in traditional units, the calculation is:
$2(Na^+ + K^+) + glucose/18 + BUN/2.8 = $ serum osmolality (mOsm/l).

Any elevation in serum osmolality >320 mmol/l (>320 mOsm/l) should be corrected cautiously. Rapid changes in an animal's serum osmolality may have disastrous consequences in the brain, and thus the components of osmolality should be monitored closely. Despite correction of serum osmolality, brain osmols, which had been formed within glial cells to counter brain dehydration, continue to persist for days. If serum osmolality is corrected rapidly, brain cells will draw water in the direction of increased osmolality, and this will result in life-threatening cerebral edema.

Once fluid therapy has been started, insulin should be administered. In unstable DKA, the primary goal of insulin administration is to reverse the production of ketones and to decrease the gluconeogenic effects of the counter-regulatory hormones. Ideally, blood glucose should be initially noted, and only small decreases obtained over the next 2–3 days. Initial blood glucose >27.75 mmol/l (>500 mg/dl) should be corrected slowly over the following 24–72 hours, to prevent rapid decreases in serum osmolality.

Table 26 Common clinical signs and historical findings in a patient with diabetic ketoacidosis

Lethargy and weakness

Dehydration and hypovolemia

Anorexia

Vomiting

Weight loss

Table 27 Diagnostic evaluation of the patient with suspected diabetic ketoacidosis

Minimum database: CBC, serum chemistry with electrolytes, urinalysis

Venous or arterial blood gas

Urine culture

Survey thoracic and abdominal radiography

Abdominal ultrasonography

Table 28 Treatment summary for the patient with diabetic ketoacidosis

1 Intravenous isotonic fluid resuscitation (correct hypovolemia rapidly, correct dehydration over 24–36 hours)

2 Administer insulin

3 Administer antibiotics

4 Correct electrolyte derangements

5 Close monitoring of blood glucose, electrolytes, urine production, and serum osmolality

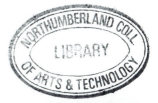

Table 29 Protocol for insulin CRI

The amount of insulin may need to be titrated up or down. The goal is to maintain a relatively steady state for blood glucose, while simultaneously providing exogenous insulin. In some patients, smaller adjustments are required as standard ones cause large swings; in other patients, an increased dose of insulin is required to maintain glycemic control. The insulin CRI protocol requires two intravenous catheters, ideally at least one of which bleeds back easily. The patient will normally receive a set fluid rate per hour of crystalloids, combined with a separate infusion of insulin. Dextrose may be added to the fluids in order to permit ongoing administration of insulin to help reverse the ketogenesis. The starting insulin CRI is made by adding 1–2 U/kg regular insulin to 240 ml of 0.9% saline. For animals with suspected insulin resistance, the CRI is started with 2 U/kg of insulin. The blood glucose is checked every 2–4 hours. The fluid rate is calculated using normal guidelines, recalling that almost all diabetics are whole body potassium depleted.

Blood glucose (mmol/l) [mg/dl]	Insulin rate	% dextrose in regular fluids
>22.2 [>400]	20/ml/hr	0%
13.9–22.2 [250–400]	10/ml/hr	0%
8.3–13.8 [150–249]	5 ml/hr	2.5%
4.4–8.2 [80–149]	0 ml/hr	5%
<4.4 [<80]	0 ml/hr	5% + bolus 1 ml/kg 50% dextrose, + alert veterinarian

Regular insulin can be administered intramuscularly, subcutaneously or intravenously, or via CRI (*Table 29*). Regardless of the route of insulin administration, blood glucose should be monitored at least every 4 hours, and the dose of insulin adjusted to maintain cautious glycemic control. Unless blood glucose drops precipitously, insulin therapy should be continued to reverse the spiral of ketone production. Dextrose infusions should be instituted and titrated with vigilant blood glucose monitoring during continuation of insulin administration.

Following initial resuscitative therapies, electrolytes should be closely monitored. During treatment, serum magnesium, potassium, and phosphorus will commonly be decreased, requiring supplementation. A complication of hypophosphatemia in cats is hemolytic anemia. Blood transfusions may be required. Concurrent disease should be identified and treated. If persistent vomiting precludes the use of enteral nutrition, TPN should be formulated according to the specific needs of the animal. Intravenous bicarbonate therapy in DKA remains controversial, and is not generally recommended unless pH falls to <7.0. Severe cases should be referred to hospitals equipped to offer 24-hour critical care management.

PROGNOSIS

The prognosis is fair. Animals that survive the initial treatment will need to receive life-long therapy. Committed owners are a necessity. Most animals that survive treatment have an excellent quality of life.

Hypoglycemia

KEY POINTS

- The most severe effect of prolonged hypoglycemia is neurological impairment.
- Hypoglycemia has many possible causes, but the most common include insulin overdosage (real or relative), neoplasia, hypoadrenocorticism, sepsis, and liver dysfunction.

DEFINITION / OVERVIEW

Many organ systems in the body utilize glucose as a source of energy, but only the brain has an obligate requirement for glucose as its energy source. Hypoglycemia is generally defined as a plasma glucose level that decreases to <2.8 mmol/l (<50 mg/dl), yet clinically hypoglycemia may not be apparent until a critically low level of glycemia occurs in the brain, defined as neuroglycopenia. Glucose uptake by the brain is a passive activity, allowing the brain to extract enough glucose from the circulation to maintain homeostasis in the face of long-term decreasing glycemia. The body accomplishes this by up-regulating the production of glucose receptors, the Glut receptors, thereby preventing life-threatening neuroglycopenia. Clinical signs of hypoglycemia are typically recognized during actual neuroglycopenia, or when brain glucose has finally reached critically low levels.

ETIOLOGY

Normal glycemia is generally maintained within a range of approximately 3.9–6.1 mmol/l (70–110 mg/dl) through regulation of combined responses in the body. The beta cells of the endocrine pancreas (islet cells) secrete insulin when blood glucose rises above 6.1 mmol/l (110 mg/dl), and functions to induce cellular uptake of glucose until blood glucose decreases to about 3.3 mmol/l (60 mg/dl). At this point, insulin secretion ceases, allowing blood glucose to rise into its considered normal range. Insulin secretion should be minimal at blood glucose levels <3.3 mmol/l (<60 mg/dl), and to maintain normal glycemia, the liver responds by increasing glucose production by breakdown of its limited glycogen stores (glycogenolysis). Additionally, the liver is the primary site of gluconeogenesis, but requires substrates including fatty acids, glycerol, and specific amino acids supplied from muscle and adipose tissue. Glucagon, secreted by

Table 30 Common causes of hypoglycemia
Insulin overdose
Neoplasia (insulinoma, leiomyoma, liver tumor)
Hypoadrenocorticism
Liver disease
Sepsis

the endocrine pancreas (alpha cells), catecholamines, cortisol, and growth hormone all function in response to hypoglycemia to regain normal glycemia.

Hypoglycemia occurs with breakdown of any of the counter-regulatory mechanisms (Table 30):

- Neonates and juveniles can have low stores of substrates for gluconeogenesis to provide normal glycemia between meals.
- Middle-aged to older animals develop neoplasms of the endocrine pancreas which continue to secrete insulin in the face of persistent hypoglycemia. Insulinomas are pancreatic islet (beta) cell tumors. Hepatic tumors or those that invade the liver, in addition to some GI tumors, may secrete insulin-like growth factors, which behave similarly to insulin. Examples include leiomyosarcoma, leiomyoma, hepatic adenocarcinoma, lymphoma, and hemangiosarcoma.
- Liver disease (portocaval shunting, microvascular dysplasia) or failure (cirrhosis) can result in hypoglycemia as the number of functional hepatocytes decreases, limiting the liver's ability to convert available substrates into glucose.
- Hypoglycemia can occur with disruption of the hypothalamus–pituitary–adrenal axis. Mild hypoglycemia is commonly found with hypoadrenocorticism, due to the lack of production of adequate levels of cortisol.

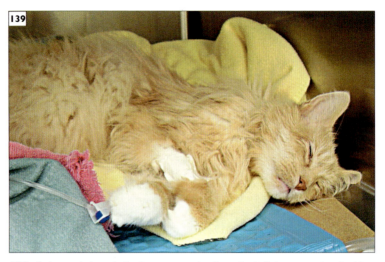

139 A domestic long-haired cat recovering from brain injury associated with relative insulin overdosage.

- Hypoglycemia in sepsis is multifactorial. Hepatic dysfunction, disregulation of gluconeogenesis, and bacterial usage of glucose all likely play a role.
- Insulin overdose (**139**) is a common cause of hypoglycemia in the poorly regulated diabetic.

If hypoglycemia progresses to severe neuroglycopenia, neuronal injury may result. The severity of injury depends on the length of time the animal remains in this state, in addition to the degree of hypoglycemia. Some animals respond to resuscitation with glucose and supportive care, and recover normal function. Others may die, or remain severely impaired with loss of vision, mental appropriateness, and ability to ambulate well, or may have persistent epilepsy.

CLINICAL PRESENTATION

Clinically, the hypoglycemic animal is seldom identified until signs of neuroglycopenia (decreased brain glucose) are recognized, including ataxia, collapse, or epileptic seizures (*Table 31*). Hypoglycemic animals may have lethargy or weakness for weeks to months prior to progression to more severe signs. Animals with blood glucose <2.8 mmol/l (<50 mg/dl) may still be able to extract enough glucose into the brain for maintenance of CNS function due to an increased production of passive glucose receptors. Once a critically low level of neuroglycopenia occurs, the animal may become obtunded, and suffer seizures which progress to status epilepticus and eventually coma.

Table 31 Common signs of hypoglycemia
Weakness
Lethargy
Seizures
Stupor
Coma

DIAGNOSIS

Any animal with acute or recent onset of central nervous signs which progress should have a blood glucose level assessed. Minimum database includes CBC, serum chemistry analysis, and urinalysis. Microcytic anemia, hypoalbuminemia, decreased BUN, ammonium biurate cystic calculi, or a history of PU/PD in a juvenile or young animal should raise suspicion for portocaval shunting or microvascular dysplasia. Continued examination with ultrasonography of the abdomen or technetium liver scan may identify the portocaval shunt. Hyponatremia, hyperkalemia, lack of a stress leukogram, and eosinophilia should suggest hypoadrenocorticism, and an ACTH stimulation test should be performed.

Signs of sepsis include fever or hypothermia, leukocytosis or leukopenia, tachycardia, and tachypnea. If sepsis is considered, a complete search for a focus of infection should be pursued, cultures obtained, and appropriate imaging carried out, including survey radiographs or abdomen ultrasonography.

In an otherwise stable middle-aged to older animal, persistent hypoglycemia should prompt the concern for insulinoma or other neoplasm. The endocrine pancreas with insulinoma is unable to function appropriately when the blood glucose decreases to 3.3 mmol/l (60 mg/dl), and continues to secrete insulin. Often, administration of dextrose will result in increased insulin secretion from the insulinoma, which should raise suspicion. An insulin level should be obtained with a simultaneously drawn blood glucose sample, when blood glucose is 2.8 mmol/l (50 mg/dl) or less. Commonly used glucometers often register slightly lower blood glucose levels, and for this reason it has been suggested to check the insulin level when blood glucose is registered at 2.2 mmol/l (40 mg/dl) on the glucometer. If hypoglycemia is due to insulinoma, insulin levels will be normal to increased when blood glucose is <2.8 mmol/l (<50 mg/dl). Examination of the abdomen with ultrasonography should be carried out in animals suspected to have hypoglycemia due to neoplasia, as most will have tumors arising in the pancreas, liver, or GI tract.

MANAGEMENT / TREATMENT

Hypoglycemia should be suspected in any animal with acute or recent onset of neurological signs and dextrose should be administered. Dextrose should not be withheld until test results are available, and it can be given orally, applied to the gums, if the animal is not comatose or in status epilepticus. Otherwise, venous access should be obtained and 50% dextrose (0.5 g/kg) should be administered as a bolus over 3–5 minutes. Although life-saving, administration of a source of glucose during prolonged brain anoxia could precipitate further brain injury which includes both neurons and glial cells (pannecrosis). Unless a central line is available, 50% dextrose should be diluted in a crystalloid solution to decrease osmolality and vascular injury.

Other therapies should be aimed at correcting underlying diseases. Septic animals should be aggressively supported with intravenous fluid and antibiotic therapy. Animals with suspected hypoadrenocorticism should be administered corticosteroid therapy and intravenous fluid therapy. Animals with suspected liver disease should be assessed for hyperammonemia as a cause for neurological signs, and treated with therapies aimed at decreasing blood ammonia if present. Animals with insulinoma or other neoplasia and persistent clinical hypoglycemia should be treated with infusions of dextrose, using up to 5% solutions. Corticosteroids should be administered (prednisone (prednisolone) 0.5–1 mg/kg/day). Although insulinomas are considered highly metastatic, surgical excision of insulinomas and identified metastases is recommended.

Diabetic animals with presumed insulin overdose should be hospitalized until blood glucose is in the normal range. Re-evaluation for glucose regulation is advised after the animal recovers. Owners of diabetic animals should be educated to the clinical signs of hypoglycemia (weakness, lethargy), and neuroglycopenia (collapse, stupor, seizures, or coma) and taught how to administer an oral glycemic agent (e.g. corn syrup) at home as emergency therapy. Follow-up for improved glucose regulation is warranted. Animals with persistent hypoglycemia or insulin overdose that are mentally appropriate should be fed frequent meals. Animals with persistent seizures despite normalized glycemia may require continued antiepileptic therapy.

Hypoadrenocorticism (Addison's disease)

KEY POINTS
- Not all animals with hypoadrenocorticism have 'classic' presentations.
- In the absence of sodium and potassium abnormalities, decreases in glucose, cholesterol, and albumin, and increases in calcium and lymphocytes support the diagnosis of hypoadrenocorticism.
- Hypoadrenocorticism is very treatable after confirming the diagnosis.

DEFINITION / OVERVIEW
Hypoadrenocorticism (adrenal insufficiency, Addison's disease) represents a failure of the adrenal glands to produce mineralocorticoids and/or glucocorticoids. This failure manifests in an inability to respond to progressive hypotension and stress. Signs of hypoadrenocorticism can wax and wane over months to years. At some time, however, the animal with hypoadrenocorticism will be faced with an insurmountable stress, such as infection, surgery, or even boarding away from home, and this inability to mount an appropriate response may result in life-threatening disease. Only the ACTH stimulation test can reliably provide a diagnosis of hypoadrenocorticism. Clinical signs, serum electrolytes, hypoglycemia, and lack of a stress leukogram will combine with an index of suspicion to identify the animal with hypoadrenocorticism.

ETIOLOGY AND RISK FACTORS
Hypoadrenocorticism is a result of reduced production of aldosterone and/or cortisol by the adrenal cortex. It may be either primary or secondary (*Table 32*).

Aldosterone is produced by the adrenal cortex, the product of the renin–angiotensin–aldosterone system. Baroreceptors located in the juxtaglomerular apparatus sense decreased circulating volume and release renin. Renin acts to begin a series of reactions involving angiotensin, which result in the production of aldosterone in the adrenal cortex. Primary hypoadrenocorticism results in a lack of production of both aldosterone and cortisol, and usually occurs as a result of autoimmune destruction of the adrenal cortex.

Table 32 Causes of hypoadrenocorticism

Primary: autoimmune destruction of adrenal cortex resulting in decreased aldosterone and cortisol production

Secondary: hypothalamic or pituitary lesion resulting in decreased production of cortisol

The consequence of secondary hypoadrenocorticism may primarily be limited to a lack of cortisol production. Although epinephrine is produced by the adrenal medulla and should not be affected by destruction of the adrenal cortex, its production is mediated by cortisol, and requires a local cortisol concentration. Therefore, epinephrine production may be additionally decreased. Secondary hypoadrenocorticism may result from lesions in the hypothalamus or pituitary, such as neoplasms, inflammation, or infection. Most commonly, however, secondary hypoadrenocorticism is caused by exogenous glucocorticoid administration. The administration of systemic or topical glucocorticoids, even short term, may suppress the hypothalamic production of CRH, or the anterior pituitary's production of ACTH. The effect of this suppression is a lack of adrenal response to a stimulus, and, potentially, adrenal cortical atrophy. With time and withdrawal of the exogenous glucocorticoid medication, adrenal function may return. However, return of adrenal function is unlikely with primary adrenal insufficiency. The implication of primary adrenal insufficiency is a potentially life-threatening inability to respond to hypotension and/or stress.

Although dogs of any breed, age or sex may develop hypoadrenocorticism, females are more likely than males to be affected, and neutered females and males are more likely to be affected than intact animals. Dogs aged 4–7 years are more likely to be affected than younger or older animals, but, again, dogs of any age may be affected. A variety of breeds have been 'listed' to have either increased risk or potential genetic predispositions. Among these are the Great Dane, Poodle (Standard, Miniature and Toy), West Highland White Terrier, Bearded Collie, Portuguese Water Dog, Leonberger, Bassett Hound and Labrador Retriever. Hypoadrenocorticism is rare in the cat.

PATHOGENESIS

The body's response to stress relies on the contributions from each of the components of the hypothalamus–pituitary–adrenal axis. The hypothalamus produces CRH, which induces the anterior pituitary to produce ACTH, which then acts on the cortex of the adrenal gland to produce mineralocorticoids, including aldosterone, and glucocorticoids, including cortisol. Adrenal insufficiency can be primary, in which the adrenal cortex is nonfunctional, or secondary, in which the hypothalamus–pituitary arms of the axis fail.

Aldosterone regulates the reabsorption of sodium and excretion of potassium. Cortisol acts on several vital systems, but mainly influences maintenance of blood glucose by regulating glycogenolysis and gluconeogenesis. Sodium retention is essential for volume control. Sodium plays a primary role in maintaining the renal medullary concentration gradient, allowing the retention of water when volume needs to be restored. Aldosterone induces the up-regulation of sodium/potassium exchange pumps, which function primarily in the distal convoluted tubule and collecting ducts, but also to a lesser degree in the proximal convoluted tubule.

Cortisol plays a vital role in carbohydrate and protein metabolism, and is involved in a variety of interactions which function to maintain vascular and cellular integrity. Cortisol also binds to glucocorticoid receptors on the hypothalamus, to provide negative feedback.

CLINICAL PRESENTATION

Although an animal with hypoadrenocorticism may have waxing and waning signs over months to years, diagnosis is not often suspected until the animal is presented in an acute crisis (*Table 33*). Dehydration and hypovolemia that respond to intravenous fluid resuscitation, lethargy and weakness, anorexia, weight loss, vomiting, diarrhea, or melena are all common signs. In severe cases of acute disease or crisis, shock and collapse, bradycardia, and weak femoral pulses may be present with hypovolemia, hypoglycemia, and life-threatening hyperkalemia. Recently, hypoadrenal function has been recognized in critically ill people and animals with a failure to respond to appropriate fluid therapy for shock/sepsis.

Table 33 Common signs of hypoadrenocorticism

Lethargy, weakness

Inappetence

Weight loss

Vomiting, regurgitation

Diarrhea, melena

Dehydration

Hypovolemia

Bradycardia

Table 34 Diagnosis of hypoadrenocorticism

ACTH stimulation test: failure to increase basal cortisol level

Complete blood test: nonregenerative anemia, lymphcytosis, eosinophilia

Serum chemistry profile: azotemia, hyponatremia, hyperkalemia, hypoglycemia, hypocholesterolemia, hypoalbuminemia, hypercalcemia, mild increase in liver enzymes

ECG: tented T waves, flattened P waves, prolonged R-R interval

Thoracic radiography: microcardia, esophageal dilation

DIAGNOSIS

A minimum database that includes a CBC, serum chemistry profile, and urinalysis should provide a number of clues which, when combined with clinical signs, signalment, and physical examination, should prompt suspicion for hypoadrenocorticism (*Table 34*). Hyponatremia and hyperkalemia are common findings in dogs with primary hypoadrenocorticism, although this derangement may be characteristic of a variety of disorders. Hypoadrenocorticism should always be considered in an animal with hypovolemia and collapse.

Evaluation of the ECG may indicate changes consistent with hyperkalemia, including tenting of T waves, flattening of P waves, and prolongation of the R-R interval. Sinus bradycardia occurs with dangerously elevated serum potassium, and warrants emergency treatment to prevent progression to cardiac arrest. The ECG is a simple monitoring aid that should be used in all dogs with cardiovascular collapse.

Table 35 Treatment of hypoadrenocorticism

Emergency intravenous therapy: shock dose 0.9% NaCl over 20–30 min, 50% dextrose (0.5 g/kg), dexamethasone (1 mg/kg)

Long-term mineralocorticoid support: DOCP, fludrocortisone

Long-term glucocorticoid support: prednisone (prednisolone)

Additionally, most dogs with hypoadrenocorticism will have azotemia, which is generally attributed to dehydration and decreased GFR (pre-renal azotemia). Comparison of BUN with serum creatinine will usually identify disparity in their elevations. Some animals will retain some urine concentrating ability, but many, due to chronic sodium loss, will lose the medullary concentration gradient and thus have isosthenuria (urine specific gravity 1.008–1.020). GI bleeding may contribute to azotemia, as blood is considered a 'high-protein meal' and will increase BUN levels.

Mild, nonregenerative anemia may be present due to a lack of cortisol and its resultant suppression of erythropoeisis. The lack of a stress leukogram (normal or decreased white blood cell count with lymphocytosis or eosinophilia) may be present. Hypoglycemia, hypocholesterolemia, mild increase in liver enzymes (from presumed liver hypoxia during hypoperfusion), mild hypoalbuminemia, and hypercalcemia may be identified on a chemistry profile. Measurement of arterial blood pressure may identify hypotension. Survey thoracic radiographs may show microcardia due to hypovolemia, or dilation of the esophagus. Mild metabolic acidosis may be present.

Although a variety of clinical signs and test results may be highly suggestive of hypoadrenocorticism, the only test to definitively provide a diagnosis is the ACTH stimulation test. The ACTH stimulation measures the animal's ability to respond to ACTH (gel) or synthetic cortrosyn by increasing its plasma cortisol level. Animals with both primary and secondary hypoadrenocorticism will invariably be unable to respond. Very rarely can an animal with hypoadrenocorticism increase its plasma cortisol above 85.53 nmol/l (3.1 µg/dl). Most animals will have no increase above basal cortisol.

TREATMENT

Treatment (*Table 35*) should be started based on index of suspicion for hypoadrenocorticism. Hypovolemia should be aggressively treated with intravenous fluids, and if indicated, at shock doses (90 ml/kg in the dog, 60 ml/kg in the cat, over 20–30 min). Because hypovolemia is often the consequence of excessive sodium loss, and because hyperkalemia is often present, the fluid of choice is 0.9% NaCl. Hypovolemia should be corrected rapidly, followed by correction of dehydration over 24–36 hours. Moderate hyperkalemia, 6.6–7.5 mmol/l (6.6–7.5 mEq/l), may readily respond to intravenous fluids; severe hyperkalemia >7.5 mmol/l (>7.5 mEq/l) may be life-threatening, and should be treated if bradycardia is severe or progressing to atrial standstill. Azotemia is usually pre-renal and responds to fluid resuscitation. Further consideration of renal disease should be pursued should azotemia persist despite achievement of effective circulating volume.

An ACTH stimulation test should be performed, and glucocorticoid therapy started prior to test results. Dexamethasone at 0.5–2 mg/kg IV q8–12hr has been suggested as a resuscitative dosage for animals in crisis. DOCP (not available in all countries) should be administered for mineralocorticoid support. These therapies can and should be administered parenterally during the emergency treatment period. Animals with hypoadrenocorticism usually respond within 24–72 hours, at which time oral medications can be administered. Oral fludrocortisone (Florinef) provides both mineralocorticoids and some glucocorticoid support, but needs to be dosed daily. DOCP is administered parenterally, approximately once monthly, but has little glucocorticoid support and may need to be supplemented with daily prednisone (prednisolone). Metabolic acidosis usually resolves with fluid resuscitation and seldom requires treatment. Gastric ulceration is sometimes severe enough to require gastric protectants or even blood transfusions.

PROGNOSIS

The prognosis for animals with hypoadrenocorticism is usually excellent, with appropriate medications and monitoring.

Disorders of calcium

KEY POINTS
- The normal calcium level in the body is tightly regulated.
- Excessive calcium will cause PU/PD and may result in calcification of vital organs.
- Hypocalcemia may result in tetany or seizures.

DEFINITION / OVERVIEW
Disorders of calcium include causes that increase or decrease serum concentrations of ionized calcium. Because calcium plays a vital role in a variety of cellular functions, a significant decrease in extracellular calcium concentration may result in a loss of cellular homeostasis and a derailing of control over neuromuscular excitability. Significant increases in extracellular calcium may be associated with vague clinical signs, and usually result in serious consequences only when coupled with increased phosphorus, or when hypercalcemia is severe enough to cause mineralization of tissues.

PATHOPHYSIOLOGY
Calcium is important to all cells. Regulation of neuromuscular activity is maintained by calcium, integrity of membrane stabilization is maintained by calcium, and a variety of intracellular functions are reliant on calcium. Any derangement resulting in decreased serum ionized calcium, the form that is physiologically active, will hence disrupt a wide range of normal cellular activities. Increased concentration of serum calcium has less of an effect on normal cellular homeostasis, but when combined with hyperphosphatemia may

result in widespread tissue mineralization and nephrotoxicity. Seldom does this development occur. Serum calcium is tightly maintained within normal ranges in dogs (total 2.3–2.9 mmol/l [9.0–11.7 mg/dl], ionized 1.12–1.42 mmol/l) and cats (total 2.0–2.6 mmol/l [8.0–10.5 mg/dl], ionized 1.1–1.4 mmol/l). Acute and chronic fluctuations are managed by the activities of PTH and vitamin D (calcitriol). Together, PTH and vitamin D function to maintain serum and extracellular calcium concentrations for cellular activities. When serum calcium levels rise, concentrations and activity of PTH and vitamin D decrease. Regulation of production and secretion of PTH and vitamin D is achieved by negative feedback of calcium. When serum calcium levels decrease, PTH is produced and secreted by the parathyroid gland and acts on bone and distal renal tubular cells. The effect is to increase serum calcium by increasing bone resorption and renal calcium reabsorption. Vitamin D is synthesized and acts on the intestine, in concert with PTH, to increase dietary absorption of calcium. When serum calcium increases, the production and activities of PTH and vitamin D decrease. A PTH-rP is produced by many tissues, and is increased by a variety of neoplastic diseases. It produces unregulated hypercalcemia that fails to respond to normal negative feedback mechanisms.

ETIOLOGY
Hypercalcemia
Hypercalcemia occurs when normal feedback and corrective mechanisms do not respond to increasing calcium concentrations (*Table 36*). The most common cause in both dogs and cats is hypercalcemia of malignancy (MAH), which results in increased amounts of circulating PTH-rP. In both dogs and cats, the most common neoplasia identified with hypercalcemia is lymphosarcoma. Other neoplasms commonly associated with hypercalcemia include apocrine gland carcinoma of the anal sac, multiple myeloma, melanoma, and other carcinomas.

A pair of parathyroid glands is associated with each thyroid gland. Hypercalcemia can result from unregulated production of PTH from a parathyroid gland adenoma, or from hyperplastic parathyroid glands. These conditions are referred to as primary and secondary hyperparathyroidism, respectively. *Primary hyperparathyroidism* commonly results in mild to moderate

---

Table 36 Common causes of hypercalcemia

Malignancy-associated hypercalcemia (lymphosarcoma, apocrine gland carcinoma of the anal sac)

Primary hyperparathyroidism (adenoma)

Secondary hyperparathydoism (nutritional, renal failure)

Vitamin D toxicosis (cholecalciferol-containing rodenticides, human psoriasis medications)

Hypoadrenocorticism

Granulomatous disease (fungal infection)

Table 37 Common causes of hypocalcemia

Parathyroidectomy
Pancreatitis
Puerperal tetany (eclampsia)
Ethylene glycol intoxication

Table 38 Common signs of hypercalcemia

PU/PD
Lethargy and weakness
Inappetence
Vomiting
Signs of ARF or CRF

increases in serum calcium, but elevated PTH will also act to depress serum phosphorus (law of mass action). Hence, it is uncommon for calcium and phosphorus to reach a level at which risk of nephrotoxicity and mineralization is high. Secondary hyperparathyroidism typically occurs as a result of chronic diets deficient in either calcium and/or vitamin D, or high in phosphorus and relatively low in calcium. Mild or moderate hypocalcemia results in chronically increased PTH and parathyroid gland hyperplasia. Parathyroid gland hyperplasia is also common with CRF, due to a variety of complications of decreased GFR and distal tubular dysfunction.

Hypoadrenocorticism, granulomatous disease (fungal infection), and vitamin D toxicosis are other but less common causes of hypercalcemia. Vitamin D toxicosis occurs secondary to ingestion of cholecalciferol rodenticides (e.g. Muritan, Quintox, and Rampage), and human psoriasis medications containing the vitamin D analogs calcipotriol and calcipotriene (Dovonex, Davionex, and Psorcutan). Excessive administration of vitamin D to cats for hypocalcemia following thyroidectomy and inadvertent parathyroidectomy has been reported to result in toxicity.

Hypocalcemia

Because of the importance of maintenance of extracellular calcium concentration for cellular function and homeostasis, the response of the parathyroid glands and production of vitamin D to correct small decreases in serum calcium is very efficient, and hypocalcemia is relatively rare.

Common causes of hypocalcemia (*Table 37*) include hypoparathyroidism resulting from parathyroidectomy, or other surgery, trauma, or disease in the area of the parathyroid glands. Hypoparathyroidism may follow after the surgical removal of a unilateral parathyroid adenoma or adenocarcinoma, as the remaining parathyroid has atrophied. Other common causes include pancreatitis, puerperal tetany (eclampsia), CRF, intestinal malabsorption, phosphate-containing enemas, and ethylene glycol toxicity (**140**).

CLINICAL PRESENTATION
Hypercalcemia
Clinical signs of hypercalcemia are typically nonspecific and include weakness or lethargy, inappetence, and vomiting (*Table 38*). If hypercalcemia is severe, interference in the ability to concentrate urine may occur, resulting in the production of dilute urine, and potentially excessive water loss. Animals may have mild or chronic hypercalcemia for weeks to months that is undetectable. Hypercalcemia may be identified only when PU/PD is observed. PU/PD is the most common presenting clinical sign with hypercalcemia.

Since the major cause of hypercalcemia is MAH, animals often present with signs more attributable to the neoplastic process. Renal failure associated with hypercalcemia results from mineral deposits, and occurs when hypercalcemia is severe or is coupled with high phosphorus levels. Signs of ARF can occur as a result of vitamin D toxicosis from ingestion of human medications containing vitamin D analogs, or

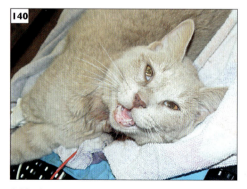

140 A cat experiencing tetany due to hypocalcemia associated with ethylene glycol intoxication.

houseplants (such as *Cestrum diurnum*, day-blooming jasmine). Clinical signs including lethargy, anorexia, hematemesis, and hemorrhagic diarrhea resulting from cholecalciferol rodenticide intoxication appear within 24–72 hours of ingestion.

Hypocalcemia

The primary clinical signs of hypocalcemia involve the nervous system (*Table 39*). Because calcium maintains cell membrane integrity, loss of control allows unregulated sodium entry into cells and membrane depolarization. Calcium also regulates the release of the neuromuscular neurotransmitter, acetylcholine. The result of decreased calcium is increasing excitability, tetany, and seizures. These are the predominant signs of hypocalcemia. Other common signs include stiffness, restlessness, facial rubbing, and inappetence. A form of latent tetany has been described, in which animals may exhibit stiffness that exacerbates to tetany with excitement and hyperventilation. Because respiratory alkalosis may worsen hypocalcemia, owners may describe intermittent tetany signs. A common cause of hypocalcemic tetany is eclampsia, which may occur with nursing. Any animal with a history of potential exposure to ethylene glycol (known exposure or roaming) and hypocalcemia should be suspected of intoxication. Hypocalcemic animals presenting with pancreatitis may have vomiting or anorexia.

DIAGNOSIS

Hypercalcemia

All animals presenting with hypercalcemia should have a minimum database including CBC, serum chemistry analysis, and urinalysis (*Table 40*). Primary hyperparathyroidism is typically determined by the presence of elevated serum total calcium and decreased phosphorus. The CBC and chemistry profile are usually otherwise unremarkable. Cervical ultrasonography is useful in localizing parathyroid gland adenomas. Surgical exploration for identification and resection has been advocated, as well.

PTH will often be decreased with MAH, resulting in relatively normal serum phosphorus. Because of the likelihood of MAH as a cause for hypercalcemia, all animals with hypercalcemia should be tested for levels of both PTH and PTH-rP. With MAH, PTH-rP should be elevated, and a complete investigation for neoplasia should be performed, including survey

Table 39 Common signs of hypocalcemia
Muscle twitching, tetany
Seizures
Stiffness
Restlessness
Inappetence

Table 40 Diagnostic testing for hypercalcemia
Minimum database (CBC, serum chemistry analysis, urinalysis)
Ionized calcium, PTH, PTH-rP
Thoracic and abdominal radiography
Rectal examination
Cervical ultrasonography
Abdominal ultrasonography
ACTH stimulation test

thoracic and abdominal radiographs and abdominal ultrasonography. A rectal examination should be performed to assess for small masses in the area of the anal sacs, and lumbar lymphadenopathy. Although hypercalcemia due to hypoadrenocorticism usually resolves with fluid resuscitation, adrenal function should be evaluated with an ACTH stimulation test. Hypercalcemia associated with renal failure is usually mild to moderate and does not require further testing.

Hypocalcemia

Diagnosis of hypocalcemia is usually made in conjunction with history, clinical signs, and demonstration of decreased serum calcium. Again, all animals should have a minimum database, including CBC, serum chemistry analysis, and urinalysis. Animals with primary hypoparathyroidism post parathyroidectomy will have decreased PTH until the remaining parathyroid glands recover functional ability to respond to hypocalcemia. Calcium depletion is probable in nursing animals, or those with pancreatitis or ethylene glycol toxicity. Abdominal ultrasonography is fairly sensitive in detecting pancreatitis in both dogs and cats. Ethylene glycol levels should be obtained in any animal with potential exposure, or other clinical signs including metabolic acidosis or renal failure.

Table 41 Treatment for calcium disorders

Hypercalcemia

Intravenous 0.9% NaCl diuresis

Furosemide

Bisphosphonates (e.g. pamidronate)

Glucocorticoids

Sodium bicarbonate

Hypocalcemia

Intravenous supplementation (10% calcium gluconate 0.5–1.5 ml/kg over 20 min)

MANAGEMENT / TREATMENT

Treatment for calcium disorders is summarized in *Table 41*.

Hypercalcemia

Hypercalcemia rarely presents as an emergency that requires immediate stabilization. Careful assessment of potential causes will guide therapy. If hypercalcemia is severe, and nephrotoxicity or other tissue mineralization is evident, intravenous 0.9% NaCl diuresis should be administered to promote calciuresis. Furosemide can also be given as an intravenous bolus or CRI to promote calciuresis. Glucocorticoids additionally promote calcium urinary excretion, but their use may interfere with diagnosis of underlying neoplasia, such as lymphosarcoma or multiple myeloma. Their use as an initial treatment, therefore, is not advised. Salmon calcitonin inhibits bone resorption and is effective in vitamin D toxicity. Alkalinization with sodium bicarbonate decreases serum calcium but requires monitoring of pH. Bisphosphonates, including pamidronate, have been used with success.

Hypocalcemia

Severe hypocalcemia can be life-threatening and requires immediate stabilization. Animals that present with seizures or tetany should be administered intravenous calcium supplementation (10% calcium gluconate 0.5–1.5 ml/kg IV slowly over 20 min) until signs resolve. Serum total calcium <1.5–1.75 mmol/l (<6–7 mg/dl) (ionized calcium 0.6–0.7 mmol/l) should be corrected until at least that value is achieved. Ideally, an ECG should be monitored during administration. Animals post parathyroidectomy should receive calcium and/or vitamin D supplementation until an ability to maintain serum calcium within a normal range can be demonstrated. Nursing animals may benefit from additional calcium supplementation, but principally owners should be directed to remove the nursing neonates. Additionally, bitches affected with eclampsia with one litter are likely to be affected again. Animals with ethylene glycol toxicity or pancreatitis should receive supplementation to maintain serum calcium levels within the normal range.

PROGNOSIS

Prognosis for diseases resulting in hypocalcemia or hypercalcemia is variable and depends on the cause.

Trauma

- **Vehicular trauma**

- **Degloving wounds**

- **Bite wounds**

- **Gunshot and stab wounds**

- **Emergency fracture management**

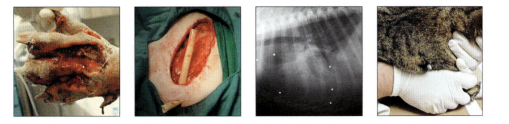

KEY POINTS
- Trauma may have multi-systemic effects.
- A systematic approach to the trauma patient will minimize the incidence of missed injuries.
- Trauma may have some effects that require as much as 12–96 hours to become apparent, and subtle signs of illness, such as lethargy or vomiting, several days following trauma should not be overlooked.

Vehicular trauma

KEY POINTS
- A primary survey consisting of rapid evaluation of cardiac, neurological, and respiratory systems should be performed and immediate therapy initiated prior to evaluation of wounds or fractures (141).
- Fluid therapy should be initiated if shock has been identified, and continued until improvements in heart rate, mucous membrane color, pulse quality, and mentation are observed.
- Thoracic radiographs should always be performed to rule out injuries such as rib fracture and diaphragmatic hernia, and to look for evidence of pulmonary contusion.

DEFINITION/OVERVIEW
Injuries that occur secondary to vehicular trauma range in severity from mild to life-threatening. In order to maximize the chances of a positive outcome, a systematic approach to the trauma patient is essential.

PRIMARY SURVEY
Examination of major body systems, including the CNS, cardiovascular system, and respiratory system should be performed immediately. The goal of the primary survey is to identify injuries which require immediate intervention, such as hypovolemic shock, respiratory distress, and head trauma.

Signs of shock include pale mucous membranes, tachycardia, weak femoral pulses, and, in some cases, altered mentation. Hypovolemic shock may result from massive sympathetic stimulation, blood loss (internal or external), or reduced venous return secondary to tension pneumothorax. Identification of shock necessitates immediate administration of intravenous fluids to restore intravascular volume. Administration of supplemental oxygen via face mask or flow-by may be beneficial in the patient with respiratory distress.

A proper history should include whether or not the animal was able to stand, bear weight on

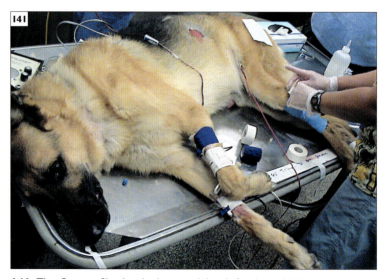

141 This German Shepherd is being stabilized after being hit by a car.

all limbs, or walk following the traumatic event. A cursory neurological examination should be performed in all animals following vehicular trauma. Scleral hemorrhage, facial abrasions, and epistaxis are all supportive of head trauma. While physical examination findings suggestive of head trauma do not require specific therapy *per se*, changes in neurological status must be noted so that therapy to reduce intracranial pressure can be instituted if necessary. In addition, facial swelling, as well as blood accumulation in the nasal passages, may lead to respiratory difficulty.

SECONDARY SURVEY

Once major body systems have been assessed and appropriate treatment has been initiated, a secondary survey can be performed to identify emergencies which are not life-threatening, such as wounds and fractures that require attention once hemodynamic stability has been restored . All wounds should be cleaned, explored, and closed, either primarily if minimal contamination has occurred, or over a drain if necessary. All penetrating wounds to the thorax and abdominal cavity warrant full exploratory surgery to assess the degree of internal injury and to remove all foreign material. If possible the animal should be encouraged to stand and walk to ensure that no obvious fractures are present. If the animal is unable to stand, then both an orthopedic and neurological examination are warranted to identify injuries, such as long bone or back fractures, that may have an impact on overall morbidity and cost of care. Fractures should be stabilized until surgical repair or casting can be performed.

DIAGNOSTIC TESTS

A minimum database consisting of PCV, total solids, dextrose, and azo-stick determination should be performed in all animals having sustained vehicular trauma. In dogs, splenic contraction and subsequent release of red blood cells into the circulation may mask the anemia associated with hemorrhage. The PCV must always be evaluated along with total solids, as total solids <60 g/l (<6.0 g/dl) should raise the index of suspicion for blood loss (in the absence of underlying disease causing hypoproteinemia). If available, lactate analysis is a helpful tool in evaluating the patient for hypoperfusion or shock. Hyperlactatemia in the trauma patient is generally due to reduced tissue perfusion

secondary to hypovolemic shock, and warrants immediate fluid therapy to restore effective circulating volume.

Thoracic radiographs are almost always indicated to identify the presence of pulmonary contusion, pneumothorax, rib fractures, or diaphragmatic hernia. Although nonspecific, the size of the cardiac silhouette and the caudal vena cava can be helpful in determining the severity of hypovolemia.

Abdominal radiographs can be helpful in identifying injuries including large-volume abdominal effusion, body wall hernia, and diaphragmatic hernia. Since radiographs are relatively insensitive for the detection of small volumes of fluid accumulation, the use of ultrasonography is preferred for the identification of abdominal effusion.

MANAGEMENT / TREATMENT

Venous access is instrumental in the management of the trauma patient. As the primary survey is being performed, a large gauge, short over-the-needle intravenous catheter should be placed in a peripheral vein for rapid fluid administration. Long catheters should be avoided due to the inability to administer large volumes in a short period of time. Baseline information, including heart rate, respiratory rate and temperature, can be recorded, and, if available, ECG leads can be placed for continuous heart rate monitoring and for the identification of cardiac arrhythmias.

Intravenous fluids in the form of crystalloids can be administered for the treatment of hypovolemic shock. A shock dose of 90 ml/kg/hr for the dog and 45–60 ml/kg/hr for the cat can be calculated, and administered in increments until improvements in heart rate, mucous membrane color, pulse quality, and mentation are observed. As many animals will require less than the calculated shock dose of intravenous fluids to restore hemodynamic stability, frequent patient re-evaluation is required to tailor fluid therapy to individual needs. In the presence of significant pulmonary contusion, hemo-abdomen, or head trauma, over-resuscitation should be avoided, as excessive fluid therapy in these cases can lead to worsening of clinical signs and the need for mechanical ventilation or blood-product administration.

Animals with pulmonary contusion may benefit from oxygen supplementation. Animals with significant pneumothorax should have thoracocentesis performed. Oxygen can be administered using nasal cannulae, or through the use of an oxygen-rich environment provided by an oxygen cage. Persistent respiratory distress despite oxygen supplementation may indicate the need for sedation, intubation, and intermittent positive pressure ventilation.

Once hemodynamic stability has been restored, supportive care, including intravenous fluids and pain medication, can be provided. Reversible agents with minimal cardiovascular depression such as opioids are preferred. Potentially nephrotoxic agents should be avoided in those animals that have recently experienced a period of hypoperfusion.

DELAYED ILLNESS

Due to the possibility of internal injuries that take several days to cause clinical signs, any animal that has experienced vehicular trauma should be monitored carefully for several weeks for signs of lethargy, inappetence, or vomiting. The two main injuries to consider for those animals showing signs of illness several days to several weeks following trauma include biliary tract rupture with subsequent bile peritonitis, and septic peritonitis secondary to mesenteric avulsion. Other injuries, such as organ-associated thrombosis, are also possible, ultimately leading to necrosis (i.e. splenic necrosis).

A complete examination should be performed in any animal with even vague signs of delayed illness following vehicular trauma, and findings such as fever or tachycardia should be investigated promptly. The finding of a fever should prompt the emergency clinician to perform diagnostic tests such as a CBC, biochemistry profile, lactate concentration, and diagnostic imaging, including thoracic radiographs and abdominal ultrasonography. Documentation of free abdominal fluid should be followed by abdominocentesis, and cytological findings of septic, suppurative inflammation (neutrophilic inflammation with intracellular bacteria) warrant an exploratory laparotomy. Bile peritonitis is also a surgical disease and prompt abdominal exploratory surgery is warranted.

Degloving wounds

Degloving wounds are common sequelae to vehicular accidents. They are so named as a large portion of skin and underlying soft tissue is sheared away from the bone (142).

MANAGEMENT

Management involves meticulous cleaning and debriding of the affected tissues. General anesthesia is mandatory. If the patient is too unstable for anesthesia due to other wounds, the wounds should be clipped if possible and covered with a sterile bandage. Most wounds require several days of wet-to-dry bandages, followed by daily bandage changes for 7–10 days, then every 2–3 days. Most wounds will actually heal very nicely despite an initial dramatic appearance (143).

PROGNOSIS

The prognosis is generally good, although there may be weeks of bandage changes before healing is complete. In some cases, due to the extent of the tissue trauma, amputation may result in a more rapid return to function at least cost to the client.

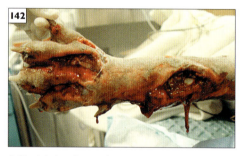

142 A Labrador with a severe degloving wound.

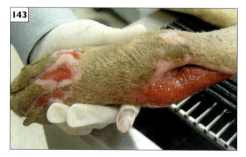

143 The same dog, 14 days later.

Bite wounds

KEY POINTS
- Bite wounds are often more extensive than they appear on the surface.
- Wounds should be thoroughly cleaned and debrided to decrease infection.
- Antibiotic therapy is warranted in dogs and cats with bite wounds.

DEFINITION / OVERVIEW
Bite wounds are commonly observed in veterinary patients, comprising approximately 10–15% of the traumatic injuries seen in dogs and cats. The actual frequency of bite wounds may be even higher, as some owners may not seek medical attention for wounds believed to be superficial. (See also Chapter 12.)

ETIOLOGY
Bite wounds are the result of animal–animal interactions. They are usually accidental, although occasionally they are malicious. It is necessary to determine the rabies vaccination status of animals in endemic parts of the world.

PATHOPHYSIOLOGY
Because dogs possess such powerful jaws, bite wounds inflicted by dogs typically cause severe crushing injury in addition to punctures and lacerations. Once the teeth penetrate through the skin, shaking and pulling frequently result in avulsion of the skin from its subcutaneous attachments and tearing of the subcutaneous tissue, muscle, vasculature, and underlying structures. The skin itself may still appear relatively intact as it tends to be more elastic and moveable than the underlying structures. For this reason, superficial-appearing skin wounds should be regarded as only 'the tip of the iceberg'.

Bacteria from the attacker's mouth, as well as hair and debris from the victim's skin, may be driven deep into the wounds, leading to contamination of devitalized tissues. The presence of dead space and accumulation of fluid or blood further contribute to the development of severe infections. Up to two-thirds of canine bite wounds in veterinary patients may become infected, frequently with multiple isolates. The most common aerobic isolates include *Staphylococcus intermedius*, *Enterococcus* spp., coagulase-negative *Staphylococcus*, and *Escherichia coli*. There tends to be a predominance of anaerobes in the oral flora of dogs and cats, and as a result, *Bacillus* spp., *Clostridium* spp., and *Corynebacterium* spp., have also been frequently isolated from dog bite wounds.

Feline bite attacks are more likely to result in small, deep puncture wounds because of their sharp, pointed teeth and lesser tendency to shake their victims. Cat-inflicted bite wounds are also more likely than dog-inflicted wounds to become infected, with *Pasteurella* spp. most commonly isolated.

CLINICAL PRESENTATION
Clinical signs attributable to dog-inflicted bite wounds typically relate to the location of injury, severity of underlying damage, and the presence or absence of infection. The neck and extremities are the most commonly reported wound locations, followed by head, chest, shoulder region, and abdomen. Frequently, multiple body parts are involved. Neck wounds may result in severe bleeding due to disruption of the jugular vein or carotid artery. Injuries to the trachea or larynx may result in airway obstruction or subcutaneous emphysema. Esophageal perforation may lead to esophagitis, abscessation, or stricture formation.

Wounds to the extremities may result in pain, lameness, hemorrhage, and swelling. Nonweight-bearing lameness should prompt suspicion of severe muscular injury, joint penetration, fracture, or abscessation. Variable degrees of skin laceration or avulsion may be present.

Wounds overlying the thoracic or abdominal cavity should always be presumed to be penetrating until proven otherwise. Thoracic wounds may result in pneumothorax, contusion, severe hemorrhage, rib fractures or flail chest, and pyothorax. Penetrating bite wounds to the abdomen may cause penetrating, tearing, or crushing injury to the GI tract, liver, spleen, pancreas, kidneys, bladder, or ureters. Abdominal wall hernias may also be present, whether or not skin penetration has occurred.

Feline bite wounds may be more difficult to identify as the small puncture wounds may contract or be hidden by fur. Lameness and fever are among the more common presenting complaints. Frequently, owners do not identify cat bite wounds until the wounds become abscessed.

MANAGEMENT / TREATMENT

Appropriate management of bite wounds consists of clipping and cleaning, wound debridement, lavage, establishment of drainage, and antibiotic therapy. All dog-inflicted bite wounds (with the possible exception of the distal extremities) should be surgically explored, as superficial skin wounds frequently hide more significant underlying damage. The practice of probing bite wounds with an instrument should not be performed as it frequently underestimates injury severity. Probes may not be able to follow the path of a bite wound through the various planes of moveable fascia and may therefore fail to identify large pockets of dead space.

The cleaning and debridement process should proceed from the outside inward (i.e. starting with the skin and wound margins before moving on to the deeper portions of the wound) in order to avoid dragging contaminated material from the periphery deeper into the wound. A #40 clipper blade works best for clipping the skin surrounding bite wounds. A small amount of sterile, water-based jelly may first be applied to the wound to prevent contamination of the deeper tissues with hair and debris. Once the wound has been clipped, the skin surrounding the wound may then be scrubbed with a surgical scrub solution, such as povidone–iodine or chlorhexidine. The interior of the wound should not be scrubbed with these preparations, as they may be irritating to delicate tissues. Hydrogen peroxide is not considered an effective antimicrobial, and its use within wounds should also be avoided.

Sterile gloves and drapes should be used for wound debridement. The contaminated wound margins should be excised, and the incision extended if needed to facilitate exploration of the wound. All devitalized tissues should be excised using a scalpel blade or Metzenbaum scissors. Lavage should be performed during the debridement process to facilitate removal of bacteria, hair, and debris from the wound. Sterile 0.9% NaCl is typically adequate for this purpose. The addition of antibiotics to lavage solutions has not been shown to be beneficial. Lavage may be performed using a bulb syringe, a plastic 1 liter bottle of sterile saline with several holes punched in the lid, or a 35 ml syringe with an 18 ga needle. This syringe may be attached by a three-way stopcock to a bag of sterile saline in cases when copious lavage is needed.

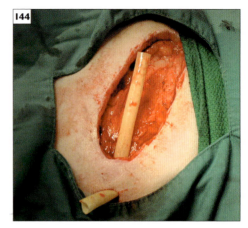

144 Placement of a Penrose drain. The drain is anchored at the dorsal aspect of the wound with a suture passed through the skin. The drain exits through a separate site ventrally, and is sutured to the skin at this site to prevent dislodgement or retraction into the wound. (Photograph courtesy of Dr B. J. Stanley)

Once a wound has been adequately debrided, the decision can then be made as to whether the wound may be safely closed or should be left open for drainage. It is *never* appropriate to close bite wounds that have not been aggressively debrided. Wounds in which all devitalized tissue has been removed, with adequate blood supply, negligible dead space, and no evidence of infection may be closed primarily. More commonly, some form of drainage is needed because of the presence of dead space, compromised blood supply, or contamination. The simplest method of providing drainage is to simply leave puncture wounds open to allow healing by second intention. This form of drainage is most effective for small puncture wounds and wounds involving the extremities. For slightly larger wounds with moderate amounts of dead space, passive drainage using 6 mm (¼ inch) or 12 mm (½ inch) Penrose drains may be employed. Following debridement, Penrose drains are anchored at the dorsal aspect of the wound and allowed to exit from a separate site ventral to the wound (**144**).

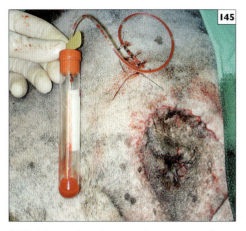

of ascending infection, and the ability to quantitate discharge. Disadvantages include expense, need for in-hospital maintenance, and possible occlusion of drains as a result of kinking or thick discharge.

When managing degloving wounds, severely infected wounds, wounds with questionable tissue viability, or wounds with excessive necrotic tissue or foreign material, staged debridement may be needed. Wet-to-dry bandages may be used to facilitate staged debridement. Following surgical debridement, sterile gauze squares are moistened and placed within the wound. These are then covered by dry gauze, another layer of absorbent bandage material, and finally by a protective porous outer layer. The moistened gauze is allowed to dry and to adhere to the contaminated wound. Each time the bandage is changed, the sponges mechanically debride the wound, pulling away necrotic tissue and foreign material. Once a granulation bed begins to form, the bandage may be replaced with a non-adherent dressing. Wet-to-dry bandages typically need to be changed as often as twice daily initially until the amount of discharge decreases, and then once daily until a granulation bed has formed.

Antibiotic use should be strongly considered for moderate to severe bite wounds in veterinary patients. Although antibiotic therapy is considered controversial in human patients with dog-inflicted bite wounds, veterinary patients are more likely to have their wounds become contaminated with fur and debris, and may be at greater risk for sepsis. Because Gram-positive, Gram-negative, and anaerobic pathogens are frequently isolated from bite wounds, broad-spectrum coverage with an antibiotic such as amoxicillin/clavulanate potassium is indicated. Alternatively, combined therapy with amoxicillin and enrofloxacin may be used. First-generation cephalosporins alone are not considered appropriate therapy as they may not be effective against anaerobes or Gram-negative bacteria, such as *Pasteurella* spp.

145 A butterfly catheter and vacutainer tube may be used to provide closed-suction wound drainage. (Photograph courtesy of Dr B. J. Stanley)

The drain should not be run directly underneath the suture line as this may decrease blood flow to the healing incision, nor should the drain exit directly from the wound.

Closed-suction drains may also be used in large wounds, or in areas such as the face and ears where even small amounts of dead space are undesirable. A 'poor man's' drain can be constructed from a butterfly catheter and vacutainer tube (**145**). The Luerlock is cut from the plastic tubing of the butterfly catheter, and the tubing is then fenestrated using a scalpel blade. The plastic tubing is inserted into the wound through a separate exit site, and is held in place with a purse-string suture. Following wound closure, a vacutainer may be attached to the butterfly needle to provide continuous suction, and may be changed each time it becomes full. Larger closed-suction drainage systems are commercially available. Advantages of closed-suction drains include the provision of drainage in areas with poor dependent drainage, the ability to keep wounds and dressings dry, a reduced risk

PROGNOSIS

Most bite wounds heal uneventfully, but severe wounds to the chest or abdomen may be life-threatening. A guarded prognosis is warranted in cases of severe injury.

Gunshot and stab wounds

OVERVIEW

Gunshot and similar wounds represent an uncommon source of injury to dogs and cats. Most dogs are injured in hunting accidents, while cats are more often shot maliciously or accidentally (146, 147). Some dogs are injured by police during attempts to apprehend their owners.

If it is unclear, it is wise to try to determine the origin of the injury. In cases of malicious intent, appropriate authorities should be alerted. In some cases, bullet fragments are found incidentally on radiographs performed for another purpose.

CARE

The basic tenet for care of the gunshot wound involves careful attention to the patient-stability, including assessment of the cardiovascular, pulmonary, and neurological systems (148). Wounds should be evaluated on a case-by-case basis. Abdominal gunshot wounds should all be explored via a celiotomy; it is impossible to

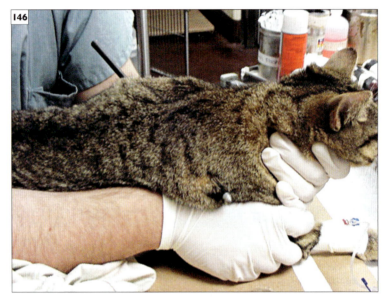

146 A cat shot with an arrow.

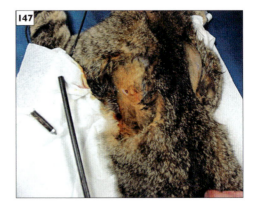

147 The arrow after removal.

exclude significant internal damage from evaluation of surface wounds. Many intra-abdominal gunshot wounds have intestinal disruption or damage. Thoracic wounds that are not accompanied by severe hemorrhage or pneumothorax *may* occasionally be treated conservatively.

Wounds to extremities are commonly accompanied by severe soft tissue trauma (**149–151**). Amputation or extensive surgical reconstruction may be required. Smaller bullet fragments or buckshot may not need to be removed.

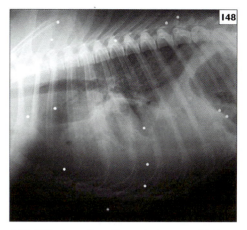

148 This thoracic radiograph shows multiple metallic densities (bullet fragments/buckshot) as well as pleural effusion. The effusion is blood, from a lacerated major vessel.

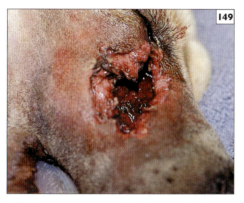

149 An entrance wound on the muzzle of a Labrador that was inadvertently shot while hunting.

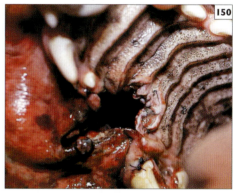

150 The exit wound in the mouth.

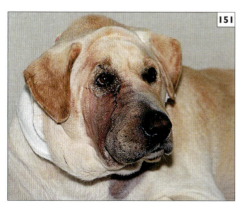

151 The dog himself.

Emergency fracture management

KEY POINTS
- Fractures should not be addressed until cardiovascular stability has been restored.
- Fractures may only be stabilized and bandaged if the joints above and below can be strictly immobilized.

OVERVIEW
Patients presenting to the emergency room with fractures and luxations have sustained significant trauma. Overall, it should be stressed that the treatment of fractures, wounds, and other orthopedic injuries is to be addressed only when the vital signs of the patient are stable. There are instances when the orthopedic injuries and wounds may be a major contributor to the patient's overall debilitated state and, if to, they may assume a higher level of importance. But in general, fractures are to be dealt with only after the patient is hemodynamically stable.

FRACTURE IDENTIFICATION AND CLASSIFICATION
Careful assessment of the trauma patient is critical in properly identifying fractures. As in any routine thorough physical examination, all parts of the appendicular and axial skeleton should be evaluated in a systematic fashion. Each limb is examined in turn from the digits to the axial skeleton articulation. Close attention is to be paid to each articulation looking for crepitus, instability, or subluxations and luxations, as well as to each long bone for any derangements, swellings, and regions of pain that suggest a fracture. The limbs are examined for neurological abnormalities at this time, and underlying neurological deficits are noted, as these can significantly alter outcome and prognosis. Vascular compromise and ischemia are to be noted in the distal limbs. As the limbs are evaluated, any open wounds should also be noted, as these will affect the classification of the fracture. The axial skeleton is evaluated next in a systematic fashion. Careful evaluation is made of the head, jaw, and cervical spine for pain or instability. The spine is palpated along the dorsum, checking for areas of malalignment along the dorsal spinous processes or areas of swelling and pain. Tail injuries are common, and tails should always be checked for fractures and injury.

Any spinal fracture takes precedence above other fractures and injuries. Immediate stabilization and restriction of activity must be imposed to prevent re-injury. Spinal fracture patients may require sedation for immobilizaton. As with any spinal trauma, patients are to be strapped to a rigid supportive structure (a back board) to minimize movement. Tape, velcro straps, or bandage material can be utilized to secure the patient to the board.

In the absence of a spinal injury, any identified fracture in the appendicular skeleton is next classified as open or closed. Open fractures comprise anywhere from 5% to 10% of all fractures that present to the emergency room, and require rapid treatment and emergency management. Open fractures are fractures in which the soft tissue covering of the bone has been compromised, allowing the bone to be exposed to the outside environment. They are rated as grade I–III depending on the severity of the soft tissue compromise and degree of bone exposure. Grade I open fractures have a small wound associated with the fracture site but no visible bone within the wound, indicating that the bone briefly penetrated the skin at the moment of injury. A grade II open fracture results when there is sufficient soft tissue trauma and compromise to allow gross exposure of the bone, but the bone is still viable and relatively clean. A grade III fracture occurs when there has been severe soft tissue loss and gross contamination, either through exposure or duration, which results in devitalization, compromise, and, often, loss of some of the bone. Shearing or degloving injuries of the extremities would fall into this final category.

RADIOGRAPHIC IMAGING
Definitive diagnosis and classification of the fracture can only be achieved with radiographic imaging. This may be painful for the patient, and requires careful positioning of the limbs, so sedation and pain medication should be considered. A *minimum* of two complementary views are required with any fracture to visualize fully the nature of the injury. If there is injury to a joint with suspected instability, stressed views of the joint to identify the specific region of instability should be obtained. The fracture can then finally be identified with specific terminology to describe the injury completely. The fracture is named based on six identifying characteristics:

- Open or closed.
- Location within the bone (diaphyseal, proximal, or distal).
- Degree of comminution.
- Degree of displacement.
- Fracture shape (spiral, transverse, oblique).
- Bone involved.

For example, a patient could be described as having an 'open, mid diaphyseal, highly comminuted, moderately displaced, spiral fracture of the right tibia'. Once the fracture has been properly identified and visualized, proper treatment and temporary stabilization can be accomplished.

OPEN FRACTURE MANAGEMENT

All open fractures are considered contaminated wounds, but are treated initially with the application of sterile dressings to protect the underlying tissues. After patient stabilization, the wounds are flushed and cleaned. Sterile lubricating jelly is placed into the wound bed to allow the hair in the area of the wound to be clipped without contamination of the wound bed. The wound can be flushed with sterile isotonic saline with or without 0.04–0.05% chlorhexidine solution to hydrate the tissues and remove any gross contaminants. An 18 ga needle used with a 20–35 ml syringe will result in an adequate lavage pressure. Highly pressurized pulsatile devices are to be avoided, as the high pressure generated can drive contaminants deeper into wounds and injure soft tissues. In serious soft tissue wounds, any devitalized tissues should be debrided and debris removed from the wound bed. A sterile, nonadherent dressing with a protective, padded layer can then be applied gently to the wound. If gross contamination is still suspected after initial debridement (as in a grade III open fracture) then a wet-to-dry bandage should be applied. A wet-to-dry bandage should consist of a moistened (not soaking), sterile, rough sponge applied into the wound bed. The 'wet' layer is only one layer thick and is applied only to the wound surface, not to the surrounding intact dermal surfaces. This initial layer is followed by successive layers of dry, sterile gauze and absorptive bandage material to 'wick' debris out of the wound and into the initial contact layer. When this bandage is changed 12–24 hours later, the changing of the now dehydrated bandage should debride the wound surface.

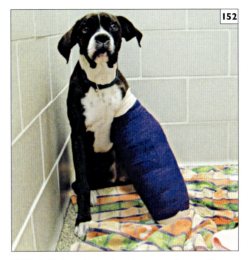

152 A Robert Jones bandage may be used to immobilize fractures of the radius and ulna.

BANDAGING / SPLINTING OF FRACTURES

The type of protection and/or stabilization used is based on the location and nature of the fracture. First, the location of the fracture/injury must be considered. Fractures may only be stabilized and bandaged if the joints above and below can be strictly immobilized. This is easily accomplished with fractures at or below the level of the elbow or stifle, but almost impossible with femoral and humeral fractures, unless specialized splints or support rods are created. Very distal physeal fractures of the femur and humerus in immature animals can be bandaged to reduce swelling and pain, but in general, bandaging of fractures of these bones should be avoided. Without stabilization of the joint above (the hip or the shoulder, in these cases) the weight of the bandage creates a fulcrum, which results in greater fracture distraction, destabilization, and pain.

The degree of soft tissue damage should be considered next. Wounds requiring a wet-to-dry bandage or those with significant soft tissue trauma and swelling are generally treated with heavy soft padded bandages alone. A Robert Jones bandage (**152**) is a large pressure bandage (usually 4–8 cm thick) using many layers of

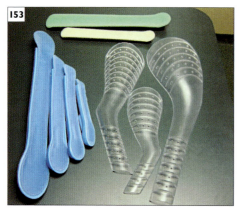

153 An emergency veterinary hospital should have an assortment of bandages and splints available for the traumatized patient.

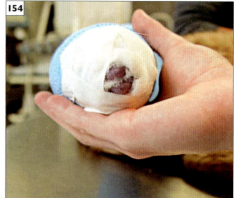

154 This bandage was applied too tightly, resulting in blue discoloration to the cat's toes.

compressible bandage material to create stability and reduce swelling and tissue edema (see Chapter 18). If minimal soft tissue trauma is present and the location of the fracture is amenable to splinting, then a modified Robert Jones bandage can be used, with a resultant thickness of 1–2 cm. If a splint is to be applied, the amount of bandage material should be just enough to protect the soft tissues and create a smooth surface for the splint to be applied. As the thickness of the supporting bandage increases, the stability provided by the splint decreases.

Splinting can be accomplished in a variety of ways to achieve stability. Splints can be prefabricated or customized, and can be made from a variety of materials, including fiberglass casting tape, hard and moldable plastics, and metal sheets or rods. There are many prefabricated splints available in a wide array of shapes and sizes to meet the needs of the emergency clinician (**153**). These commercially available splints are very easy to use and apply, but have limitations. Not all prefabricated splints will be appropriate for all animals. Chondrodystrophic, excessively long-limbed, or juvenile patients can be difficult to fit properly with these ready-made splints. For these patients, a customized splint made with bent support rods or thermodynamically moldable plastics will usually be superior. The most rigid

structure for external coaptation is the full cast, created with encircling layers of fiberglass casting tape. A full cast is custom-designed to fit the patient's own anatomy, is very rigid when used in several layers, and is lightweight and comfortable when properly applied. The full cast should always be bivalved (cut along the sides) at the time of placement to create a clamshell effect. This will allow for soft tissue swelling underneath the bandage and facilitate future bandage changes.

All bandages are placed from the distal extremities (digits) and continued proximally to the area of interest (**154**). A bandage is never placed just over the area of interest, as this creates a tourniquet-like effect. All bandages should be created with three basic layers. The first layer, the contact layer, is composed of a non-adherent sterile material, and is applied to any wound surface. Then the padding and compressive layer is applied, which is created with soft cotton to create the padding and followed by roll gauze applied with steady even pressure from the distal limb moving proximally to distribute even tension over the area. The third and final layer, the tertiary layer, is applied to provide protection of the underlying layers. This layer is not to be applied with any tension, but is simply a supportive layer applied with at least 50% overlap of the material as it is applied.

Reproductive emergencies

- **Dystocia**

- **Pyometra**

- **Neonatal emergencies**

- **Male reproductive emergencies**

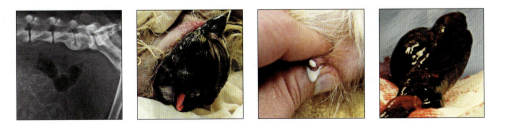

Many of the reproductive abnormalities that present as emergencies are straightforward and relatively easy to resolve. Treatment of these diseases, however, requires knowledge of the underlying pathophysiology as well as the options available for dealing with such emergencies. Many breeders are well informed about the latest developments and expect their veterinarians to be as well. This chapter will discuss the most common reproductive diseases that present to the emergency veterinarian and provide treatment options and recommendations for each.

KEY POINTS

- Early C-section is a valuable tool for maximizing neonatal survival.
- Pyometra should be ruled out in all intact females that present with signs of systemic illness.
- Medical treatment of pyometra may be successful in dogs without signs of systemic illness.

Dystocia

OVERVIEW

Appropriate management of dystocia requires that the client be well educated and able to recognize signs of impending problems (**155**). Once dystocia does occur, there is typically a small window of opportunity to save the unborn puppies or kittens. An algorithm for the general approach to dystocia is given in **156**.

The first question to be answered is 'What is the expected whelping/kittening date?' Ninety-nine percent of dogs whelp 63 days after ovulation (the day progesterone rises above 15.9 nmol/l [5 ng/dl]). By establishing this date, the owner can be appropriately prepared for whelping and the timing of an elective C-section, if desired, can be established. As the expected whelping date nears, the owner should take the bitch's temperature once or twice daily. A fall in temperature to below 37.2°C (99°F) indicates that the bitch will begin labor within 24 hours. Owners, particularly first-time breeders, should be instructed how to prepare a whelping area and how to deal with a normal uncomplicated whelping.

SIGNS OF FETAL DISTRESS
Vaginal discharge
Off-colored discharge (green, red, or brown) from the vagina *prior* to labor is a sign of fetal distress. If discharge is seen an emergency C-section should be performed if the goal is to have as many live puppies or kittens as possible.

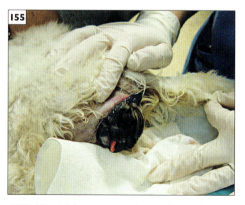

155 This Maltese was inadvertently bred to a Labrador. The resulting fetal–dam size mismatch contributed to dystocia.

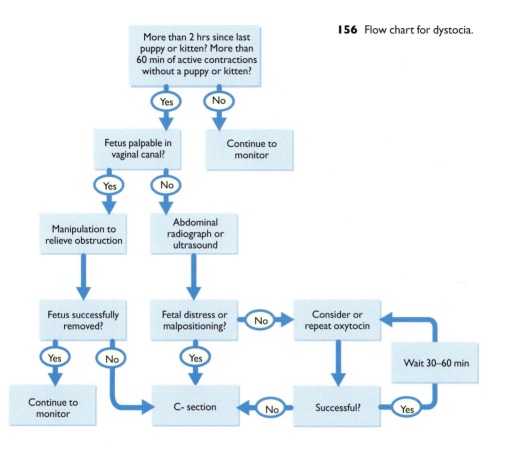

156 Flow chart for dystocia.

Time delay between stage 1 and 2 labor

If the dam takes longer than 2 hours between the initiation of labor and the birth of the first puppy or kitten, a C-section should be considered.

Time delay between puppies or kittens

It is not unusual for cats to take several hours between kittens, but a pause of more than 4 hours is a cause for concern and the queen should be examined. If a bitch is in active labor and more than 1 hour passes between puppies, the bitch should be examined to determine if a puppy is malpositioned or any other problems exist.

Fetus lodged in the birth canal

A small birth canal can result from healed pelvic fractures, vaginal strictures, vaginal prolapse, and so on. The puppies or kittens may be too big to pass through a normal-sized canal. In some dog breeds, such as the Bulldog, the conformation of the breed is such that the wide-bodied, wide-headed pups frequently cannot pass through the pelvis. Bulldogs also have poor uterine contractility. C-section is routinely done in these breeds. When litters are very small (one or two pups or kittens) the feuses may grow to be too large to pass easily through the canal. Fetal monsters and anasarcous fetuses may also cause problems.

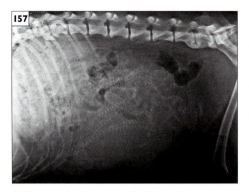

157 Lateral radiograph of a bitch with uterine inertia showing a fetus positioned at the pelvic inlet without signs of fetal distress.

DIAGNOSIS

A physical examination should be performed in order to identify any systemic illness that might contribute to a difficult birthing, such as anemia from torn uterine vessels or sepsis from a uterine rupture. A digital vaginal examination should then be performed in order to detect obstructions or the presence of a wedged fetus. Radiographs may be helpful to evaluate fetal size and number, and any possible abnormalities of the pelvic canal. Serum calcium and glucose should be measured to detect low concentrations which may prevent adequate contractions, although these are uncommon causes of dystocia.

Dystocia due to failure of the uterus to push the fetus into the birth canal can be divided into primary uterine inertia and secondary uterine inertia. Primary uterine inertia is recognized by lack of abdominal press. In some instances when the litter is small, parturition does not occur normally. It is hypothesized that there is not enough hormonal stimulation from the small number of fetuses to induce the normal process of parturition. Diagnosis of primary uterine inertia is based on the failure of parturition to occur within the expected period, or better, or the failure of labor to follow a drop in temperature within 24 hours. Secondary uterine inertia follows a period of apparently normal labor, which then ceases. Diagnosis is based on the lack of labor, without problems involving the birth canal (no impingements or stuck puppies or kittens) (**157**).

TREATMENT

If there is absolute fetal oversize or inadequate pelvic diameter, a C-section should be performed. If there is only one large baby or fetal monster wedged in the canal, one can try to manipulate it. In some cases gentle traction and the addition of lubrication will allow the fetus to pass. However, in many cases this approach is unsuccessful.

Bitches and queen cats with primary uterine inertia are usually healthy with normal calcium concentrations. Oxytocin (see Appendix 3) is the first line of treatment, however most animals with primary uterine inertia will not respond to oxytocin. C-section is indicated and is usually successful if done within 24 hours of the drop in rectal temperature.

In cases of secondary uterine inertia, plasma glucose and calcium should be measured, if possible, to find out whether there is a deficiency. Supplementation should only be given in cases with a documented deficiency. Treatment is administration of oxytocin. If no active contraction is seen within 20 minutes, the dose can be repeated. If no puppy or kitten is born after two doses of oxytocin then a C-section is indicated. Oxytocin should not be used in cases of narrowed birth canal, fetal malpositioning, and fetal oversize.

Pyometra

Pyometra is an endocrine-related disease in the female, less common in cats than dogs. Although a bacterial infection is involved, it is the presence of progesterone (during diestrus) that has allowed the disease to occur. Pyometra occurs almost exclusively in bitches in the 2 months following estrus (during the luteal phase). The cause is related to progesterone-induced excess glandular activity, low myometrial activity, and cervical closure, causing accumulation of secretions that allow bacterial overgrowth. The most common bacteria involved is *Escherichia coli*. The source of infection is probably the vagina, as *E. coli* is a common vaginal inhabitant. Estrogen enhances the effects of progesterone and may increase the chances of pyometra.

CLINICAL PRESENTATION

Pyometra is most commonly seen in older bitches, but may occur in young bitches. The pertinent history is that the bitch was in heat within the last 2–3 months. Signs can occur as early as the end of estrus. Bloody or purulent discharge is usually noted by the owner. In some cases, there is no discharge (closed-cervix pyometra). In these cases, the bitch presents not as a reproductive problem (vulvar discharge) but as a medical problem (systemically ill). The most common clinical sign is PU/PD. Pyometra should always be ruled out in any intact female that is ill. The bitch may not show any systemic signs of disease, or depression, anorexia, PU/PD, or vomiting may be observed. Clinical signs of illness are more common in a closed-cervix pyometra. Fever is variable, as temperature may be normal or even low. Depending on the severity of the disease, the bitch may also be anemic and dehydrated. Untreated, pyometra leads to worsening dehydration, endotoxemia, shock, coma, and ultimately death.

DIAGNOSIS

Ultrasonography is diagnostic; a fluid-filled uterus is seen dorsal to the bladder and extending into the abdomen (158). Radiology is less sensitive, but may document the shadow of a large uterus (159). White blood cell count is usually elevated, often $>30 \times 10^9/l$ ($>30,000$ cells/mm^3). In some cases of open-cervix pyometra, the WBC count can be normal. Since these bitches also may appear healthy, the ultrasound examination is useful in differentiating pyometra from a severe vaginitis.

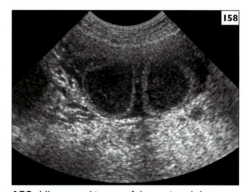

158 Ultrasound image of the canine abdomen demonstrating a fluid-filled uterus consistent with pyometra.

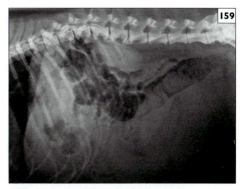

159 Lateral radiograph of a dog with pyometra showing a large fluid-filled uterus.

TREATMENT

The treatment options for pyometra are the same for both cats and dogs, except medical management is not recommended for cats.

Fluid therapy should be instituted in order to correct dehydration or shock, if present. OHE is the treatment of choice. In the severely ill animal, the uterus is the source of the endotoxemia, and must be removed as soon as possible (**160**). Surgery should be performed as soon as the animal is rehydrated and is cardiovascularly stable.

If the animal's reproductive potential is of great importance to the owner, medical management may be attempted. Medical management should not be attempted in the severely ill bitch. Additionally, medical management is not as successful and has a higher complication rate in bitches with closed-cervix pyometra. It is generally recommended to limit medical management to those bitches with open-cervix pyometra that are not systemically ill.

Medical management involves the use of PGF$_2$ alpha. Bitches in the second month of diestrus (>30 days after estrus) will respond to treatment better, as the corpus luteum is more mature and thus more easily lysed.

Recommended procedure:
- The bitch should be placed on broad-spectrum systemic antibiotics.
- The bitch is given PGF$_2$ alpha (only the natural salt, e.g. Lutalyse®, should be used); 0.25 mg/kg SC q24hr for 3–5 days.

This dosage causes side effects including panting, salivation, trembling, vomiting, and diarrhea. The side effects lessen after repeated doses as the bitch appears to become refractory. Pre-treatment with atropine or glycopyrrolate (glycopyrronium bromide) can greatly diminish the side effects while maintaining the effectiveness of treatment. Walking the dog for 10–15 minutes after treatment may help alleviate side effects as well. Following medical management, the general attitude of the bitch should start to improve quickly. The bitch is re-evaluated 2 weeks after treatment. The amount of fluid in the uterus should be markedly decreased or absent, the white blood cell count should be decreased and there should be no discharge or only a serous or clear mucus discharge. If these signs of resolution are not present, the bitch should go through the series of injections a second time or an OHE should be performed.

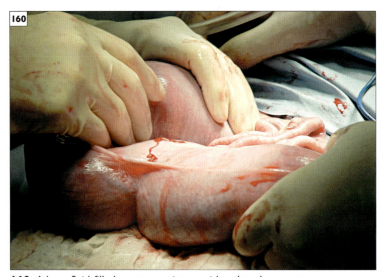

160 A large fluid-filled uterus consistent with a closed pyometra.

Neonatal emergencies

KEY POINTS
- Malnutrition is common in fading puppies and kittens.
- Normal neonatal body temperature is lower than adults and overheating should be avoided (*Table 42*).
- Neonates have greater fluid needs than adults.

OVERVIEW
Puppies and kittens are considered neonates from birth until 3 weeks of age. Animals in this age group can make very challenging patients due to the difficulties associated with examining, obtaining blood samples, and establishing vascular access in such small fragile patients. Most neonates present to the emergency clinician for 'fading' or doing poorly. An underlying reason for this failure to thrive is never identified in the vast majority of cases.

Trauma has been reported to account for up to 30% of these cases. Other possible causes include congenital defects, such as a cleft palate, infectious disease, such as herpes virus, and poor husbandry. A complete history will aid the veterinarian in differentiating between these causes. The owner should be specifically questioned about whether or not the neonate successfully nursed, since failure to do so could indicate inadequate colostrum intake. If a single puppy or kitten is presented for examination, the status of the rest of the litter should be ascertained.

In many cases no underlying disease process will be identified, and the care provided will be strictly supportive in nature.

HYPOTHERMIA
Neonates rely upon transfer of environmental heat in order to maintain body temperature. Normal neonatal temperature is 35.6°C (96°F) during the first week of life and increases by approximately 0.5°C (1°F) per week until normal adult body temperature is attained. Puppies and kittens with a temperature <34.4°C (<94°F) will stop feeding and heat-seeking behavior (**161**). Many neonates that fail to thrive do so due to inadequate heat in the whelping box.

Hypothermic neonates should be warmed using a heating pad or circulating warm water blanket. Care must be taken not to overheat the neonate. This is best achieved by providing a 'warm' and a 'cool' area of the cage and allowing the neonate to move between them as needed.

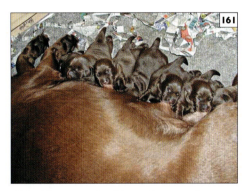

161 All puppies should stay close together. An isolated puppy may be prone to hypothermia, and may rapidly fade.

Table 42 Normal heart rate, respiratory rate, and temperature for neonatal puppies			
Age	Heart rate (bpm)	Respiratory rate (breaths/min)	Temperature °C [°F]
0–24 hours	200–250	15–35	34.4–36 [94–96.8]
1 week	220	15–35	36.1–37.2 [97–99]
2 weeks	210	15–35	36.4–37.2 [97.5–99]
3 weeks	190	15–35	37.2–37.8 [99–100]
4 weeks	150	20–35	37.8 [100]
5 weeks–adult	100–130	20–24	38.3–39.2 [101–102.5]

FAILURE OF PASSIVE TRANSFER

In cases where there is a suspicion of inadequate transfer of maternal antibody, additional antibodies should be provided in the form of either plasma or serum. The serum or plasma can be administered either subcutaneously or intraperitoneally at a dose of 20 ml/kg. In the first 24 hours after birth, serum or plasma may also be administered orally at the same dose to provide immunoglobulins.

HYPOGLYCEMIA

The normal neonatal blood glucose can be as low as 2.22 mmol/l (40 mg/dl). Because of their limited glycogen stores and immature liver, newborns can become hypoglycemic after just 2–3 hours without food intake. Clinical signs of hypoglycemia can include flaccidity, weakness, or coma. The severity of signs does not always correspond to the degree of hypoglycemia.

Treatment should consist of rapid intravenous infusion of 25% dextrose followed by a CRI of 5% dextrose. Additionally, the underlying reason for the hypoglycemia should be aggressively sought.

DEHYDRATION/HYPOVOLEMIA

If it is not possible to establish intravenous access, an intraosseous catheter may be placed. This is most easily performed using a hypodermic needle placed into the medullary cavity of the femur. It should be remembered that neonates have higher fluid requirements than adults. Maintenance fluid rate for neonatal puppies and kittens is approximately 90 ml/kg/day. In addition to providing for maintenance needs, fluid rate should be adjusted to replace any ongoing losses or dehydration. Fluids may be given subcutaneously in more mildly affected neonates (162). It should be noted that heart rate is not an indicator of cardiovascular status in puppies and kittens since heart rate is dependent upon body temperature. Bradycardia may be associated with hypothermia regardless of the volume status.

NEONATAL ISOERYTHROLYSIS

This syndrome is rare in puppies, but can occur if the bitch received a blood transfusion prior to pregnancy or has whelped previous litters. Type A kittens born to a type B queen can also develop neonatal isoerythrolysis. Breeds particularly at risk include Cornish Rex, British Short-hair, and Scottish Fold. The neonate is born healthy, but develops severe hemolytic anemia within a few days of nursing due to colostrum-derived antibody attack on red cells. Treatment consists of removing the neonate from the bitch or queen and providing a blood transfusion if required. Additionally, pre-emptive efforts may avoid the complication in breeds of cat considered at risk.

MALNUTRITION

Malnutrition is a common cause of neonatal death. Puppies and kittens may lose weight in the first 48 hours after birth, but they should steadily gain weight thereafter. In many cases, the puppies or kittens will be seen to nurse, but there is inadequate milk production to meet the needs of the litter (163). In this case, the malnourished puppies will not sleep after nursing, but will continue to cry. The bitch should be examined for signs of mastitis since this can lead to decreased milk production.

Puppies and kittens that are being bottle fed frequently become malnourished due to inadequate caloric intake. Owners who are bottle feeding should be especially diligent about weighing neonates. Tube feeding may be a valuable tool since it will save the caregiver time, as well as ensuring the neonate is consuming the desired volume of formula. A small (8–10 Fr) red rubber catheter should be passed down the left side of the oropharynx into the esophagus to the level of the last rib. The tube should be palpated next to the trachea to ensure it has not been inadvertently passed into the trachea. The desired volume of milk replacer can then be slowly fed through the tube.

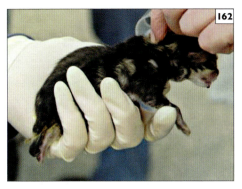

162 This neonatal kitten is receiving subcutaneous fluids for mild dehydration.

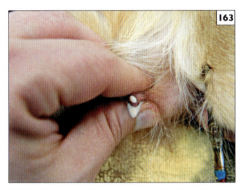

163 Mammary glands can be milked in order to inspect for adequate milk production.

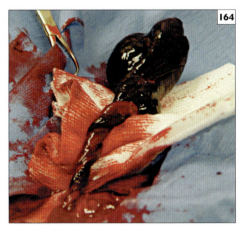

164 A testicular torsion may present with acute abdominal pain and is considered a surgical emergency.

Male reproductive emergencies

PROSTATE

An enlarged prostate gland may result in dysuria and difficulty in defecation. In dogs that are intact (entire), differential diagnoses include prostatitis/prostatic abscess, benign prostatomegaly (BPH) and neoplasia. Dogs with prostatitis or an abscess are typically very painful on digital prostate examination and often show signs of systemic inflammation or infection. In BPH, the prostate gland is symmetrically enlarged and generally not painful, while in neoplasia, the prostate is typically very irregular on palpation and often accompanied by regional lymph node enlargement. Diagnosis is based upon sonographic appearance and histopathology and/or bacterial culture results. Infections respond best to drugs than penetrate the prostate, including fluoroquinolones, trimethoprim-sulfa and chloramphenicol. Some dogs with large abscesses require surgical exploration and marsupialization or omentalization. Most dogs should be surgically castrated to prevent hormonal influences. In neutered dogs, prostatomegaly is almost always neoplasia.

TESTICLES AND SCROTUM

Deep bite wounds to the testicles are most often treated with castration. Occasionally, dogs with paraplegia develop ulcerative lesions on their testicles due to trauma with the ground. Testicular torsions (**164**) appear extremely painful and present with signs of severe abdominal pain. Testicular tumors are common, and typically benign. They will rarely present on an emergency basis.

PENIS

Penile emergencies are commonly divided into trauma, which is often associated with jumping over objects too high for the dog, or priapism (persistent erection). Trauma to the penis should be treated as any other injury, with the caveat to try to maintain the dog in a relatively sedated state as excessive excitement may result in hemorrhage. Priapism in dogs in commonly pseudopriapism, with entrapment and subsequent engorgement of the penis by long fur, or may be due to spinal cord lesions. The penis should be well lubricated and replaced within the prepuce during diagnostic evaluations.

CHAPTER 12

Environmental emergencies

- **Bites and stings**

- **Heatstroke**

- **Hypothermia**

- **Smoke inhalation**

- **Burn injury**

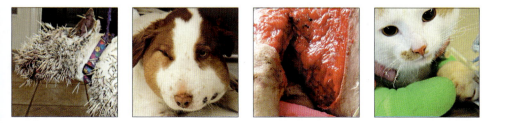

- Prevention of many environmental injuries may be accomplished by good husbandry.
- Rapid restoration of normothermia is critical in heatstroke.
- Hypothermia results in a slowed metabolic rate.
- Carbon monoxide toxicity is common following house fires and supplemental oxygen is advised.

See also Chapter 5 (Toxicological emergencies) for information on poisonous plants.

Bites and stings

OVERVIEW

Inquisitive animals are liable to come across others that would rather be left alone (**165**). Snakes, spiders, scorpions, bees, wasps, and so on, even if not of naturally aggressive species, will strike out in self-defence. Bee stings are more common during warm weather when the insects are active. Spiders and scorpions are more usually encountered in the fall and winter when they move indoors in response to cooler weather. Sick animals frequently present with no known history of a sting or bite. Instead, they present for clinical signs associated with an allergic reaction. Severity of these signs will depend upon the type of venom, location and number of the stings or bites, and sensitivity of the patient.

Local reaction associated with an immunologic response is the most common finding. This may include a swollen head/face (**166**) or diffuse urticaria (**167**). Cases with severe facial swelling can develop respiratory distress from airway occlusion. Less commonly, an animal may develop anaphylaxis. Symptoms of anaphylaxis will develop within 15 minutes of a sting. Anaphylaxis in dogs is manifested as vomiting, defecation, urination, muscular weakness, respiratory depression, and convulsions. Cats most often show signs of pruritis, dyspnea, salivation, incoordination, and collapse. Animals with massive envenomation may show signs of acute respiratory distress syndrome or disseminated intravascular coagulation.

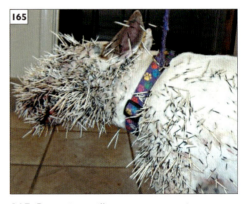

165 Porcupine quillings are common in many parts of North America. The veterinarian should recall the porcupine is *never* the aggressor.

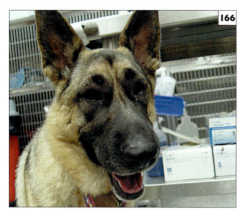

166 Bee stings may result in facial edema and hives (urticaria).

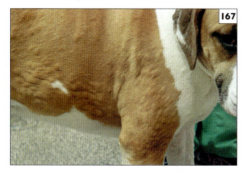

167 A Boxer-x with severe hives (urticaria) secondary to insect hypersensitivity.

Bite wounds from other dogs are common. Some breeds of dogs may be more likely involved in fights, but it should be recalled that any breed of dog may bite. Diagnosis of dog-bite wounds is usually straightforward as most attacks are witnessed.

General treatment for stings
Facial edema/urticaria
- Remove stinger, if present.
- Diphenhydramine 1–2 mg/kg IM.
- Dexamethasone SP 0.2 mg/kg IV slowly.

Anaphylaxis
- Epinephrine 0.01 mg/kg IV.
- Intravenous fluid support.
- Diphenhydramine 1–2 mg/kg IM.
- Dexamethasone SP 0.2 mg/kg IV slowly.

General management of bites
Management of a bite wound involves clipping and cleaning the wound and then determining the appropriate surgical therapy. In all but mild cases, sedation or general anaesthesia is warranted to be able to accurately evaluate the wound. Bite wounds are often much deeper than they may appear from the surface. Wounds with pockets of dead space, except on the distal extremities, should be opened and copiously flushed and debrided. It is common to find hair and debris several centimeters into the wound. Bite wounds over the chest cavity in small animals almost always penetrate the chest, although usually at several intercostal spaces removed from the site of the puncture. Similarly, intra-abdominal wounds may damage the intestines or other internal organs. Pets with abdominal bite wounds should have an abdominal exploratory performed as soon as possible to resect and repair damaged organs. Passive (Penrose) or active drains should be used as needed. Bite wounds should never be closed entirely without a drain due to the high likelihood of contamination. Broad-spectrum antibiotics are warranted. See also Chapter 10.

SNAKE BITES
Most venomous snake bites occur in tropical and subtropical regions, often in agricultural settings where people work barefoot; Southeast Asia, India, Brazil and Africa are heavily represented. Four hundred thousand venomous snake bites are reported annually, and of these, 40,000 result in death.

In the USA, 45,000 snake bites are reported each year, of which 7,000 to 8,000 are venomous. Of these, six to 15 result in death. Of all fatalities resulting from venomous animal bites, 30% are due to snakes; 52% to insects (mostly bee stings), and 13% to spiders. Most snake bites in people occur between the months of April and October, when people (and snakes) are outdoors and more active. This corresponds to a report of dogs with rattlesnake bites.

To be venomous an animal must possess specific glands for producing venom, connected to an apparatus for venom delivery. This is in contrast to animals that are poisonous following ingestion, such as tree frogs or some shellfish.

Venomous snakes

Of the 3,000 known species of snake, 10–15% have been identified as venomous. There are 14 families of snakes, with five containing venomous species. These five families are the Colubridae (boomslang and bird snake), Hydrophidae (sea snakes), Elapidae (cobras, kraits, mambas and coral snakes), Viperidae (true vipers), and Crotalidae (pit vipers including rattlesnakes, water moccasins, copperheads, bushmasters, fer-de-lance). Snakes are found worldwide, with the exception of the Arctic and Antarctic zones, New Zealand, Madagascar, Ireland, and many small islands. Sea snakes are found in the Pacific and Indian Oceans.

Crotalidae (pit vipers)

The most prevalent of venomous snakes in the USA, pit vipers are native to every state except Maine, Alaska and Hawaii. Of the 120 species of snakes indigenous to the USA, 20 are venomous and, except for the coral snake, all are pit vipers.

The pit vipers are classified into 3 main groups: (1) *Crotalus* or true rattlesnake, (2) copperheads and water moccasins, and (3) pygmy and massasauga rattlesnakes.

Pit vipers have a heat-sensing pit between the eye and nostril on each side of the head, which enables the snake to locate its prey. They typically have elliptical pupils, retractable, canalized fangs, and triangular-shaped heads. *The pit is the 100% consistent identifying feature of the pit viper.*

Viperidae (true vipers)

The true vipers are found in Africa, Europe, the Middle East, the Indian subcontinent, and Southeast Asia: they are distinguished from the pit-vipers in that they have no heat-sensing pit.

Elapidae

The Elapidae are found in the tropical and warm temperate zones. They include the cobras, mambas, kraits, coral snakes, and the most venomous snakes of Australia. They have short, fixed fangs and inject their venom in a succession of chewing motions.

The coral snake resembles the non-venomous kingsnake, common in the southern United States. The nose of the coral snake is black, and they have adjacent red and yellow bands. These red and yellow bands are separated by a black band on the kingsnake, hence, the key identifying phrase: red next to black—friend of Jack, red with yellow—deadly fellow.

Identification

The venomous snake can be distinguished from the non-venomous snake by its triangular-shaped head, elliptical pupils, heat-sensing pits, presence of fangs, and characteristic single row of subcaudal plates on the anal plate. Rattlesnakes also have a rattle.

Venom

A traditional classification of venom as hematotoxic or neurotoxic is considered antiquated and not recommended. Major determinants of the pathophysiology of venom include the toxic properties of the venom in addition to the victim's response to it. Most venoms have both hematotoxic and neurotoxic properties. Further classification is based on toxic components, and whether their effects are local or systemic. Proteins comprise 90–95% of venom. The Elapidae and Hydrophidae venoms produce mostly systemic effects, whereas the Colubridae, Viperidae, and Crotalidae produce predominantly local effects.

Major exceptions include the Mojave rattlesnake, which has minimal local effects and deadly systemic effects, and the cobra, that has extensive local tissue destruction.

Local effects are due to a combination of enzymes acting on cellular and noncellular tissues. Examples of systemic effects include coagulation disorders, hemorrhage, hemolysis, and mitochondrial dysfunction. Phospholipase A is found in the venoms of Hydrophidae, Elapidae, Viperidae and Crotalidae; it inhibits electron transfer, hydrolyzes phospholipids in nerve axons, breaks down acetylcholine vesicles at neuromuscular junctions, and results in myonecrosis and hemolysis. Polypeptides are smaller and rapidly absorbed; these account for most of the systemic effects, including changes in pre- and post-synaptic nerve membranes and other distant organs such as the kidneys.

Some venoms may have both local and systemic effects, depending on the snake. Some local syndromes can result in systemic conditions including disseminated intravascular coagulation, pulmonary edema and shock. The victim's response is important, as many venoms contain enzymes that release bradykinin, histamine or serotonin, and may result in anaphylactoid reactions. Effects may be observed for a period lasting from minutes to days, which is why patients are often hospitalized for at least 12–24

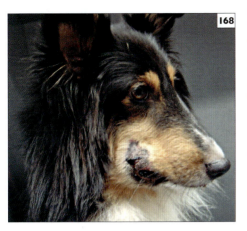

168 A Shetland sheepdog with a necrotic wound from a snake bite. Dogs are almost invariably bitten in the face, while cats receive bites to the belly as they spring backwards.

hours following envenomation. Signs can range from mild erythema or swelling to multi-organ dysfunction and death. Venom is produced in venom glands, and transported via venom ducts and delivered via hollow or grooved fangs. The pit vipers have large maxillary anterior teeth that are hollow and rotate out from resting positions to strike. Alternatively, the coral snakes have hollow maxillary teeth but these are stationary and smaller than those of the pit viper. This differentiates the pit viper, which strikes its prey, from the coral snake that traps its victim and then chews to inject its venom.

Clinical signs and presentation
Signs are based on several factors. In addition to the victim's size, age and overall health, the snake's age, size and overall health are important considerations. Snakes can usually control the amount of venom released, but often this control is lost if the snake is frightened. Also, the fangs are replaced periodically, and their condition may be important. Additionally, the location of the bite (**168**) may influence the effect. In all, the clinical response of the victim may be the only way to judge the severity of the snake bite.

Pit vipers
Following initial burning pain at the area of the bite, subcutaneous edema (**169**, **170**) spreads rapidly. Compartmentalism may occur with massive tissue injury, along with petechiae, ecchymoses, serous or hemorrhagic bullae and skin necrosis. Systemic signs of pit viper envenomation include weakness, vomiting and hypotension. Death can occur and is usually due to DIC, endothelial cell damage and permeability, hypotension, pulmonary edema and multi-organ failure.

Coral snakes and Mojave rattlesnakes
Little pain or swelling is usually noted at the site, and weakness and paralysis result from blockade of acetylcholine receptors. Death occurs as a result of direct inhibition of cardiac and skeletal muscle and respiratory failure. Ptosis is common, and other signs include lethargy, salivation, and nausea. Signs may take up to 12 hours to become apparent.

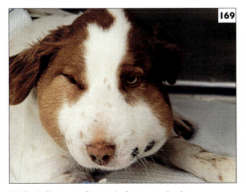

169 A Brittany Spaniel after a snake bite.

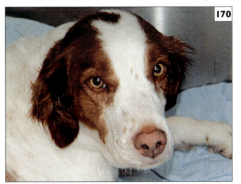

170 The same dog five days later.

Assessment and stabilization

Initial assessment and stabilization are critical, and venomous snake bites should be considered a high-priority emergency. The initial 6–8 hours post-bite are critical, and treatment during this period decreases morbidity and mortality. The type and extent of pre-hospital stabilization rely on the distance between the attack and the nearest hospital. Pre-hospital care is directed at limiting the spread of venom by using techniques that impede lymph flow but not arterial flow. Application of ice or incision into the wound are NOT advised. These have been shown to increase tissue destruction and have been associated with negative side effects. Venom suction is recommended if arriving at the ED within 15 minutes of the attack. Intravenous fluids are recommended for cardiovascular support. Respiratory support should be given if indicated. A complete history, including prior allergic reactions, should be obtained. If possible, the snake should be identified. Sequential neurological examinations should be performed. The area of snake bite should be marked and monitored for spreading tissue destruction. A minimum database including a CBC, serum chemistry profile, coagulation profile and blood type should be obtained. Care in the ED centers on the decision to administer antivenin. A scoring system and algorithm have been developed to assist in this decision. The scoring system grades bites from zero (snake bite is suspected but there are no overt signs of envenomation) to IV (very severe envenomation).

Antivenin therapy

An equine-derived antivenin (Antivenin (Crotalidae) Polyvalent (ACP)) has been the mainstay of therapy for venomous snake bites for 35 years, and it has been used to treat 75% of venomous snake bites in humans annually. It is highly antigenic, and its use may be as dangerous or more so than the snake bite itself. Allergic reactions in people ranged from 23% to 56%, and that rate is even greater for the development of delayed serum sickness. A new ovine-derived antivenin (CroFab) received US FDA approval in 2000 and is now replacing ACP. Ideally, antivenin should be given within 4 hours of the snake bite. Indications include:

- All victims of eastern coral snake bites.
- All victims of Mojave rattlesnake bites.
- All victims of exotic snake bites.
- Others based on the envenomation score.

Antivenin is also recommended for snake bite victims with coagulopathy, rather than the transfusion of blood products, as continued supply of substrate maintains circulation of the venom. Complications of antivenin include serum sickness – a type III hypersensitivity reaction typically occurring 7 to 21 days following completion of therapy. Serum sickness usually responds to a tapering dose of glucocorticoids.

SPIDER AND SCORPION BITES

Spiders and scorpions belong to the phylum Arthropoda – animals with segmented bodies and jointed appendages – which contains 80% of all known species. Of the 12 classes, two – Arachnida and Insecta – contain venomous species. These account for a greater number of human deaths than do snakes, and they are active in both warm and cold months. They can be found indoors, and can be active 24 hours per day. The result is millions of envenomations annually, and often death is due to an autopharmacologic response (anaphylactic reaction) by the victim rather than venom intoxication. Arthropods deliver their venom by stinging, biting, secreting through pores or hairs, or some combination of these.

Arachnids (spiders and scorpions) account for the largest number of venomous species known, with about 20,000 species of venomous spiders, and 1,400 species of venomous scorpions. In the USA, only some 50 species of arachnids are known to cause illness, and this is likely due to limited ability to deliver venom via short fangs or stings. Almost all spider venoms have evolved to paralyze prey, and most cause only minor injury such as local skin necrosis.

Widow spiders (*Latrodectus* spp.)

Five classes of widow spiders are found in the USA, in every state except Alaska. The black widow spider (*Latrodectus mactans*) is the most well-known, but the venom of the brown widow is the most potent. The female black widow is twice as large as the male, and more capable of envenomation. The mature black widow female has a leg span of up to 5 cm (including body), and a body length of 1.5 cm. She has a shiny black color with a red marking on the abdomen that resembles an hourglass. The smaller, harmless male is brown. These are shy spiders, and are found in woodpiles, ground cover, crevices, garages/barns, and outhouses.

Venom

The venom is released from the digestive glands via the venon apparatus (chelicera). It is composed of both protein and non-protein compounds, and it serves to paralyze its prey and liquefy tissue for digestion. The primary active compound is alpha latrotoxin, and it results in an initial pre-release of neurotransmitters from nerve endings, and eventually results in their depletion. Both sensory and motor nerves are affected.

Clinical signs

Clinical signs may be evident within 1–8 hours of envenomation. There may be an initial faint sensation followed by minimal local swelling and redness; two fang marks may be identified. Generally more systemic signs are seen, with cramping pain spreading from the extremities to either the chest or abdomen, depending on whether upper or lower extremities are involved. Cats seems to be more affected than dogs. Other signs that may follow include ataxia, restlessness, nausea/vomiting, dyspnea, and ptosis. Hypertension, cardiac dysrhythmias, and pulmonary edema may occur in severe cases, with fatalities in very small or debilitated patients.

Diagnosis and treatment

Those animals suspected of lactrodectism (widow spider envenomation) should have emergency assessment. The suspected spider should, if possible, accompany the patient (in a container). Many harmless spiders resemble venomous ones, and *vice versa*. A minimum database includes CBC, serum chemistry analysis, urinalysis, coagulation profile, electrocardiogram, and arterial blood pressure. Those patients suspected to have serious envenomation should be considered for lactrodectus antivenin (Lyovac antivenin, Merck, Sharp and Dohme). Patients should be tested prior to administration for sensitivity, and then the vial diluted with normal saline and infused slowly over 15 minutes. Relief of signs is usually obtained within 30 minutes of administration. Supportive care and measures to control hypertension are clearly indicated. Other therapies, including muscle relaxants and benzodiazepines, have no proven efficacy over antivenin but may provide some temporary relief.

Recluse spiders (*Loxosceles* spp.)

Many species of recluse spiders (also known as violin or fiddleback spiders) are venomous and up to five of these are found in the USA: the best known is the brown recluse spider (*Loxosceles reclusa*). As their name implies, these spiders are shy – found in woodpiles, under rocks, in attics or closets. Their bites can become ulcerated or necrotic, and two forms are recognized: 1) cutaneous, and 2) viscerocutaneous. *Loxosceles* bites are the only known cause of necrotic arachnidism. Unless the offending spider is available for identification by a competent arachnologist, a necrotic wound attributed to a spider bite in a non-endemic area should be suspect. Many bites of brown recluse spiders are self-limited, and unwitnessed or unproven spider bites may detract from consideration of more accurate and likely differentials. There is no proven effective therapy for brown recluse spider bites.

Identification

Brown recluse spiders have a pigmented, violin-shaped pattern on the cephalothorax, which helps distinguish them but is an inconsistent feature in young spiders and thus an unreliable identifying trait. A more important distinguishing feature is that they have six eyes arranged in pairs (dyads) with one median and two lateral pairs, rather than eight as in other spiders.

Venom

Although the composition of *Loxosceles* venom is largely undetermined, envenomation is considered a consequence of both the effects of the toxins and the victim's immune response. The primary toxin is sphingomyelinase D. The venom causes an intense thrombosis of the small capillaries, resulting in depletion of coagulation factors and hemorrhage.

Clinical presentation and signs

In the cutaneous form, there is an initial burning followed 3–4 hours later with pain. The area of necrosis progresses from a small, bull's-eye lesion to a small bleb with an eschar in the center. As the bleb sloughs, a slow-healing ulcer remains. In the viscerocutaneous form, systemic signs including hemolytic anemia, thrombocytopenia and DIC are not uncommon. Death can occur from shock, DIC and multi-organ failure including severe pulmonary edema and renal failure. The victim's immune response plays a role in this form.

Diagnosis

Diagnosis depends on a witnessed account of the spider in the act, and/or positive identification of the spider by a trained arachnologist. Differential diagnoses include other infections, immune-mediated processes, and neoplasms.

Treatment

General first aid and supportive care including intravenous fluids, pain management and muscle relaxants remain the mainstay of treatment. First aid includes elevation and immobilization of affected limbs, application of ice and local wound care. There is no consensus on the efficacy of other reported therapies.

Scorpions

Arachnids that resemble crustaceans, scorpions are amongst the oldest terrestrial animals, and are found throughout the world. Many species are found in the southwestern USA, but only one, *Centruroides exilicauda*, found in Arizona, is known to be dangerous. Most scorpions are nocturnal and predatory, and spend their day under rocks, logs, floors and in crevices. *Centruroides exilicauda*, also known as the bark scorpion, is often found on or near trees.

Venom

The last six segments of a scorpion's abdomen form a tail-like structure, with the last segment containing two venom glands. The toxicity of scorpion venom varies among species, with the more dangerous venoms causing more systemic reactions with minimal local reactions. Like other venoms, scorpion venom contains enzymes that cause hemolysis, and others that act as neuro-toxins. *Centruroides exilicauda* contains a neuro-toxin.

Clinical presentation and signs

Common clinical signs include restlessness, fever, nausea/vomiting, hypertension, salivation, seizures, hemiplegia, cardiac dysrhythmias, syncope and respiratory arrest. Some signs can occur in waves over 24 hours, whereas other patients can suffers toxicity severe enough to result in respiratory arrest within 30 minutes.

Treatment

Treatment is largely supportive once in the emergency department, with application of ice to the area of the bite prior to arrival at the hospital. Supportive care includes intravenous fluids and other therapies directed at controlling seizures, cardiac arrhythmias, etc. Antivenin is available for severe *Centruroides exilicauda* envenomations. Patients should be observed for 24 hours.

Heatstroke

KEY POINTS

- Rapid cooling is associated with better outcome. Clients should be instructed to try actively to cool over-heated animals prior to transport.
- Brachycephalic dogs are more commonly affected.
- Early summer days before heat acclimatization may be more deadly.
- Heatstroke can result in DIC, multiple organ failure, and death.

DEFINITION/OVERVIEW

Heatstroke is a nonpyrogenic form of thermal tissue injury that occurs when the internal body temperature rapidly increases (often >41°C [>106°F]) because the imposed heat load overwhelms the body's mechanisms to dissipate the heat. If not rapidly identified and treated it often progresses to a life-threatening state. The condition occurs in warm environments and is therefore most common in the summer months, especially following exercise or confinement to an enclosed area with poor ventilation, such as an automobile.

ETIOLOGY

Factors known to increase the risk of heatstroke include warm humid environments, especially when there is a history of exercise, excitement, or confinement in an enclosed, poorly ventilated area. It has been demonstrated that dogs require a period of up to 20 days for acclimatization to warmer weather and without it there is an increased risk of heatstroke. Lack of this transitional period prior to commencing active exercise may account for the increased number of heatstroke cases seen in the early summer. Restricted access to water and pre-existing medical conditions that prevent proper heat dissipation, such as cardiac disease, laryngeal paralysis, upper airway disease, and neurological disease, may also increase the risk of animals developing heatstroke. A predisposition for brachycephalic, obese, long-haired, and dark-coated animals has been reported. Finally, certain drugs that interfere with heat dissipation and prior episodes of heatstroke may increase the risk of developing heatstroke. Although dogs are more commonly affected than cats, accidental confinement to the clothes dryer is a reported cause of heatstroke in cats.

PATHOPHYSIOLOGY

The pathophysiology of heatstroke is complex and not fully understood. The basic mechanism is that the heat load on the body is greater than the body's ability to dissipate the heat. The source of heat can be exogenous, endogenous, or, most often, a combination of the two. Regardless of the cause, the ensuing rise in body temperature results in a complex interaction of acute physiological alterations associated with hyperthermia (increased metabolic demand, circulatory failure, and hypoxia), direct thermal tissue injury, and inflammatory and coagulation responses. With the initial acute physiological and direct thermal tissue injury there is an alteration in the microcirculation and consequent damage to vascular endothelium of tissues throughout the body, leading to multiple organ dysfunction syndrome. An increase in intestinal permeability may occur due to gut ischemia (most of the cardiac output is diverted to exerting muscles and peripheral organs, such as the skin, in an effort to dissipate heat); this may lead to endotoxemia and the overproduction of inflammatory cytokines and subsequent development of SIRS. Insufficient fluid intake may increase an animal's susceptibility to heatstroke as it can lead to volume depletion and the body attempting to maintain a normotensive state by delivering less blood to the skin, which results in less dissipation of heat and a more rapid rise in body temperature. Cardiac insufficiency also predisposes animals to heatstroke because of an inability to dissipate heat adequately.

CLINICAL PRESENTATION

Clinical signs may be seen as a direct result of thermal injury to the tissues, as a result of physiological responses by the animal to dissipate heat or as a secondary consequence of advanced heatstroke leading to endotoxemia from GI translocation or DIC through activation of the coagulation cascade. Animals usually present with excessive panting (in an effort to increase evaporative cooling), collapse, ataxia, altered mental status, and hypersalivation. The rectal temperature is often >41°C (>106°F), although it is also possible to have a normal or low temperature with advanced stages of shock or if the owner has attempted efforts at cooling the animal prior to presentation. Physical examination findings include hyperemic mucous membranes (due to peripheral vasodilation to promote heat loss), panting, hypersalivation, and tachycardia in the early phases of the disease, which are the consequences of the animal trying to dissipate the excessive heat. Dehydration, reflected by a prolonged skin tent and dry mucous membranes, may also be present.

With more advanced stages of heatstroke signs of multiple organ dysfunction may be present, manifesting as altered mental status, lethargy, cortical blindness, seizures, stupor or coma, abnormal cardiovascular function (weak irregular pulses), cutaneous or mucosal petechiae, vomiting, diarrhea (often bloody), icterus, oligurea, and pale mucous membranes. Secondary activation of the coagulation system or translocation of bacteria from the GI tract may result in concurrent symptoms associated with sepsis or DIC.

DIFFERENTIAL DIAGNOSES

It is important to differentiate heatstroke from diseases that cause fever, such as infection (bacterial or viral), immune-mediated conditions, and neoplasia. As the fever in these patients is the result of an alteration of the set point in the thermoregulatory center of the hypothalamus, these animals often display behaviors that tend to increase the body temperature, such as shivering. They do not usually have a history of heat exposure (e.g. locked in a car, shipping on a hot day, excessive exercise) or display heat-dissipating behavior, such as panting and salivating. In addition, the majority of animals with fever are ambulatory while those with heatstroke are weak, ataxic, and may be unable or unwilling to rise. Endogenous forms of heatstroke include tremorogenic toxins and eclampsia, which can be differentiated from exogenous heatstroke based on a recent history of toxin exposure or whelping, respectively.

DIAGNOSIS

Heatstroke should be suspected in animals that have a temperature >41°C (>106°F), that have a supportive history, and in which other causes of hyperthermia have been excluded. There will often be a history of excessive panting, ataxia, and collapse. The physical examination will usually reveal CNS abnormalities and other signs of multiple organ involvement, including cardiac, pulmonary, liver, renal, and GI dysfunction.

Diagnostic tests

There is no specific test that will confirm a diagnosis of heatstroke. Emergency point-of-care testing should be performed at the time of presentation and should include evaluation of the PCV, total solids, blood glucose, and BUN level (dipstick).

The PCV and total solids are often elevated as a result of hemoconcentration secondary to dehydration, although anemia can also occur as a result of GI blood loss or, possibly, hemolysis secondary to direct thermal injury. The total solids may also be decreased, especially in more advanced stages of heatstroke, as protein may be lost in association with vasculitis, GI injury, and renal injury. Hypoproteinemia at the time of presentation has been reported to be associated with a poor outcome.

Azotemia is common and may be pre-renal or renal in origin. Direct thermal injury to renal tubules, hypoperfusion and microvascular thrombosis may all contribute to renal azotemia. Blood glucose levels may be high, normal, or low. The finding of hypoglycemia is fairly common and has been associated with a poor prognosis. The arterial blood pressure is often low in advanced stages and the ECG may reveal arrhythmias secondary to direct thermal injury to the myocardium or as a result of hypoperfusion and ischemia.

The CBC will often reveal nucleated red blood cells, which may be the result of direct thermal injury to the bone marrow. The platelet count may be low secondary to consumption, especially with concurrent DIC. The white cell count is usually increased, although more severely affected dogs may be leukopenic.

Many chemistry profile values (i.e. renal and liver enzymes) may worsen over the first 24–48 hours and a serum biochemistry profile establishes the baseline values at presentation and helps guide further therapy and diagnostics. Most patients will have an elevation in liver enzymes, which may be a direct result of thermal injury or potentially the result of hypoperfusion. Elevations in creatinine and BUN are also common for reasons discussed above. Electrolyte values are variable depending on the volume status, degree of muscle damage, and the presence of vomiting, diarrhea, and renal injury. It is therefore important to recheck electrolyte values frequently. As DIC can be a serious complication of heatstroke the coagulation system should be evaluated, including at least the PT, aPTT, platelet count, fibrinogen levels, and FDPs.

The blood lactate level can also be evaluated to help detect the degree of hypoperfusion and guide response to fluid therapy. Normal blood lactate levels in the dog are <2.5 mmol/l (<22.6 mg/dl), and values >5 mmol/l (>45 mg/dl) usually indicate significant hypoperfusion if other causes have been eliminated (e.g. seizures or certain drugs and cancers). A significantly elevated blood lactate level that fails to respond to appropriate initial fluid therapy is often associated with a poor prognosis.

A urinalysis is also important to help detect potential renal injury through the presence of proteinuria, hematuria, or casts. Myoglobinuria may also be detected and may indicate rhabdomyolysis.

Other diagnostic tests should be performed on an individual basis, depending on the status of the patient. Thoracic radiographs are indicated in the presence of respiratory compromise and may aid in the diagnosis of pulmonary infiltrates secondary to edema, ARDS, PTE, pneumonia, or pulmonary hemorrhage. A blood gas analysis is also helpful to assess respiratory function and to determine the acid–base status which may reveal an alkalosis, acidosis, or mixed disorder.

MANAGEMENT/TREATMENT

Cooling the patient is critical and should be started immediately. Ideally the cooling efforts should be completed within the first 30 min of arrival. Cooling can be divided into external and internal techniques. External techniques include the application of cold water or soaked cold towels to the skin, the use of a fan to improve convective losses, and the application of alcohol to the footpads, axilla, and groin. The easiest and most important form of internal cooling is the administration of room temperature intravenous fluids (171). Not only does this help decrease the patient's temperature but it also provides continued intravascular support, which is warranted in almost all heatstroke patients. If these techniques fail to decrease the temperature within 30–45 min, more aggressive therapy, such as the use of cool water enemas, gastric lavage, or peritoneal lavage should be considered. It should be borne in mind that cool rectal enemas will interfere with ability to monitor temperature. To avoid hypothermia, cooling efforts should be discontinued when the temperature reaches 39.4°C (103°F) and the temperature should be rechecked frequently to detect recurrence of hyperthermia or the development of hypothermia.

Iced water baths should be avoided as they may result in peripheral vasoconstriction and

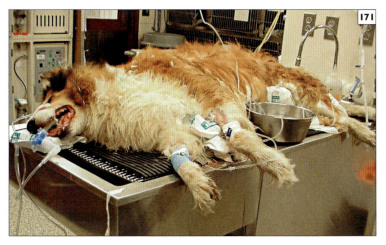

171 Administration of intravenous fluids for heatstroke.

shivering which impede cooling of the animal. In addition, ice water baths may decrease cutaneous blood flow and promote capillary sludging, which can contribute to DIC. Antipyretics, such as aspirin, flunixin meglamate, and ketoprofen, are also contraindicated to decrease body temperature as they are ineffective in cases of heatstroke and may contribute to morbidity and mortality.

In animals that present with signs of shock (hypotension, tachycardia, and weak peripheral pulses), isotonic crystalloids, including lactated Ringer's solution and 0.9% sodium chloride, given at a shock rates (60–90 ml/kg/hr) intravenously until signs of shock are reversed, are good initial fluids. Colloids may be preferable in patients with hypoalbuminemia and decreased COP, as the risk of pulmonary and peripheral edema formation may be lower when colloids are used in these patients. If the symptoms of shock persist after appropriate initial resuscitative fluid therapy, positive inotropes and vasopressors should be considered. These agents should not be used until adequate volume resuscitation has been attempted.

Due to the risk of GI hypoperfusion, ischemia, and bacterial translocation, broad-spectrum antibiotics should be administered. GI protectants, such as an H2 blocker and sucralfate, can also be administered.

In patients that present with seizures, intravenous diazepam or phenobarbital should be given. If the neurological status continues to deteriorate despite initial resuscitative efforts, mannitol can be given to try to decrease cerebral edema; it should be kept in mind, however, that mannitol could potentially increase intracranial bleeding. Steroids have been suggested for the treatment of patients presenting with heatstroke to improve neurological function and guard against some of the concerns with multiple organ dysfunction. However, given the lack of evidence to support any benefit from the administration of steroids in animals or humans suffering from heatstroke, and the enhanced risk of GI bleeding and infection that is associated with steroids, they should be used cautiously.

In patients in which hypoglycemia is documented, a bolus of glucose (1 ml 50% glucose diluted to 25% in saline given intravenously) followed by administration of fluids containing 2.5–7.5 % dextrose is recommended to maintain normal glucose levels.

Oxygen is warranted in most critically ill patients to maximize oxygen delivery, especially if respiratory compromise is present.

In oliguric patients (urine production <1 ml/kg/hr) or in cases where anuric renal failure is suspected, furosemide administration as a bolus or as a CRI may be started to promote diuresis. It is important to be sure the animal is well hydrated and has an adequate intravascular volume prior to administering furosemide, as oliguria is a normal physiological response in dehydrated animals and giving furosemide to these patients can further compromise the intravascular volume and decrease tissue perfusion.

As arrhythmias are not uncommon in severely affected heatstroke patients and the heart rate is often reflective of intravascular volume status, frequent or continual ECG monitoring may be beneficial in the initial resuscitative phase and for ongoing care. If a ventricular arrhythmia develops which is significant enough to affect perfusion (weak pulses, pulse deficits, sustained tachycardia >180 bpm, pale mucous membranes, or generalized weakness), a bolus of lidocaine at 2 mg/kg IV can be given followed by a CRI (40–80 μg/kg/min) if a response is noted.

In patients that display signs consistent with DIC, fresh frozen plasma and standard or low-molecular-weight heparin can also be administered.

The medical state of heatstroke patients can change very rapidly during resuscitation and over the first 24–48 hours of therapy; it is therefore necessary to monitor these patients closely. Depending on the state of the patient, monitoring during initial resuscitation should include:

- Assessment of rectal temperature (continually or every 10 min during the first 1–2 hours of resuscitation).
- Heart rate, capillary refill time and pulse strength (to judge initial response to fluid therapy).
- Blood pressure (may need further fluids or vasopressors if <90 mmHg systolic), CVP (to help determine intravascular volume status and response to initial fluid therapy).
- Urine output (to detect development of oliguric or anuric renal failure).
- Continuous ECG (to detect arrhythmias and help monitor heart rate in response to fluid therapy).
- Serial PCV/total solids, serial blood lactate, serial electrolytes, and serial blood gases.

PROGNOSIS

The prognosis varies with the severity of tissue injury and the presence of any underlying disease that may have contributed to the development of hyperthermia. There is a high risk of serious complications and in patients with evidence of multiple organ involvement the prognosis is poor. However, it has been reported that most animals that die from heatstroke do so in the first 24 hours of the incident, while animals that improve over the first 48 hours have an excellent prognosis, with most making full recoveries.

Hypothermia

KEY POINTS
- Most severe hypothermia is environmental in origin.
- The underlying cause for the hypothermia should be addressed.
- Prognosis is dependent upon extent of underlying disease and severity of hypothermia.

DEFINITION

Hypothermia is defined as a core body temperature <37.5°C (<99.5°F). Hypothermia may be a sign of systemic illness, as a result of inability to maintain the basal metabolic rate, or result from exposure to low environmental temperature.

ETIOLOGY

Severe hypothermia results from exposure to low environmental temperature, such as occurs when an animal is accidentally left outside during extremely cold weather or a fall through of ice. Animals with poor perfusion, such as may accompany CHF, may be hypothermic. Additionally, neonates are often unable to thermoregulate and may rapidly develop hypothermia (**172**). Hypothermia may be protective, as oxygen consumption is reduced.

PATHOPHYSIOLOGY

Mild hypothermia, a core temperature between 35°C and 37.5°C (95°F and 99.5°F), can result from sedation, anesthesia, or short-term exposure to low environmental temperatures. More severe hypothermia results from prolonged

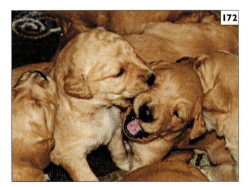

172 Neonates are at great risk for the development of hypothermia.

exposure to low environmental temperatures. When the rectal temperature falls below 27.8°C (82°F), animals lose their ability to return their body temperature to normal, even when brought into a warm environment.

CLINICAL PRESENTATION

Clinical signs will vary widely depending upon the degree of hypothermia. Altered mental states ranging from depression to coma are common. Animals will also frequently exhibit bradycardia and hypotension until the core temperature begins to return to normal. ECG analysis may document a J-wave (Osborn wave), which is a deflection seen at the QRS-ST junction of patients with hypothermia. Additionally, a 'cold diuresis' due to hyperglycemia may be observed. Shivering is common, but will be absent if the core temperature is <31°C (<88°F).

MANAGEMENT/TREATMENT

The patient should be actively warmed using warm intravenous fluids as well as external rewarming with warm towels or blankets. Warm-water bottles may be used, but care should be taken to ensure they do not result in cutaneous burns.

More aggressive rewarming may be indicated in patients with severe hypothermia. Options include warm colonic or gastric lavage as well as peritoneal lavage of warm fluid through a peritoneal dialysis catheter.

Once a patient's temperature has returned to normal, the patient should be evaluated for any other injuries, since animals found outside have frequently sustained some form of trauma that prevented them from seeking shelter.

Animals that are hypothermic due to systemic disease should be treated based upon their underlying condition. For example, animals with CHF may benefit from diuretics and positive inotropes, in addition to being placed in an oxygen-rich and warm environment. Neonates, in particular, should be placed in a warm, oxygen-rich environment to anticipate changes in metabolic rate associated with rewarming.

PROGNOSIS

Animals with mild hypothermia generally have an excellent prognosis. Animals with severe hypothermia that can be successfully warmed to a normal body temperature typically make a complete recovery.

Smoke inhalation

KEY POINTS

- Irritation and swelling of the upper airway are common. Tracheostomy may be required.
- Antibiotics should be avoided unless infection is clearly present.
- Pulse oximetry and arterial blood gas analysis are inaccurate in the face of elevated carboxyhemoglobin concentrations.

DEFINITION

Smoke inhalation results from exposure to burning materials. In companion animals, this most often is due to house fires (**173**).

ETIOLOGY

The effects of smoke inhalation can vary widely depending upon the intensity and duration of exposure as well as the specific toxins inhaled. The exact toxins present in smoke are determined by the type of material that is burned, the amount of heat generated, and the amount of oxygen available for combustion. Smoke inhalation can be associated with tissue hypoxia, thermal injury, and pulmonary irritation/ damage or infection.

PATHOPHYSIOLOGY

Tissue hypoxia occurs due to a decreased inspired oxygen concentration, decreased ability of the blood to carry oxygen (carbon monoxide poisoning), and disruption of the cells' ability

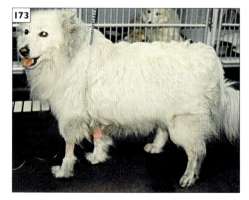

173 A Samoyed which was trapped in a house fire. The fur has been discolored by soot and smoke.

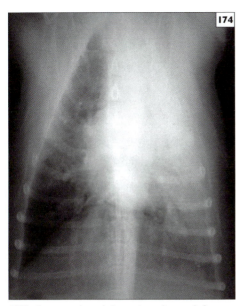

174 A ventrodorsal thoracic radiograph from the dog shown in **173**. There are pulmonary infiltrates and consolidation in the left lung lobes.

CLINICAL PRESENTATION

Clinical signs depend upon the severity of exposure as well as the products burned. Many animals will have only mild clinical signs. Those with severe clinical signs may exhibit loss of consciousness, cough, or dyspnea. The remainder of the physical examination findings will reflect the degree of hypoxia/tissue injury present.

Injury to the cornea and conjunctiva is common and may be manifest as conjunctivitis, rubbing at the eyes, or corneal ulceration. Animals may have cutaneous burns that require appropriate treatment.

Many animals with moderate to severe smoke inhalation will have upper airway swelling that presents as inspiratory stridor. The upper airway swelling can progress over the first 24–48 hours after injury. Animals may be tachypneic or dyspneic on presentation. Those that are dyspneic for >48 hours may have a worse prognosis.

DIAGNOSIS

Evaluation of a minimum database including a PCV, serum total protein, blood glucose, and dipstick for BUN is indicated in all cases.

It should be remembered that pulse oximetry will provide erroneous values in patients with carbon monoxide poisoning. Additionally, arterial blood gas analysis will not accurately reflect true hemoglobin saturation with oxygen. Co-oximetry, if available, will provide direct measurement of carboxyhemoglobin and methemoglobin levels.

Animals with ocular signs should be examined for corneal or conjunctival foreign bodies and the cornea stained to look for ulceration.

Thoracic radiographs are useful to characterize the degree of pulmonary compromise and monitor changes over time. Numerous radiographic changes can be observed, including interstitial, bronchial, and alveolar changes (**174**). It should be remembered that radiographic changes will tend to lag behind changes in clinical status.

to utilize oxygen (cyanide toxicity). Carbon monoxide is the most common toxin produced during combustion. It results from the incomplete combustion of carbon-containing compounds and can be associated with a 75% decrease in the inspired oxygen concentration. In addition, carbon monoxide binds hemoglobin 200 times more tightly than oxygen, resulting in decreased oxygen-carrying capacity. Cyanide is produced by the combustion of numerous natural and synthetic products. Cyanide inhibits oxidative phosphorylation by disrupting the mitochondrial electron transport chain. As a result, cells must rely upon anaerobic metabolism.

Direct thermal injury to the tissue lining the oropharynx and airways results in severe swelling and exudation. There are numerous chemical irritants in smoke, including sulfur dioxide and chlorine gas. These irritants cause direct injury to the airway as well as causing bronchoconstriction.

MANAGEMENT/TREATMENT

The treatment of smoke inhalation is largely supportive. Any patient exhibiting tachypnea or dyspnea should receive oxygen supplementation. Increasing the inspired oxygen concentration will also hasten the elimination of carboxyhemoglobin. Animals with severe upper airway swelling may require tracheostomy. Prophylactic antibiotics are not indicated and all antimicrobial therapy should be based upon clinical indication of pulmonary infection and antimicrobial culture and sensitivity testing.

Bronchoconstriction can be a major clinical component in animals with smoke inhalation. Bronchodilators, such as beta-2 agonists and aminophylline/theophylline, may improve clinical signs. Animals will also benefit from nebulization and coupage in an effort to moisten and dislodge pulmonary secretions. Ocular injuries should be treated as indicated.

PROGNOSIS

In general, animals that are not severely dyspneic on presentation and those that show improvement within 48 hours have a good prognosis. A delayed neurotoxicity has been described in some dogs and cats. Thus, any altered mentation following initial recovery should prompt serious concerns.

Burn injury

KEY POINTS

- Burns may result in substantial fluid losses.
- Meticulous wound care is essential to good outcome.
- Infected burns should be treated with antibiotics effective against *Pseudomonas* spp.

DEFINITION/OVERVIEW

Burn injuries can result from thermal injury, acidic or alkaline household chemicals, or electrical current. Most cases of high-temperature burns, such as from a house fire (**175**) or scalding liquid, result in injury that is immediately evident. Injury from less intense sources, such as a heating pad (**176**) or low voltage electrical cord, may take several days to become evident.

CLASSIFICATION OF BURNS

The severity of burns is determined by evaluating the depth of injury and percentage of the total body surface area affected. Burns are classified as first degree or superficial, second degree or partial thickness, and third degree or full thickness. Superficial burns affect only the uppermost epidermal layers and are characterized by redness, mild swelling, and pain. Partial thickness burns affect the deeper layers of the epidermis but leave the subdermis intact. They are extremely painful and characterized by blistering and exudation. Full thickness burns involve both the epidermis and subdermis. The skin will have a charred appearance. These burns are not painful since the underlying nerve fibers have been destroyed.

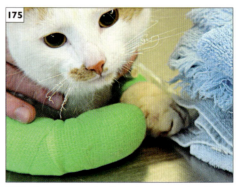

175 A cat recovering from burns sustained in a house fire. The whiskers have been burned and the bandages are covering wounds on the paws.

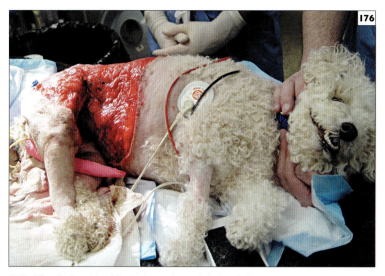

176 This Bichon Frisé had a large dermal defect following surgical resection of a widespread area of burned skin. The burn was the result of a heating pad injury.

PATHOPHYSIOLOGY
Local burn injury

Burns occur when tissue is exposed to a source of thermal injury. The temperature of the heat source, the duration of contact, and the ability of the tissue to dissipate heat all affect the severity of injury. The most severely affected tissue will undergo necrosis. The area adjacent to the necrosis is characterized by reduced blood flow and ischemia. This may also progress to necrosis over 24–48 hours. The tissue farthest from the injury has damage similar to that seen in a superficial burn.

Chemical injury

The injury caused by chemical exposure will vary widely depending upon the specific chemical, its concentration, and the duration of exposure. Most caustic chemicals cause coagulative necrosis and can directly denature proteins. Common caustic chemicals include cleaning agents, paint solvents, furniture strippers, and concentrated flea and tick products.

Electrical injury

Electrical current causes injury by converting current into heat. This results in tissue coagulation. The severity of the injury depends upon several factors including voltage, amperage, duration of contact, and tissue resistance. The injury will be most severe at the point of contact. Electrical injury in North America is most often encountered in small animals when the animal chews through the cord to a household appliance. Burns to the mouth, lips, and gums are common. Electrical injury may also be associated with the formation of NCPE, which typically develops within 24 hours of injury and has a caudodorsal distribution on thoracic radiographs.

Systemic effects

Burns that affect more than 20% of the TBSA will have effects beyond the local injury and can include changes in the cardiac, respiratory, and immune systems. Patients with severe burns are likely to have massive fluid shifts and hypoalbuminemia due to exudation across the damaged dermis. If left uncorrected, these fluid shifts can cause severe cardiac compromise due to hypovolemia. Patients with severe burns are also likely to have smoke inhalation injury, which can compromise respiratory function.

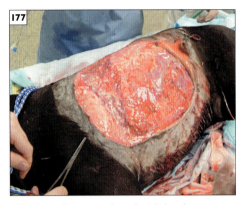

177 Large burn in a chocolate Labrador Retriever due to a heating pad injury. The eschar has been removed, revealing healthy tissues. Eventual wound closure required 6 weeks of wound care.

debridement is likely to be necessary. Removal of the eschar is a key step in preventing bacterial colonization of the wound and subsequent sepsis (**177**).

Large volumes of fluid may be required in patients with severe burns. Fluid guidelines are to infuse fluid volumes as needed to compensate for losses. Additional fluid may be necessary in order to achieve cardiovascular stability.

Antimicrobial therapy is not indicated unless there is evidence of infection. If antimicrobial therapy is instituted an agent with activity against *Pseudomonas* spp. should be selected.

Chemical burns should be copiously lavaged in order to return the skin pH to normal. Solvents and petroleum products can be removed with dishwashing detergent. Tar requires a surface active agent, such as polyoxyethylene, which is present as an emulsifying agent in many commercial triple antibiotic ointment preparations.

DIAGNOSIS

Following stabilization of the major body systems, the first step in patient evaluation is to determine the depth and extent of burns. The clinician should remember that the true extent of the injury may not be apparent for several days as further tissue dies. A minimum database including a PCV, serum total protein, CBC, and serum biochemistry analysis should be obtained. Increases in PCV or serum sodium concentration will reflect loss of fluid due to exudation with subsequent hypovolemia. Thoracic radiographs may document an interstitial or alveolar pattern consistent with smoke inhalation.

MANAGEMENT/TREATMENT

If the patient is seen within 2 hours of injury cold water or saline should be applied to the wound for at least 30 min. This will help to prevent further necrosis. Extremities may be completely submerged in cold water. Tissue should not be packed in ice since this will compromise circulation. After cooling, the wound should be gently clipped of hair and reassessed. Superficial and small partial thickness burns can be covered with triple antibiotic ointment and covered with an occlusive dressing. Deeper or more extensive injury is typically treated without a dressing. Silver sulfadiazine is the most commonly used agent for this purpose. Necrotic tissue will tend to separate from the underlying tissues and serial

PROGNOSIS

Superficial and mild partial thickness injuries typically resolve with supportive care. Patients with burns affecting 20–50% of their TBSA have a guarded prognosis while those with injuries affecting >50% of the TBSA have a poor prognosis.

PART 2

Critical care

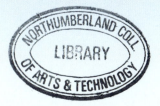

Care of critically ill animals

Major advancements in the care of critically ill animals have been made through improvements in diagnostic, therapeutic, and monitoring techniques. Successful recovery of many patients depends on careful monitoring and attentive adjustments to therapeutic measures. In some patients, recognizing changing trends of particular parameters, rather than simply the actual values, are more useful in evaluating improving or deteriorating status. Another essential aspect of critical care is effective communication among caregivers. The importance of cohesive cooperation among doctors and technicians cannot be overly emphasized. Careful documentation of vital parameters as well as the overall impression of the staff regarding a patient should be communicated whenever primary care is transferred from one team of caregivers to the next.

This section gives an overview of techniques and concepts commonly employed in the care of critically ill patients. Fluid therapy, nutritional support, transfusion medicine, monitoring, and analgesic and anesthetic considerations are the cornerstones of veterinary critical care medicine and each is discussed in its own chapter. These principles are applicable to almost all aspects of critical care and should assist critical care clinicians in formulating the best possible plan for their patients. We continually improve our ability to provide optimal care to our patients through ongoing growth of our understanding of disease processes and through technological advancements (**178**).

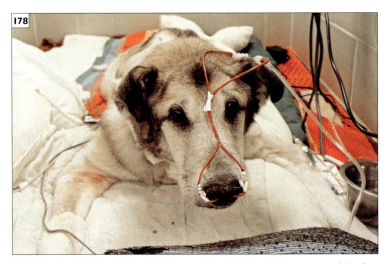

178 A critically ill dog recovering from pneumonia and a laminectomy. Nasal oxygen is used to improve oxygen saturation and patient mobility.

Monitoring critical care patients

- **Monitoring of cardiac function**

- **Monitoring of respiratory function**

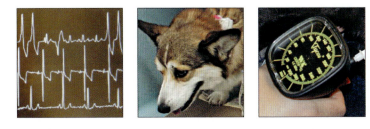

Monitoring of critically ill patients is essential in the evaluation of improving or deteriorating status and allows early interventions to be performed as necessary. A variety of parameters may be monitored using noninvasive techniques. In the most fragile patients changes in vital organ function can occur rapidly, and frequent assessment is absolutely necessary. Continuous monitoring tecniques, such as ECG and pulse oximetry, have become indispensable in many intensive care units. However, all of the techniques discussed are prone to inaccuracies, and therefore they should always be performed in conjunction with careful assessment of the patient by other means, such as by physical examination and blood work analysis. The monitoring techniques outlined should be used to guide clinical decisions, but should not replace other mechanisms of patient evaluation (179).

Monitoring of cardiac function

Monitoring parameters of cardiovascular function provides a great amount of information regarding overall cardiac function, vascular tone and volume, as well as reflecting changes in other systems, such as red blood cell concentration, respiratory function, and blood electrolyte concentrations. Cardiovascular function can be assessed by monitoring heart rate, pulse quality, mucous membrane colour, and by the use of ECG and blood pressure monitors.

ECG MONITORING

ECG monitoring in critically ill patients provides a means to monitor heart rate and rhythm, and placing a continuous ECG monitor greatly improves the early detection of arrhythmias and heart rate changes (180). ECG analysis may provide an indicator of tachyarrhythmias due to hypovolemia, anemia, hypercapnia or hypoxemia; bradyarrhythmias may indicate elecrolyte abnormalities, such as hyperkalemia, or increased vagal tone (e.g. due to elevation in intracranial pressure). Cardiac rhythm abnormalities also frequently occur in intensive care patients; for example, ventricular tachycardia is commonly observed in dogs following surgery for splenectomy, GDV, or septic peritonitis. Even if the arrhythmias are not severe enough to require anti-arrhythmic therapy, continuous ECG

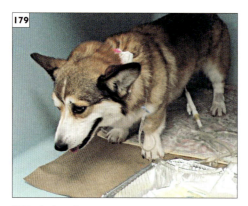

179 A closed urinary system may be used to monitor urine production to help titrate fluid therapy. This Corgi is in the polyuric phase of renal failure and has produced >1000 ml of urine in the previous 4 hours.

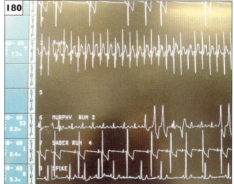

180 A centrally located telemetry unit may provide information on the ECG of a number of patients at one time. In this picture, the ECG tracings from five separate patients may be monitored simultaneously.

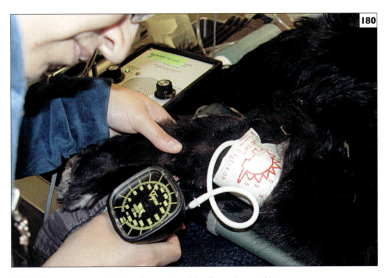

181 Blood pressure being determined by Doppler technique.

monitoring of these patients is beneficial, allowing early detection of worsening of arrhythmias. This may provide an indication that the patient has become hypovolemic, has developed an acid–base abnormality, or has disease recurrence, therefore prompting further diagnostic tests. ECG rhythm abnormalities often precede other clinical signs of patient deterioration and therefore facilitate early interventions before the patient's health deteriorates further.

Although ECG analysis is valuable for following heart rate and rhythm changes, it is important to remember that this is not a good indicator of cardiac contractility. ECG monitoring should therefore always be performed in conjunction with other means of assessing cardiac output and systemic perfusion. This is most easily accomplished by evaluating end-organ perfusion, such as by assessing peripheral pulse quality, urine output, mucous membrane color, and capillary refill time. Most continuous ECG monitors provide a reading of the heart rate, however the ECG tracing should always be evaluated to avoid inaccurate heart rate interpretation. The displayed value of the heart rate is generally obtained by averaging the readings from the previous 5–15 s, and therefore periods of heart block or tachycardia lasting only a few heart beats may not alter the displayed heart rate, despite a significant abnormality occurring that may require further intervention. In addition, the displayed heart rate

is calculated from the rate of generation of R waves. Artifacts, such as muscle twitching or electrical devices, may be mistakenly counted as R waves by the computer, or may result in R waves being indistinguishable from background noise. Other abnormalities, such as large T waves, may also result in an inaccurate heart rate, if the T waves are counted as additional heart beats. In these examples, the displayed and real heart rates may be widely different.

ARTERIAL BLOOD PRESSURE MONITORING

Arterial blood pressure is a major force driving tissue perfusion, and therefore is an important parameter to measure in critical patients. During excessive hypotension (mean arterial pressure <60 mmHg) or hypertension (mean arterial pressure >145 mmHg) decreases in perfusion to major organs may occur. Changes in blood pressure result from changes in stroke volume and vascular tone, and therefore monitoring blood pressure also provides an indication of plasma volume, vasodilation/vasoconstriction, and heart function. Blood pressure may be monitored by:

- Noninvasive techniques, such as automated oscillometric blood pressure measuring devices, or sphygmomanometer and Doppler ultrasonography (**181**).
- Invasive techniques, using an arterial catheter.

The simplest way to measure arterial blood pressure is by the use of a sphygmomanometer and return of flow technique; this includes measurement using Doppler ultrasonography. Other methods of blood flow detection, such as pulse oximetry, stethoscopy, or even manual pulse palpation, can also be used. An inflatable cuff is placed around a limb, and the device being used to detect blood flow is placed distally, for example over one of the digital arteries. If the Doppler technique is being used, clipping the hair and applying a coupling gel prior to placing the Doppler transmitter over the artery aid in the detection of blood flow. The cuff is inflated using the sphygmomanometer, until blood flow is no longer detectable. Further inflation to a greater pressure is unnecessary and may cause pain and increased risk of complications, such as peripheral neuropathy. The cuff is then deflated slowly, using a hand-held manometer as a guide, until return of blood flow is detected, either as an audible signal from a Doppler monitor, as a visible pulse oximeter waveform, or as a palpable pulse. The pressure at which return of blood flow is first detected is a good estimate of systolic arterial blood pressure. Diastolic and mean arterial pressures are less easily measured, but they can be estimated in some patients using Doppler technique. The sounds generated by arterial blood flow vary according to the extent of arterial occlusion: as occluding pressure is decreased to diastolic pressure the sounds generated become more continuous.

Measuring blood pressure by this method is dependent on peripheral blood flow. Erroneous measurements therefore occur in individuals in whom peripheral blood flow is compromised, e.g. due to excessive vasoconstriction or poor cardiac output. This may occur secondary to hypovolemia, vasopressor use, hypothermia, or severe heart failure. Poor peripheral blood flow attenuates sound generation and results in underestimation of blood pressure. Poor compliance of tissues underneath the cuff, for example due to muscle spasm or rigidity, results in an increased cuff pressure required for blood flow occlusion and therefore overestimates blood pressure. Selecting an inappropriate cuff size is a common cause of inaccuracy and, therefore, when measuring blood pressure repeatedly in the same patient, it is pertinent to use the same size cuff for all measurements. The cuff width should be 40–50% of the diameter of the patient's limb, if the patient lies between two cuff sizes it is preferable to use the larger cuff as use of a cuff that is too small results in incomplete transmission of cuff pressure to the underlying artery and overestimation of blood pressure. A cuff that is too large generally produces less error. Cuff deflation rate also contributes to inaccurate readings, especially in bradycardic patients. This occurs even if the low heart rate is normal for the individual, such as in healthy large-breed dogs. The cuff should be deflated slowly enough that the first pulse sound is detected at the correct pressure reading, as rapid deflation will likely result in underestimation of blood pressure. The best accuracy is reportedly achieved when the cuff is deflated at a rate of 2 mmHg per heart beat.

Automated noninvasive blood pressure monitoring techniques produce values for systolic, diastolic, and mean arterial pressures, can be programmed to perform measurements at regular intervals, and reduce the human error associated with rapid cuff deflation rate. However they remain dependent on peripheral blood flow, often failing during severe vasoconstriction or hypotension, and produce inaccurate readings when an incorrect cuff size is used. It is often not possible to obtain oscillometric blood pressure measurements in small patients (e.g. <7–8 kg). These devices function by detecting oscillations in cuff pressure resulting from arterial pulsations. As cuff pressure is decreased and arterial blood flow returns, tiny oscillations in cuff pressure occur which are detected by the blood pressure monitor. The greatest oscillations occur at the mean arterial blood pressure, values for systolic and diastolic pressures are then calculated from this reading. Of the three pressures, the diastolic is the most prone to inaccuracies when measured by this technique.

Direct blood pressure monitoring involves the placement of an arterial catheter (often into the dorsal pedal artery), which is connected by a fluid-filled extension line to a pressure transducer and then to the output monitor. The output monitor then displays an arterial pressure wave tracing in addition to measured values for systolic, mean, and diastolic blood pressures. This method produces the most accurate blood pressure readings, the presence of an arterial catheter also permits blood sampling for arterial blood gas analysis. Inaccurate blood pressure readings may occur if the arterial catheter has become partially occluded by a blood clot, however this generally results in dampening of the waveform on the monitor, and therefore can be easily recognized and corrected by flushing the catheter with heparinized saline. Frequent catheter flushing is necessary as arterial catheters are more prone to occlusion than venous catheters. Other sources of error include the presence of air bubbles within the line connecting the catheter to the pressure transducer; this also tends to dampen the blood pressure waveform and narrow the recorded systolic–diastolic pressure difference.

Disadvantages of direct arterial blood pressure monitoring include technical difficulty associated with arterial catheter placement, especially in small dogs, cats, and patients with poor peripheral perfusion. Continuous blood pressure readings require the availability of monitors designed to measure direct arterial blood pressure. Complications of arterial catheterization are few, however hemorrhage may occur, particularly in patients with severe coagulopathy or if the catheter becomes disconnected from the transducer, leaving it open to the environment. As with any vascular catheter, infection and thrombosis are also possible complications. The arterial catheter should be clearly labelled to prevent accidental intra-arterial injection of intravenous medications.

CENTRAL VENOUS PRESSURE MONITORING

Monitoring CVP provides an indication of intravascular fluid volume, specifically venous blood volume and cardiac preload. Because CVP is also dependent on cardiac output, a high CVP in conjunction with a low cardiac output indicates heart failure. Increasing CVP measurements suggest that the patient is at risk of fluid overload or right-sided heart failure. Conversely a low CVP reading indicates the patient is hypovolemic. CVP measurements are therefore extremely useful in patients that are at risk for both hypovolemia and heart failure (e.g. a patient with hypovolemia secondary to sepsis that also has a history of heart disease). They are also useful in patients whose fluid volume status is confusing, such as a patient that is polyuric or one that is effusing a large volume of fluid into its abdomen, such as in pancreatitis or following certain abdominal surgeries. In patients such as these,

with large ongoing fluid losses, greater intravenous fluid rates than expected are often required to prevent hypovolemia, and utilization of CVP monitoring can help guide fluid therapy.

Normal values for CVP are $0–5\,cmH_2O$. Hypovolemic patients have a CVP $<0\,cmH_2O$, while patients with values $>10\,cmH_2O$ are likely to be volume-overloaded (or have right-sided heart failure). Following the CVP trends is often more useful than single measurements: if a patient has progressive increases or decreases in CVP, or has a sudden change when previous measurements have been constant, this may reflect a change in fluid volume status that requires intervention, even if the CVP value remains within the normal range.

CVP measurements are performed using a central venous catheter, which is introduced via the jugular or femoral veins, and must be of sufficient length to reach either the junction of the right atrium (for jugular venous catheters) or caudal vena cava (for catheters entering the femoral veins). Correct positioning of the catheter is necessary for accurate CVP measurement, and can be verified by thoracic radiography. Once placed, the catheter is connected via a saline-filled extension line and three-way stopcock to a fluid manometer. The manometer is calibrated by positioning the base of the manometer at the height of the right atrium (approximately at the level of the manubrium of the sternum), with the patient positioned in lateral recumbency. During calibration, the three-way stopcock is set to be switched off to the patient's catheter, and open to the manometer and environment. When positioned at the level of the right atrium, the fluid level in the manometer is then set as zero. To take a CVP measurement, the three-way stopcock is then switched on to the patient and manometer, and off to the outside, without moving the manometer. The fluid in the manometer will then move to a new level, corresponding to the patient's CVP. Small fluctuations in CVP occur during the respiratory cycle: the reading should be taken at the end of expiration. Possible sources of error during CVP measurement include incorrect placement or occlusion (by catheter kinking or clot formation) of the catheter, variable patient positioning, and failure to allow enough time for the fluid in the manometer to equilibrate and reach a constant level.

Monitoring of respiratory function

A great deal of information regarding patient respiratory function can be frequently obtained from the physical examination, with increased respiratory rate and effort being commonly associated with abnormal respiratory function. However, additional information regarding respiratory function and the possible sites of pathology (lung parenchyma, upper airways, respiratory musculature, CNS respiratory control centers) can be obtained using monitoring devices detecting arterial oxygen and CO_2 levels. This information is most accurately determined by obtaining an arterial blood gas analysis, which requires an on-site blood gas analyzer.

The functions of the respiratory system are to deliver inspired oxygen into the blood, and remove waste CO_2 from the blood into the lungs. Abnormal function of the respiratory system therefore results in hypoxemia (low arterial oxygen pressure) or hypercapnia (elevated arterial CO_2 pressure). However under certain circumstances, hypocapnia may also indicate abnormal respiratory function, caused by increased respiratory rate and effort as a result of hypoxemia. *Table 43* summarizes the changes in arterial oxygen (PaO_2) and carbon dioxide ($PaCO_2$) pressure that may occur during various respiratory diseases. In the absence of blood gas analysis, these can be evaluated using pulse oximetry and capnography.

PULSE OXIMETRY

Pulse oximetry is performed by placing a light-emitting probe across a peripheral tissue, such as ear pinna or digit. The probe emits light at two wavelengths (red and infra-red), which cross the tissue and are absorbed in varying degrees by arterial blood, venous blood, and other tissues. The remaining light is then detected, and the absorbance calculated. The two light wavelengths used are absorbed by oxyhemoglobin and deoxyhemoglobin and the ratio of the two is calculated to produce the percentage of oxygen-saturated hemoglobin in the blood. No measurement of oxygen dissolved in plasma (usually only a small fraction of the total oxygen content of the blood) is made. Calculation of arterial instead of venous oxygen saturation occurs because of the pulsatile nature of arterial blood. The pulse oximeter detects the oxygen saturation of only the pulsatile components of the light-absorbing tissues, and so displays a value for arterial oxygen saturation (SaO_2). The value for arterial oxygen hemoglobin saturation obtained by pulse oximetry is commonly termed SpO_2 to distinguish from values obtained by arterial blood gas analysis.

Because of the need to detect and distinguish arterial blood, correct functioning of the pulse oximeter is dependent on the detection of pulsatile blood. Under conditions of severely decreased cardiac output, poor peripheral perfusion, or abnormally enhanced venous pulsations, pulse oximeter monitors fail to produce a reading, or display an inaccurate (usually low) SpO_2 value. Many pulse oximeter monitors display a pulse waveform in addition to the SpO_2 reading. This is valuable when attempting to interpret the SpO_2 value displayed, because if the waveform is poor or absent, this suggests poor detection of arterial pulses and therefore increases the likelihood that the value displayed is inaccurate. The quality of the pulse waveform displayed may also be of value in estimating cardiovascular function, since poor cardiac output and/or poor peripheral perfusion result in a poor quality waveform. In the intubated patient, this waveform can additionally be used as an indicator of intravascular volume status, as positive pressure ventilation often results in dampening of the waveform in patients with hypovolemia.

Other sources of error when performing pulse oximetry include skin pigmentation, which may result in poor detection of unabsorbed light, and increased ambient lighting, which can falsely increase the SpO_2 reading. Patient motion may also result in inaccurate readings, however many newer pulse oximeters are designed to function during patient movement. The presence of abnormal hemoglobin species, such as methemoglobin (which tends to produce an SpO_2 reading approaching 85%) and carboxyhemoglobin (which produces a false SpO_2 elevation) also produces inaccurate results. The use of hemoglobin substitutes, such as Oxyglobin®, reportedly do not influence pulse oximeter readings when used at clinically relevant concentrations. The accuracy of pulse oximeters decreases variably as arterial oxygen saturation decreases, with most monitors producing inaccurate readings at SpO_2 values <60–70%. In such severe cases of hypoxemia, blood gas analysis is recommended.

Table 43 Changes in arterial oxygen and carbon dioxide pressures in common respiratory diseases

Respiratory abnormality	Arterial oxygenation	Arterial carbon dioxide
Lower airway disease, e.g. pneumonia, asthma, pulmonary edema, lung collapse (pneumothorax, pleural effusion)	Decreased	May increase (most severe pulmonary compensatory hyperventilation to increase oxygenation), or remain normal
Upper airway obstruction, e.g. laryngeal paralysis	Decreased	May increase, decrease, or remain normal
Hypoventilation, e.g. CNS disease, anesthesia, neuromuscular disease	Decreased (severe respiratory depression) or normal	Increased

CAPNOMETRY

Capnometry measures the amount of CO_2 in expired air (end-tidal CO_2), providing an estimate of the CO_2 pressure in arterial blood. The amount of CO_2 in the air passing through the upper airways varies during the respiratory cycle. During inspiration, low-CO_2 air is inhaled, and therefore the capnograph reads zero. As expiration begins, the amount of CO_2 passing through the upper airways begins to increase, as waste CO_2 is exhaled. This rapidly reaches a peak as CO_2-rich alveolar air is exhaled, giving a value for alveolar CO_2 (end-tidal CO_2) that approximates arterial blood. For end-tidal CO_2 to be detected and accurately reflect arterial CO_2, venous blood must be delivered to the lungs, CO_2 must fully diffuse into the alveolar air sacs, and the expired breath must be a full expiration, such that alveolar air, and not just tracheal and bronchial air (dead space), is detected. Falsely low values of end-tidal CO_2 compared with arterial CO_2 therefore occur if cardiac output is severely impaired, in the presence of severe lung disease or alveolar collapse, or if the patient is panting (dead space ventilation).

To measure end-tidal CO_2 a capnograph monitor lies directly in the stream of expired air (mainstream capnograph), e.g. attached to the end of an endotracheal tube, or continuously samples air from the respiratory circuit (sidestream capnograph). Both monitor types can be placed on a tight-fitting facemask, however greater accuracy is generally achieved by placement on an endotracheal tube, and therefore capnometry is most frequently performed on anesthetized patients. The capnometer monitor is connected to a digital monitor, which displays a value of end-tidal CO_2, with or without a CO_2 waveform.

In patients with healthy lung tissue, the end-tidal CO_2 reading provides a good estimate of arterial CO_2 and therefore is valuable in detecting respiratory depression, e.g. due to CNS depression, neuromuscular disease, or anesthesia. It is also valuable in guiding mechanical ventilation, to avoid either hypo- or hyperventilating the patient. In patients with severe lower airway disease, the difference between end-tidal CO_2 and arterial CO_2 (obtained by blood gas analysis) is helpful in estimating the degree of lower airway pathology. A large difference (greater than 5–10 mmHg, or 15 mmHg in an anesthetized patient) indicates severe lung disease or severe hyperventilation.

Anesthesia and analgesia for critical care patients

- **General anesthetic approach to the critically ill patient**

- **Anesthetic and analgesic agents**

- **Analgesia for critically ill patients**

- **Summary**

Anesthesia for critically ill patients is a subspecialty encompasses a diverse group of patients with varying disease processes that result in increased risk for general anesthesia. The risk may arise for a variety of reasons (*Table 44*). Patients in the intensive care unit often require anesthesia as an emergency, resulting in less time for diagnostics and planning and, often, fewer available personnel. This increases the patient's anesthetic risk, as demonstrated by the increased ASA status given to emergency cases. This scoring system is used to grade patients according to their risk of fatal complications resulting from general anesthesia:

- Category 1. Normal healthy patient. General anesthesia carries minimal risk.
- Category 2. Mild systemic disease, e.g. localized infection, compensated heart disease.
- Category 3. Severe systemic disease, e.g. fever, anemia, mild hypovolemia.
- Category 4. Severe systemic disease which is a threat to life – patient is not expected to survive without procedure, e.g. cardiac decompensation, septic shock.
- Category 5. Life-threatening disease. Patient not expected to survive 24 hours with or without procedure, e.g. extreme shock, severe trauma, terminal malignancy or infection.
- E. Given to emergency cases, increases patient's ASA category 1 level.

(*Adapted from Thurmon JC, Tranquilli WJ, Benson GJ (eds) (1996) Considerations for General Anesthesia. In: Lumb and Jones' Veterinary Anesthesia, 3rd edn. Williams and Wilkins, Baltimore, pp. 3–54.*)

KEY POINTS

- Safe anesthesia requires careful monitoring and strong knowledge of the impact various anesthetic agents have on different organ systems.
- Preparation and anticipation of possible complications are helpful to assure a good outcome.
- Analgesic therapy of critically ill patients should be individualized as there is a highly variable response to analgesics.
- The safest approach to analgesia in critically ill patients includes the selection of readily reversible agents and careful titration.

General anesthetic approach to the critically ill patient

When anesthetizing a critically ill patient, one should consider the patient's individual requirements and, therefore, it is not possible to describe a single critical care anesthesia protocol applicable to all patients. However, a number of principles apply to the anesthesia of all increased-risk patients.

STABILIZATION OF THE PATIENT

The patient must be stabilized as much as possible prior to anesthesia. Many anesthetic agents depress cardiovascular and respiratory function. This causes decreased perfusion and oxygenation of tissues, such as the liver, kidneys, heart, and brain, and is responsible for many adverse events resulting from general anesthesia. In a healthy patient, with intact cardiorespiratory function, anesthetic-induced cardiorespiratory depression does not lead to significant patient compromise. However, when oxygen delivery is decreased prior to anesthesia (e.g. heart disease, anemia, pulmonary disease, or electrolyte abnormalities) or when the function of a failing organ results in the inability to regulate its own blood flow (e.g. renal failure or traumatic brain injury), the added depressant effect of the anesthetic agents may lead to marked reduction of tissue oxygenation.

Optimization of the patient prior to administration of anesthetic agents is therefore essential. This may include intravenous fluid therapy, infusion of red blood cells, correction of electrolyte abnormalities, and improvement of pulmonary function by draining pleural effusions and pneumothorax. Other strategies that should be employed to stabilize the patient prior to anesthesia include reduction of pre-existing elevated intracranial pressure, warming hypothermic patients, treatment of hypoglycemia, and the use of fluid therapy to reduce azotemia in patients with renal failure.

DRUG SELECTION: CARDIAC AND RESPIRATORY FUNCTION

Drugs should be selected that minimally impair cardiac and respiratory function. In addition to promoting tissue perfusion prior to anesthesia, patient compromise can be further minimized by avoiding those anesthetic agents that cause the greatest myocardial, vascular, and respiratory

Table 44 Factors that may increase the risk of complications occurring during anesthetic management

Condition	Effect of condition
Cardiac disease	Decreases ability to compensate for anesthetic-induced cardiovascular depression and maintain cardiac output
Respiratory disease	Decreases ability to compensate for anesthetic-induced respiratory depression and maintain oxygenation. Upper airway disease may complicate endotracheal intubation
CNS disease	Decreases ability of brain to support perfusion during anesthesia
Hepatic dysfunction	Decreases metabolism of certain anesthetic agents, especially infusions of injectable agents
Anemia	Decreases oxygen carrying capacity of blood, and therefore decreases tissue oxygen delivery – this is already compromised by the cardiovascular depressant effects of most anesthetics
Electrolyte changes	Muscle weakness (particularly respiratory muscle), cardiac arrhythmias, and decreased cardiovascular function, hypotension
Hypoglycemia	Decreased muscle function (e.g. cardiac, respiratory), decreased thermogenesis, decreased CNS function
Hypoproteinemia	Decreases protein binding of many anesthetic agents, therefore increases anesthetic and adverse effects
Hypovolemia	Decreases cardiac output, therefore enhances cardiovascular depressant effects of anesthetics. Increases proportion of cardiac output directed to the brain, therefore decreases dose of anesthetic required
Coagulopathy	Increases risk of blood loss resulting from surgery, therefore hypovolemia, anemia, hypoproteinemia may occur during anesthetic period
Hypothermia	Decreases concentration of inhaled anesthetics required; decreases cardiac and respiratory function, increases coagulopathy and infection risk
Hypoadrenocorticism	Decreased ability to tolerate stress, therefore decreased catecholamine release in response to cardiovascular depression; exogenous steroids may be required during anesthetic period
Trauma	Respiratory dysfunction (e.g. pulmonary contusion, diaphragmatic hernia), cardiac arrhythmias, neurological dysfunction (head trauma), hemorrhage may be present
Neuromuscular disease	Neuromuscular weakness (e.g. myasthenia gravis) exacerbated by inhalant anesthetics, may increase respiratory or motor dysfunction after administration of anesthetics
Obesity	Decreases respiratory function, especially when placed in dorsal recumbency, complicates venous access
Neonatal patient	Decreased metabolism of anesthetic agents, increased loss of body heat, decreased development of cardiovascular system, and decreased ability to compensate for cardiovascular depression, risk of hypoglycemia
Small body size	Increases loss of body heat, complicates placement of monitoring equipment
Pregnancy	Decreases respiratory function due to increased intra-abdominal pressure, decreases concentration of inhaled anesthetics required, increases importance of maintaining cardiac output to support fetal perfusion

depression. Agents that best preserve cardiovascular and respiratory function include the opioids (e.g. morphine, fentanyl), benzodiazepines (e.g. midazolam, diazepam), ketamine, and etomidate. In contrast, decreased cardiac contractility, vasodilation, and hypoventilation result from administration of agents such as propofol, thiopental, and most volatile anesthetics (e.g. halothane, isoflurane, and sevoflurane). Except in the presence of severe patient depression, opioids, benzodiazepines, etomidate, and ketamine are unlikely to provide acceptable anesthetic depth when used alone. However when used in combination with additional anesthetic maintenance agents (e.g. volatile anesthetics), the dose of the maintenance agent required can be reduced. Reduction of the dose administered reduces the resulting cardiovascular and respiratory depression.

DRUG REVERSIBILITY

The ability to reverse anesthetic agents enables the removal of any anesthetic-induced patient compromise. Although agents such as opioids, benzodiazepines, and ketamine cause minimal adverse effects, in the presence of severe cardiovascular, respiratory, or neurological depression even these agents may lead to patient instability or prolonged sedation. The use of opioids (reversed using an opioid antagonist such as naloxone) and benzodiazepines (reversed using flumazenil) is therefore beneficial in the most severely compromised patients. Dosing of the reversal agent often needs to be repeated, as both naloxone and flumazenil have relatively short plasma half-lives and are likely to be outlasted by the opioid or benzodiazepine agonist administered. Administration of the reversal agent should always be performed slowly and titrated to desired effect, despite the temptation to administer such agents rapidly when a patient's status is deteriorating. Naloxone in particular is associated with adverse cardiovascular effects if administered too rapidly or at a higher dose than is required for reversal of opioid agonists. Preparing a 1:10 dilution of the reversal agent by dilution in saline facilitates slow intravenous administration of otherwise small drug volumes.

DOSE AND ROUTE OF ADMINISTRATION

Many critically ill patients have increased sensitivity to anesthetic agents. This may occur in shock states, in which a greater proportion of the cardiac output is directed to the brain. The brain, therefore, receives a greater proportion of administered drug, and, in the presence of blood–brain barrier disruption, anesthetic drugs more readily enter central neurons to produce CNS depression. In hypoproteinemia, protein-binding of drugs is reduced and therefore the unbound, active form of the drug is increased. The dose of anesthetic agent required is therefore decreased, however, the amount of dose-reduction required is difficult to predict. For this reason, administration of drugs 'to effect' is advisable. This influences both the drug choice (not all agents may be given gradually, for example the barbiturates are administered as a bolus injection) and the route of administration. Intravenous drug administration allows drugs to be given slowly, until the desired level of sedation or anesthesia is reached. This contrasts with subcutaneous or intramuscular anesthetic induction, when the selected dose is administered completely, increasing the risk of inadvertent patient overdose.

PLANNING FOR POSSIBLE COMPLICATIONS

Complications may result as a direct effect of the anesthetic agent (e.g. hypotension, bradycardia, hypoventilation, hypothermia), from the surgical procedure (e.g. hemorrhage, arrhythmias, pain), or from the patient's disease (e.g. hypoglycemia, electrolyte abnormalities, upper or lower airway disease). Once potential complications have been determined, plans should be made to monitor and treat for their occurrence, and the monitoring apparatus, medications, and other equipment required should be made readily available. Examples of potential complications and the supplies to be provided are given in *Table 45*. Emergency drugs should always be available in the event CPR is required. *Table 46* provides a list of recommended drugs and equipment for an emergency box or crash-cart, which should always be present where anesthesia is performed. This should be checked frequently to ensure medications have not been used or expired.

Table 45 Provisions for possible peri-anesthetic complications

Complication	Examples	Ensure availability of
Hemorrhage	Hepatic surgery, cardiovascular surgery	Blood products, multiple intravenous catheters, intravenous fluids, fluid administration sets
Hypotension	Sepsis	Vasopressors, e.g. dopamine (pre-calculate dose and dilution required), intravenous fluids, multiple intravenous catheters, blood pressure monitor
Cardiac arrhythmias	GDV, splenectomy	Anti-arrhythmic in pre-calculated dose suitable for suspected arrhythmia, e.g. lidocaine if ventricular tachycardia anticipated
Hypoventilation	Thoracotomy, obesity, abdominal distension	Mechanical ventilator, monitors of respiratory function, e.g. blood gas analysis, capnograph, pulse oximeter, supplemental oxygen prior to and after intubation
Difficult tracheal intubation	Brachycephalic airway, laryngeal obstruction	Small endotracheal tubes, tracheostomy kit, supplemental oxygen prior to intubation
Hypoglycemia	Insulinoma, diabetes mellitus	Dextrose infusion, blood glucose monitoring
Intracranial pressure elevation	Head trauma, brain tumors, craniotomy	Mannitol, positive pressure ventilation (to enable hyperventilation)
Hypothermia	Small patient size, prolonged anesthesia	Surface heating devices, e.g. circulating warm-water blankets, forced air devices, hot-water bottles, warm intravenous fluids; thermometer
Pneumothorax	Chest trauma, positive pressure ventilation	Equipment for thoracocentesis: long needle pre-attached to syringe, clippers, and supplies for surgical skin preparation
Hyperkalemia	Urinary obstruction	ECG, serum electrolyte analysis, calcium gluconate, reduction of serum potassium: dextrose, insulin, sodium bicarbonate
Hypocalcemia	Infusion of blood products	Serum electrolyte analysis, calcium gluconate, ECG
Cardiac arrest	Any critically ill patient	Epinephrine, atropine (precalculated doses), intravenous fluids, multiple intravenous catheters, ECG and blood pressure monitors, positive pressure ventilation

Table 46 Contents of the anesthesia emergency box

Emergency drugs	Fluid therapy	Intubation
Epinephrine (0.01–0.2 mg/kg IV)	Crystalloids: lactated Ringer's, 0.9% saline	Additional endotracheal tubes
Atropine (0.01–0.04 mg/kg IV)	Collids: e.g. etherified starch (hetastarch)	Ambubag
Lidocaine (2 mg/kg IV)	Fluid administration sets	Laryngoscope
Dopamine (5–10 µg/kg/min IV)	Administration sets for blood products	Drugs for rapid intubation, e.g. bottle of propofol, etomidate
Sodium bicarbonate (0.3 × body weight (kg) × bicarbonate deficit, IV)	Additional intravenous catheters	
Calcium gluconate (75–150 mg/kg IV)	Pressure bag for rapid fluid administration	
Dextrose (0.25–0.5 g/kg IV)		
Syringes and needles in a variety of sizes. Pre-attached needles useful for rapid drug administration		
Fluid or syringe pump, for administration of precise fluid rates for drug infusions		

All increased-risk patients undergoing anesthesia should have a secured airway and intra-venous access. In the presence of cardiorespiratory depression, administration of supplemental oxygen is necessary to improve tissue oxygen delivery. Patients may also require assisted ventilation and therefore endotracheal intubation should always be performed at the start of anesthesia. Intravenous access is necessary in case the patient requires emergency drug administration, and also permits fluid therapy during anesthesia. Most increased-risk patients benefit from the placement of multiple intravenous catheters, facilitating the administration of fluids, blood products, agents for blood pressure support, and injectable analgesics and anesthetic adjuncts.

CARDIOVASCULAR AND RESPIRATORY MONITORING TECHNIQUES

Parameters that are typically monitored in critical patients undergoing anesthesia include heart rate, respiratory rate, and blood pressure. These parameters allow an estimate of the adequacy of cardiac output, plasma volume, and respiratory function. In addition the use of pulse oximetry, to detect decreases in arterial oxygenation, and capnometry, to give an estimate of arterial CO_2 pressure, provide further indications of respiratory function. Measurement of body temperature is also beneficial, due to adverse effects on cardiac and respiratory function and decreased anesthetic requirement that result from hypothermia. Monitoring these parameters not only enables the anesthetist to follow patient cardiac and respiratory function, but also may provide an early warning of complications, such as hypovolemia, hemorrhage, or lung collapse (e.g. due to pneumothorax or accumulation of pulmonary effusion). The provision of an ECG, although in general less beneficial in assessing cardiac function than assessments of cardiac output (such as pulse quality, mucous membrane color, and blood pressure), is essential when arrhythmias or electrolyte abnormalities may occur. Other monitoring devices that may be required for some patients include urinary catheterization for assessment of renal function, central venous catheterization for CVP measurement, and blood gas and electrolyte analysis.

Anesthetic and analgesic agents

SEDATIVES, ANALGESICS, AND PRE-ANESTHETIC AGENTS

The sedative most commonly selected for compromised patients is a combination of an opioid (e.g. morphine or fentanyl) with a benzodiazepine (e.g. diazepam or midazolam). Both of these drug classes have the advantages of being reversible and having minimal detrimental effects on cardiovascular or respiratory function at clinically used doses. They have a rapid action, and so can be easily administered to desired effect by slow intravenous injection, thus avoiding inadvertent overdose. In patients that have pre-existing cardiovascular or central nervous depression, satisfactory sedation for minor procedures (such as radiographs or thoracocentesis) can be obtained by administering an opioid/benzodiazepine drug combination. This also produces excellent pre-medication prior to anesthetic induction, providing both sedation to decrease the required dose of anesthetic induction and maintenance agents, and pre-emptive analgesia for surgery or other painful interventions. This sedative combination also has few contraindications; in cases of marked CNS depression opioids may cause hypoventilation that is sufficient to produce intracranial pressure elevation, and so respiratory function should be closely monitored in such patients.

When sedation for minor procedures is required, certain patients may not reach an adequate level of sedation from an opioid/ benzodiazepine combination. Examples of situations when this is particularly problematic are patients that are aggressive, but with poor health status, and many cats. Available agents that provide more reliable sedation include acepromazine, which causes vasodilation and hypotension, and alpha-2 agonists, which cause cardiac and respiratory depression. Achieving sufficient sedation for intravenous catheterization is the goal in these patients, after which agents such as propofol or additional opioid can be slowly administered intravenously to achieve the desired depth of sedation. If an opioid/benzodiazepine combination does not produce sufficient sedation to allow intravenous catheterization, a low dose of intramuscular ketamine can be added. This mixture should not be used in cats with hypertrophic cardiomyopathy however, due to the risk of ketamine-induced tachycardia, diastolic failure, and worsening of cardiac function. With the exception of uncompensated heart failure, these cats can usually tolerate a low dose of acepromazine in combination with an opioid, which usually results in sufficient sedation for intravenous catheterization and administration of propofol or etomidate, if necessary for additional sedation.

AGENTS FOR ANESTHETIC INDUCTION

The injectable anesthetic agents that can be used to induce anesthesia include propofol, thiopental, etomidate, and a ketamine/benzodiazepine combination. Pure agonist opioid agents can also be used to induce sufficient anesthetic depth to permit orotracheal intubation; doses greater than those used for analgesia and sedation are required in more healthy patients, however in depressed patients induction of anesthesia may result from administration of a significantly reduced dose. Induction of anesthesia in compromised patients should always be performed by slow intravenous drug administration, in order to avoid anesthetic overdose. Mask induction by volatile anesthetics is also not recommended, due to the difficulty in monitoring depth of anesthesia and high dose of anesthetic required, resulting in marked cardiovascular depression.

Propofol and thiopental are frequently used anesthetic induction agents, however they are of limited value in critically ill patients due to the cardiovascular depression they produce. An exception to this is patients that have CNS disorders; barbiturates, such as thiopental, produce beneficial reduction in brain activity and reduction of intracranial pressure and can therefore be used to enhance brain oxygen delivery in patients with evidence of cerebral ischemia. In other patients alternative induction agents should be selected.

The dose of induction agent required should always be reduced by administration of a premedication agent. Ketamine/benzodiazepine combinations are beneficial anesthetic induction agents in most patients due to lack of cardiovascular depression, however this strategy is contraindicated in patients with CNS disease and cats with hypertrophic cardiomyopathy. Etomidate is also devoid of any effects on cardiovascular or respiratory function, and is therefore

Table 47 Examples of anesthetic protocols for ICU patients

Condition	Pre-anesthetic	Anesthetic induction	Maintenance
Gastric dilation–volvulus	Hydromorphone (0.05–0.1 mg/kg) + diazepam (0.1–0.2 mg/kg) IV or IM	Ketamine (5 mg/kg) + diazepam (0.25 mg/kg) administered IV to effect	Isoflurane + infusion of fentanyl (0.3 µg/kg/min)
Aggressive cat, heart murmur detected, needs radiographs	Oxymorphone (0.05–0.1 mg/kg) + acepromazine (0.02–0.05 mg/kg) IM	Titrate propofol 2–4 mg/kg IV to achieve desired sedation	
Dog requiring C-section	Butorphanol (0.2–0.4 mg/kg) + midazolam (0.1–0.2 mg/kg) IV or IM	Propofol (4 mg/kg) IV	Epidural morphine (0.1 mg/kg) + sevoflurane or isoflurane
Dyspneic dog requiring tracheal intubation (laryngeal obstruction)	Acepromazine (0.02–0.05 mg/kg) IV	Propofol (2–4 mg/kg) IV	Isoflurane + buprenorphine (0.01–0.02 mg/kg) (if surgery)
Cat with severe heart failure requiring surgery for pyometra	Oxymorphone (0.05–0.1 mg/kg) + midazolam (0.1–0.2 mg/kg) IV	Etomidate (0.5–2 mg/kg) or oxymorphone (0.2 mg/kg) IV to effect	Isoflurane + infusion of fentanyl (0.3 µg/kg/min)
Dog hit by a car, pulmonary contusions, surgery for fractured pelvis*	Morphine (0.5–1 mg/kg) + midazolam (0.1–0.2 mg/kg) IM	Ketamine (5 mg/kg) + diazepam (0.25 mg/kg) administered IV to effect	Isoflurane + ketamine infusion (0.6 mg/kg/hr)

*Analgesia for this patient: Morphine (0.1 mg/kg/hr) IV infusion, medetomidine (3 µg/kg/hr) IV infusion

suitable for use in most critically ill patients. In the most severely compromised patients, when an anesthetic technique that is totally reversible is required, induction using opioid agonists should be performed.

AGENTS FOR MAINTENANCE OF GENERAL ANESTHESIA

Maintenance of general anesthesia is usually performed using volatile anesthetic agents, such as halothane, isoflurane, and sevoflurane. Although these agents produce significant myocardial depression (halothane) and vaso-dilation (isoflurane, sevoflurane), these adverse effects can be minimized by reduction of the concentration administered. This is achieved by prior administration of analgesics and sedatives in the anesthetic premedication, administering infusions of additional opioids or ketamine during surgery, use of local nerve blocks, and administration of epidural opioids or local anesthetics. Infusion of propofol provides an alternative to volatile anesthetics, however the degree of cardiovascular depression produced is comparable and therefore this technique generally provides few advantages. If total intravenous anesthesia is selected, the patients will likely benefit from supplemental oxygen administration and assisted ventilation, and therefore tracheal intubation should still be performed. *Table 47* provides some examples of anesthetic techniques used for critical care patients.

Analgesia for critically ill patients

Analgesia for critically ill patients is usually obtained using pure agonist opioids, because of the high potency of analgesic action, reversibility, and low incidence of adverse effects. It is important to individualize analgesic regimens for critically ill patients because disease states can markedly affect drug responses. In the most severely compromised patients, administration of pure agonist opioids may result in unacceptable levels of sedation or cardiorespiratory depression. In these patients the dose of opioid should be reduced. Effective analgesia can still be achieved with a reduced dose by the co-administration of analgesic adjuncts, such as low doses of ketamine, low-dose infusion of medetomidine, or use of local anesthetics. Wound-soaker catheters are useful for local analgesia (**182**). Epidural administration of opioids also provides an effective method of providing analgesia without the adverse effects of systemic administration. The use of NSAIDs can also be considered in patients with adequate tissue perfusion. When used as an adjunct analgesic, an NSAID may allow the use of reduced doses of opioids. Mixed opioid agonists/antagonists, such as buprenorphine and butorphanol, should be used cautiously in critically ill patients, as they are not readily reversible.

Summary

The diverse nature of intensive care patients is reflected in their widely variable anesthetic requirements. However, by optimizing the patient prior to anesthesia, avoiding depression of cardiac and respiratory function, and planning carefully for possible complications, the risk of general anesthesia is reduced. Vigilant patient monitoring during the anesthetic period allows early detection of complications and enables the anesthetist to correct problems as they occur. Optimal analgesia of critically ill patients requires appropriate risk assessment, careful selection of analgesics, and an individualized approach. Despite the many challenges encountered in the treatment of critically ill patients, the astute clinician can provide safe and effective anesthesia and analgesia without compromising patient stability.

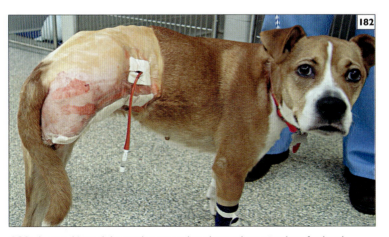

182 A mixed breed dog with a wound-soaker catheter in place for local analgesia following amputation.

CHAPTER 15

Fluid therapy

- **Determining the need for fluid therapy**

- **Choosing the appropriate fluid type**

- **Appropriate routes for fluid therapy**

- **Determining the rate and duration of fluid therapy**

- **Fluid additives**

- **Monitoring and possible complications**

- **Summary**

Fluid therapy is the cornerstone of supportive care. Various disease processes lead to imbalances in fluid, electrolyte, and acid–base homeostasis. Fluid therapy can replace excessive fluid losses, restore organ perfusion, and correct metabolic disturbances. The emergency and critical care clinician should be adept at identifying conditions requiring fluid therapy, choosing the appropriate type and route for administration, and determining the amount, rate, and duration of fluid therapy.

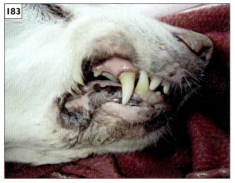

183 Severe dehydration is evident in this dog, as demonstrated by the failure of the tissues to return to their normal positions.

Table 48 Estimation of percentage of interstitial dehydration

Clinical finding	Estimated dehydration
History of fluid loss, slight dry mucous membranes	4–5%
Dry mucous membranes, mild loss of skin turgor	6–7%
Dry mucous membranes, considerable loss of skin turgor, retraction of ocular globe	8–10%
Extremely dry mucous membranes, complete loss of skin turgor, severe ocular globe retraction	>12%

Determining the need for fluid therapy

In the emergency situation, physical examination findings consistent with hypovolemic shock (e.g. tachycardia, bounding pulses, and delayed capillary refill time) necessitate rapid infusion of intravenous fluids. This is commonly referred to as shock resuscitation, and the major goal of this intervention is restoration of tissue perfusion. Physical examination findings consistent with dehydration (e.g. decreased skin turgor, dry mucous membranes) (**183**, *Table 48*) merit more gradual replacement of fluids. In some cases, hypovolemia and dehydration occur simultaneously and this is more frequently encountered in cats. While rapid restoration of volume is achieved by administration of a fluid bolus, rehydration requires more prolonged fluid therapy.

Just as important as physical findings, observations made by the owners are often instrumental in determining the need for fluid therapy. Patients with PU/PD, vomiting, and diarrhea are prone to excess fluid losses, which can result in interstitial dehydration and volume contraction.

Laboratory findings, such as elevated hematocrit, total solids, azotemia, and increased concentrations of electrolytes, are also suggestive of fluid losses and indicate the need for fluid therapy. Demonstration of hypotension in the absence of cardiac failure also warrants fluid resuscitation.

As the primary disease process responsible for fluid losses becomes apparent to the clinician, adjustments to fluid therapy may become necessary. Certain diseases impose obligatory fluid losses which must be accounted for in the therapeutic plan. Animals with vomiting and diarrhea are obvious examples of patients requiring increased amounts of fluid therapy. Other less obvious cases include patients with diabetes, exudative conditions, respiratory distress, and overt anxiety (i.e. excessive pacing and panting). Fluid therapy for these animals must not only restore existing fluid deficits, but also meet continued fluid losses. The amount of additional fluids needed by these patients is not trivial; underestimation of fluid requirements can result in severe electrolyte abnormalities in hospitalized patients, despite fluid therapy.

Choosing the appropriate fluid type

The numerous preparations of fluid types reflect the wide array of fluid-balance disturbances encountered in critically ill patients. Knowledge of the characteristics of the different fluid types is critical in formulating an appropriate therapeutic plan. Fluids are described by their electrolyte content (hypertonic, isotonic, hypotonic), by the presence of large particles (crystalloids, colloids), the nature of the particles present (natural versus synthetic colloids), and by their physiological purpose (replacement, maintenance). The main characteristics of crystalloid fluids commonly used in small animals are listed in *Table 49*.

As the particular abnormalities are identified for a given patient, fluids with particular characteristics may be necessary. For example, fluid-balance disturbance in vomiting animals with severe hypochloremia and metabolic acidosis may be more rapidly corrected with the use of 0.9% NaCl than with lactated Ringer's solution.

Generally, the different fluid types are classified as either crystalloids or colloids. The defining distinction between these solution types is the size of particles dissolved in the solution. Fluid solutions containing only small particles, such as electrolytes, glucose, and buffers, irrespective of their relative concentrations, are defined as crystalloids. These solutions are freely permeable through capillary membranes and distribute largely by diffusion. Fluids containing particles larger than 30 kDa (plasma proteins, synthetic polymers) are defined as colloids. These particles are largely restricted from diffusing through capillary membranes. The importance of these larger particles is that they impart an oncotic pressure which influences fluid dynamics. This pressure, also known as COP, impacts on the flow of fluid

Table 49 Characteristics of commonly used crystalloid solutions

Crystalloid	Na⁺ (mmol/l; mEq/l)	Cl⁻ (mmol/l; mEq/l)	K⁺ (mmol/l; mEq/l)	Ca²⁺ mmol/l (mg/dl)	Mg²⁺ mmol/l (mEq/l)	Osmolarity (mmol/l; mOsm/l)
Plasmalyte A	140	98	5	0	1.5 (3)	294
Plasmalyte 56	40	40	13	0	1.5 (3)	111
Normosol R	140	98	5	0	1.5 (3)	294
Lactated Ringer's solution	130	109	4	0.75 (3)	0	272
0.45% saline	77	77	0	0	0	155
0.45% saline + 2.5% dextrose	77	77	0	0	0	288
0.9% saline	154	154	0	0	0	310
7% saline	1200	1200	0	0	0	2400

distribution in the body almost independently of simple diffusion. Circulating plasma proteins, particularly albumin, generate a COP of 20 mmHg. Colloids commonly used in veterinary medicine have COP ranging from 20 mmHg to 70 mmHg (*Table 50*). While crystalloids distribute rapidly among all fluid compartments when administered intravenously, colloids tend to persist within the intravascular space longer, and therefore achieve more effective and longer lasting intravascular volume expansion. Crystalloids can also dilute the concentration of natural colloids (albumin, immunoglobulins) and so can lower the patient's plasma COP, which decreases the host's ability to retain fluid within the intravascular space.

Advantages of colloid therapy include preserving or even increasing plasma COP, which increases intravascular fluid retention, and necessitating smaller volumes of fluids required for resuscitation. However, colloids are more expensive and are not without complications. Whole blood and plasma are typically described as the natural colloids available for veterinary use. Packed red blood cells exert little oncotic pressure (approximately 5 mmHg) and are not expected to affect plasma COP. While human albumin solutions (5%, 25%) are in fact natural colloids,

the potential for causing anaphylactic reactions with repeated use limits their utility in veterinary patients. However, the successful one-time use of concentrated human albumin solutions in dogs has recently been reported. Synthetic colloids are much more frequently used in North America as a means of increasing COP in veterinary patients, e.g. hetastarch, dextrans, pentastarch, and hemoglobin-based oxygen carrying fluids (Oxyglobin®).

An important characteristic of all synthetic colloids is that they are heterogeneous mixtures of molecules of various molecular weights, including molecules <30 kDa which are permeable through membranes and are rapidly excreted by the kidney. Colloids containing molecules of particularly large sizes (>100 kDa) have better intravascular expansive properties and longer intravascular persistence. Although colloids are commonly described by their average molecular weight, this is not necessarily the best way to predict their effect. The COP of a solution is actually related to the number of colloidal particles (all molecules >30 kDa), rather than simply the size of the colloidal particles found in the fluid. The larger colloid particles are also responsible for coagulopathies associated with colloid use.

Table 50 Characteristics of commonly used colloid solutions

Colloid	Na+ (mmol/l; mEq/l)	Cl- (mmol/l; mEq/l)	K+ (mmol/l; mEq/l)	Average molecular weight (kDa)	Osmolarity (mmol/l; mOsm/l)	COP (mmHg)
Whole blood	150	110	5	N/A	300	20
Packed red blood cells	150	110	5	N/A	300	5
Plasma	150	110	5	69	300	18
6% Dextran 70	154	154	0	70	309	62
6% Hetastarch	154	154	0	450	308	33
10% Pentastarch	154	154	0	264	326	40
5% Human albumin	145	145	0	69	290	20
25% Human albumin	145	145	0	69	290	>200
Oxyglobin	150	118	4	200	300	42

While Oxyglobin has been licensed in the United States as a treatment for anemia in dogs, it perhaps should be more appropriately described as a potent colloid (COP of 42 mmHg) with the benefit of oxygen-carrying ability. Given these characteristics, some authors have recommended the use of Oxyglobin as an ideal resuscitative fluid. However, recent results suggest that this strategy may be detrimental in some cases. It is clear that further research is warranted before better recommendations can be made. Furthermore, on a per ml basis, Oxyglobin is significantly more expensive than crystalloids.

Much of the controversy regarding the use of colloids versus crystalloids stems from the fact that while there are many theoretical advantages of colloids, there is a lack of convincing evidence that their use results in improved outcome. In fact, there is some evidence that colloids may be harmful in certain circumstances. Despite this controversy, colloids are commonly used for shock resuscitation, and in patients with low plasma proteins and low COP. The continual decrease in plasma COP can result in the development of peripheral edema and even persistent hypovolemia.

Another major categorization strategy is to distinguish fluids by their therapeutic intent: replacement versus maintenance. Fluids usually used for rehydration and shock resuscitation (crystalloids and colloids) contain electrolyte concentrations similar to normal plasma concentrations and are referred to as 'replacement fluids'. Patients requiring replacement of daily sensible and insensible water and electrolyte losses alone are given 'maintenance fluids', which typically contain half of the sodium content of plasma. Because these fluids are hypotonic compared with normal plasma, dextrose is added at a 2.5% concentration, restoring the tonicity to normal. As the animal metabolizes the dextrose, these fluids essentially deliver a greater amount of free water. Animals with true free water deficits (e.g. a polyuric, polydipsic animal denied access to water), will usually require a combination of replacement and maintenance fluid therapies.

Fluids with supraphysiological concentrations of electrolyes (7% saline) or other osmotically active particles (20% mannitol, 50% dextrose) are referred to as hypertonic solutions. The high concentration of osmotically active particles also imparts a high osmotic pressure and drives fluid shifts from the intracellular and interstitial compartments to the intravascular compartment. For this reason, hypertonic saline is commonly used in resuscitation of severely hypovolemic animals with normal interstitial hydration (e.g. trauma patients). Similarly, patients with intracranial hypertension or cerebral edema may benefit from hypertonic fluids, such as 20% mannitol or 7% saline, which shift fluids to the intravascular compartment and they are later excreted by the kidneys.

Appropriate routes for fluid therapy

Rapid correction of intravascular volume requires intravenous access. A short, large-bore catheter allows rapid infusion of fluids. In most patients, placement of a peripheral venous catheter is adequate for resuscitative therapy. However, the use of peripheral veins, such as the lateral saphenous or femoral veins, is not ideal in some situations, e.g. in a patient with GDV. In very small patients, such as neonates, placement of an intraosseous catheter also allows rapid fluid infusion. Placement of a short intravenous catheter, normally intended for peripheral use, into a jugular vein of a very small patient may also be useful.

Restoration of hydration is also preferably achieved with the use of intravenous catheters. However, under certain circumstances fluid therapy administered subcutaneously may also be used. Patients that do not require hospitalization and are not overtly deemed dehydrated (not >5% dehydrated) (Table 48, page 232), can be treated with subcutaneous fluid therapy. Patients with chronic, increased fluid losses beyond their ability to consume their fluid requirements voluntarily, e.g. cats with advanced CRF, may also be treated with subcutaneous fluid therapy.

Determining the rate and duration of fluid therapy

The dose of fluid therapy required for resuscitation is not set at a specific value, although it is commonly cited as 90 ml/kg/hr in the dog and 55 ml/kg/hr in the cat. In reality the dose of fluids administered should be titrated to achieve desired resuscitation end-points. As tachycardia and weak or bounding peripheral pulses are common indications for the administration of fluid boluses, the return of these parameters to more acceptable ranges may serve as indicators of adequate resuscitation.

A useful strategy for treating medium to large-sized dogs with hypovolemia is to administer a 15–30 ml/kg bolus, followed by 10–15 ml/kg boluses as guided by reassessment every 15 min.

In hypovolemic cats, a bolus of 10–20 ml/kg followed by another 5–10 ml/kg bolus 30 min later, as guided by reassessment, is usually adequate. Animals that cannot be cardiovascularly stabilized with this strategy require closer scrutiny for possible causes of nonresponsive shock.

Recommended dosages of colloids include 5–20 ml/kg boluses for resuscitation and 20 ml/kg/day for supporting oncotic pressure. These dosages result in considerable intravascular volume expansion in most patients and minimal coagulation abnormalities in patients with an intact coagulation system. Dosages approaching 40 ml/kg/day have been described in dogs, but such high volumes merit clinical monitoring of plasma COP as well as judicious monitoring of volume status (e.g. CVP, echocardiography).

Administering fluid therapy to dehydrated animals is not limited to a specific fluid dose and must be titrated to the individual. Daily maintenance fluid requirements of normal animals are commonly estimated as 40–60 ml/kg/day. A common practice is simply to multiply this 'daily fluid requirement' by a multiplier, e.g. 1.5–3 × maintenance fluid rates for critically ill patients. This is often not ideal and can result in under- or over-hydration of many patients. A preferable way to calculate fluid therapy may be to account for the hydration deficit of the patient, the sensible and insensible fluid losses, as well as ongoing (contemporary) fluid loses (e.g. vomiting, diarrhea, polyuria). Table 51 describes the required calculation for this fluid replacement

Table 51 Calculation of rehydration fluid therapy

A Replacement requirement (hydration deficit):

Body weight (kg) × percentage dehydration as decimal = deficit in liters

B Maintenance requirement:

Sensible losses (urine output): 27–40 ml/kg/day

Insensible losses (fecal, respiratory): 13–20 ml/kg/day

C Ongoing fluid losses:

Vomiting, diarrhea, polyuria, wound exudates

Percent dehydration is estimated as described in Table 48

These quantities (**A** + **B** + **C**) amount to the daily fluid requirement for a given patient and should be adjusted according to changing clinical parameters

Fluid additives

A frequent finding in animals requiring fluid therapy is the presence of severe electrolyte abnormalities. The correction of electrolyte imbalances often requires choosing fluids with an electrolyte composition similar to the desired physiological effect. For example, patients with hyperkalemia should be treated with fluids containing little to no potassium. In other instances, patients with significant electrolyte deficits require supplementation that can be added directly to their intravenous fluids. The most common fluid additive is potassium chloride. The recommended amounts of potassium to be added to intravenous fluids in order to correct hypokalemia are listed in *Table 52*. With severe imbalances, the ability to monitor potassium concentration in a timely fashion, i.e. having access to a blood gas analyzer or a biochemical analyzer on-site, is desirable. Phosphorus and magnesium infusions, similar to aggressive potassium therapy, require access to a biochemical analyzer on-site.

Drugs such as insulin, opioids, vitamin B complex, metoclopramide, and catecholamines can also be combined with intravenous fluids and administered as continuous infusions, but it is imperative that their compatibility with particular solutions and other medications is carefully evaluated beforehand.

strategy. Continual reassessment of hydration status is critical in determining the duration of required therapy for dehydrated patients. As rehydration of the interstitium is achieved and ongoing and sensible losses are controlled, fluid therapy should be adjusted. Discontinuation of fluid therapy is initiated when the animal voluntarily consumes enough water to meet its fluid requirement and maintain adequate hydration.

Table 52 Sliding scale for potassium supplementation

Serum potassium (mmol/l; mEq/l)	KCl to add to 250 ml of fluid mmol (mEq)	Maximal infusion rate of fluid* (ml/kg/hr)
<2.0	20	6
2.1–2.5	15	8
2.6–3.0	10	12
3.1–3.5	7	17
3.6–4.0	5	24

*Maximum infusion rate of potassium-containing fluid should not exceed the delivery of 0.5 mmol/kg/hr (0.5 mEq/kg/hr)

Monitoring and possible complications

As with any therapy, the administration of fluid can result in complications. The most common and potentially most detrimental is volume overload (i.e. CHF). While patients without cardiac disease can accommodate large amounts of fluid therapy, patients with even mild to moderate compensated cardiac dysfunction can progress into overt heart failure with fluid therapy. Patients with identified fluid deficits and concurrent cardiac insufficiencies require judicious fluid therapy and close monitoring. Sequential and frequent body weight assessment is the simplest and perhaps the most useful monitoring tool of fluid therapy. Unexpected and significant weight gain merits prompt evaluation and adjustment of therapy. Monitoring of urine production is also a useful clinical tool in gauging fluid therapy in critically ill patients. Restoration of adequate urine production may be a useful resuscitation endpoint. Measurement of blood pressure is another important aspect of reassessing patients for adequate resuscitation. Patients that fail to normalize blood pressure despite adequate administration of fluids may require vasopressors, such as dopamine or norepinephrine (noradrenaline). Frequent monitoring and characterization of the patient's respiratory rate and effort are also important parameters in all patients receiving fluid therapy, especially those with identified cardiac insufficiencies.

For patients requiring careful titration of fluid therapy, a more objective measure of intravascular fluid status is the measurement of CVP. Jugular venous distension and pulsations are also indicators of elevated CVP and require judicious use of fluid therapy. Overt signs of excess or intolerance of fluid administration include chemosis, peripheral edema, and respiratory distress. The development of any of these abnormalities should prompt complete re-evaluation of fluid therapy.

As colloids exert a greater effect in expanding the intravascular space, they also carry a greater risk of creating fluid overload. The use of a colloid typically requires adjustment of concurrent crystalloid therapy and frequent monitoring for signs of cardiovascular and respiratory compromise. The infusion of large amounts of fluids (in excess of a blood volume) can also lead to a dilutional coagulopathy; this can be seen with excessive crystalloid or colloid use. Additionally, certain synthetic colloids (e.g. Dextran 70, hetastarch) may interfere with platelet and von Willebrand interactions and exacerbate existing coagulation disturbances. Patients with known coagulation disorders should be administered synthetic colloids with caution. As with other synthetic substances, there is also the potential of hypersensitivities and anaphylactoid reactions, although these are less commonly described in animals than in humans.

Summary

While fluid therapy is frequently indispensable in the care of emergency and critical care patients, determining the ideal type, rate, route, and duration of these fluids is sometimes challenging. The emergency and critical care clinician must integrate the pathophysiological processes afflicting the patient, the patient's ever-changing physiological responses, and an understanding of the characteristics of the fluids available. Furthermore, as severely injured and critically ill patients often have a multitude of physiological disturbances, it is increasingly important frequently to reassess these patients for the continued need for fluid therapy. Despite these challenges, appropriate fluid therapy remains instrumental in the successful recovery of most critically ill patients.

Transfusion medicine for critical care patients

- **Blood products**

- **Synthetic blood substitutes**

- **Blood types**

- **Administration**

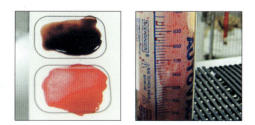

The transfusion of blood products to treat acute blood losses, coagulopathies, and severe anemia has become indispensable in the care of critically ill veterinary patients. As with any therapy, the risks, cost, and potential benefits associated with the use of blood products must be carefully considered and every effort should be made to minimize the occurrence of adverse effects. The critical care clinician should be familiar with the various forms of blood products available, their indications, proper use, and their potential side effects. As the importance of blood products continues to grow as an essential part of the therapeutic regimen available to treat critically ill patients, clinicians should strive to incorporate the various transfusion modalities into their practice environment.

Blood products

An important advancement in transfusion medicine was the recognition that not all patients required whole blood to treat their condition. As a matter of practicality, administration of whole blood to a patient that requires only plasma or pRBC is probably not harmful but could be considered wasteful. As techniques designed to extend the viability of blood products were developed further, the concept of blood component therapy was born. This not only resulted in improving resource management practices, but also diminished unnecessary risks to patients receiving blood products. By the administration of only the desired portion of blood, patients are not subjected to the possible complications of receiving the other components. Additionally, each unit collected may help more than one animal.

The common blood products available for transfusion to veterinary patients include pRBC, FFP, FP, cryoprecipitate, fresh whole blood, and synthetic blood substitutes, such as Oxyglobin®.

COMPONENT THERAPY
Packed red blood cells
Commercial veterinary blood banks routinely supply units of pRBC that are prepared by extracting most of the plasma and its associated clotting factors. The resultant product contains red blood cells and a small amount of plasma and anticoagulant. A full unit of canine pRBC is approximately 200–250 ml, and contains the same oxygen-carrying capacity as 1 unit of whole blood (450 ml). Because pRBC contains only a small amount of plasma proteins, its COP is approximately 5 mmHg. This relatively low COP, compared with that of whole blood (20 mmHg), makes pRBC a reasonable choice for transfusing anemic, normovolemic animals (e.g. dogs with hemolytic anemia, nonregenerative anemia). The recommended dosages for transfusions using pRBC are in the range of 6–10 ml/kg.

Some commercial veterinary blood banks are now supplying feline units of pRBC. The typical feline unit of pRBC contains 30–35 ml. Cats with a limited capacity to tolerate large volumes of fluids (e.g. cats with heart disease) but in need of transfusion may benefit from the administration of pRBC rather than whole blood.

Fresh frozen plasma

From a unit of whole blood, plasma is extracted after refrigerated centrifugation. Fresh plasma contains all clotting factors, and albumin. If immediately frozen at −30°C, all clotting factors retain their activity for 1 year. The main indications for use of FFP include inherited and acquired coagulopathies. Animals demonstrating prolonged clotting times and expected to undergo invasive diagnostics, such as liver biopsy, should receive particular consideration for FFP transfusion. The use of FFP specifically to treat hypoalbuminemia is impractical for several reasons. Increasing a patient's serum albumin concentration by 10 g/l (1 g/dl) may require the administration of as much as 45 ml/kg of FFP. With the exception of very small patients, this would be cost prohibitive. While FFP has a COP of approximately 20 mmHg, increasing a patient's COP would also require large volumes and the efficacy of such therapy is unknown. The use of FFP for resuscitation of hypovolemic patients is controversial and also currently not recommended. For the treatment of coagulopathies, FFP is administered at a starting dose of 10 ml/kg. This, however, should serve only as a guideline and some patients may require greater amounts of FFP.

Another proposed use of FFP is to replace depleted concentrations of AT to patients with conditions such as pancreatitis and DIC. Unfortunately, studies have not supported the efficacy of such measures in improving outcomes in human patients. Even when AT concentrates were used, administering supraphysiological amounts of AT did not significantly improved outcome. In light of these findings, there is little support for using FFP to treat these conditions in veterinary patients.

Frozen plasma

On occasion, a unit of FFP is inadvertently thawed for a patient but not used. If this unit is refrozen it is referred to as 'frozen plasma'. The activity of all clotting factors except for factors V and VIII are preserved in frozen plasma. Plasma obtained from centrifuging stored whole blood also loses the labile clotting factors and is, therefore, used for making frozen plasma. The use of frozen plasma for treating patients with ACR toxicity is adequate and effective. Patients with hemophilia or von Willebrand's disease may not be adequately treated using frozen plasma. Some commercial veterinary blood banks are now supplying feline units of plasma. If frozen, these units can be stored for up to 1 year and are also referred to as frozen plasma. The typical feline plasma unit is approximately 20 ml.

Cryoprecipitate

A commonly held misconception is that a unit of cryoprecipitate contains more clotting factors than a unit of FFP. In reality, a unit of cryoprecipitate is actually prepared from a unit of FFP and therefore contains approximately the same amount (or less) of clotting factors (there is some loss of clotting factors during processing). The advantage of cryoprecipitate is that it is a *concentrated* source of von Willebrand's factor, fibrinogen, and factors VIII and XIII. Units of cryoprecipitate are prepared by thawing FFP units to temperatures between 0 and 6°C, allowing a white precipitate to form, centrifuging the unit, and extracting the plasma (referred to as cryopoor plasma). The remaining portion is considered a unit of cryoprecipitate. The administration of desmopressin (DDAVP) to blood donors before blood collection may enhance the yield of von Willebrand's factor in the blood collected and therefore in the unit of cryoprecipitate made from that blood. By concentrating these factors, a patient can receive multiple units of cryoprecipitate without the risk of becoming volume overloaded. Cryoprecipitate is commonly used in dogs with von Willebrand's disease that require surgical interventions or are undergoing treatment for acute hemorrhage. Recommended dosage for cryoprecipitate is 1 unit per 10 kg body weight.

PLATELET-CONTAINING BLOOD PRODUCTS

Platelet-containing blood products include fresh whole blood, platelet-rich plasma, and platelet concentrates. By centrifuging whole blood at lower speeds, platelets can be extracted into the plasma with greater efficiency, yielding platelet-rich plasma. While the administration of platelet-containing blood products to animals undergoing hemorrhage as a result of severe thrombocytopenia would seem ideal, there are several logistical and practical factors which make such practice difficult. To maximize the viability of platelets, fresh whole blood must be collected and administered within 8 hours without refrigeration. This requires a practice to have blood donors readily available and the ability to collect and process blood expediently. While administration of platelet-containing blood products may control bleeding in some patients, it is unlikely significantly to increase platelet numbers. Actively hemorrhaging patients will require several units of platelet-containing blood products that make such practice cost prohibitive.

Patients that may benefit from fresh whole blood transfusions include severely thrombocytopenic patients requiring surgery (e.g. patients with splenic hemangiosarcoma), and patients developing dilutional coagulopathy as a result of massive fluid therapy. Administration of platelet-rich products to dogs with ITP is likely to be unrewarding as it has been shown in people that platelets are destroyed within minutes in such patients. Platelet-containing blood products have also been administered to human patients with neoplastic bone marrow diseases while they are undergoing either chemotherapy or radiation therapy. The efficacy of platelet transfusion in veterinary patients undergoing similar therapy is unknown.

Whole blood

In many practice environments, whole blood is the only blood product available. It contains red blood cells, all of the clotting factors, plasma proteins, platelets, and anticoagulants. A typical unit of canine whole blood contains approximately 450–500 ml of blood + 63 ml of anticoagulant (CPDA-1). Dosages of whole blood to dogs are in the range 10–22 ml/kg.

For cats, a typical unit of whole blood contains 54 ml of blood and 6 ml of CPDA-1 or another anticoagulant, such as ACD. Most blood transfusions administered to cats are whole blood transfusions, although some commercial veterinary blood banks are providing feline component blood products. Cats are commonly transfused a single unit, although some cats may require additional units. If multiple units of blood are administered to cats, careful monitoring for volume overload is required.

Synthetic blood substitutes

The introduction of a synthetic hemoglobin-based oxygen-carrying fluid (Oxyglobin®) to the veterinary market has dramatically changed transfusion medicine. The use of Oxyglobin® does not require blood typing or cross-matching, it has a long shelf-life, and can be used in dogs or cats (not licensed). Disadvantages are high cost, inconsistent availability (currently), interference with biochemical analyzers, and a short *in vivo* half-life. Once removed from its light-protecting pouch, Oxyglobin® should be administered within 24 hours. The dosages of Oxyglobin® for dogs are in the range 10–30 ml/kg and for cats, 3–5 ml/kg. The potent colloidal effects of Oxyglobin® (COP 42 mmHg) merit close monitoring of volume status in both dogs and especially cats being administered this blood substitute.

Blood types

A crucial aspect of transfusion medicine revolves around the safety of the recipient. It is useful to think of blood transfusion as a form of organ transplantation, where a tissue (blood) is infused from a donor into a new host and is subjected to similar processes akin to tissue rejection. This is particularly important in administering blood to cats, where use of the incorrect blood type can result in death. Red blood cells of dogs and cats express specific markers or antigens, which define their blood type. In dogs, many different DEAs have been identified. Of these, DEA 1.1 is considered to be most important in respect to transfusion medicine. In cats, the recognized blood types include type A, type B, and type AB.

The importance of these red cell antigens is that animals are usually tolerant of transfused cells expressing the same antigens they possess. Transfusion of cells expressing different red cell antigens can result in shortened life-span of red cells, acute hemolysis, and even death. The degree of reaction is dependent on whether the recipient was primed against the transfused blood type previously or on the presence of natural antibodies specific to the other blood type. The latter is particularly important in cats. Type A cats possess anti-type B antibodies, type B cats possess large quantities of anti-type A antibodies, and

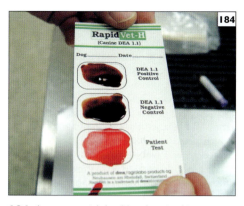

184 A commercial dog blood typing kit.

the recipient immune system to subsequent transfusion of cells expressing similar antigens. Within 10 days of being transfused, the recipient's immune system will be programmed to react if ever exposed to similar antigens. For this reason, once a patient receives a blood transfusion, a cross-match is required for all subsequent transfusions after approximately 10 days following the first transfusion. Cross-matching allows the *in vitro* demonstration of gross incompatibility between donor and recipient. However, lack of gross agglutination on a cross-match does not guarantee that no transfusion reaction will occur. A step-by-step description of performing a cross-match is listed in *Table 53*.

type AB cats possess no antibodies against either red cell antigen. For this reason, all cats either receiving or donating blood should be typed and only receive type-specific blood, with the exception of AB-type cats, which tolerate transfusions from type A cats as well.

In dogs, administration of type-specific blood is more important from a resource management point-of-view than medical necessity. Of the many different recognized canine blood types, DEA 1.1, 1.3, and 7 are the only ones believed to play any significant roles, with DEA 1.1 being the most important. Most dogs either receiving or donating blood are screened for DEA 1.1 antigens. Blood units from dogs not expressing DEA 1.1 are highly sought after, because they can be administered to almost any dog, regardless of their blood type. Dogs that are DEA 1.1 positive are typically administered blood of the same type, but could also receive blood that is DEA 1.1 negative. From a practical stance, DEA 1.1 negative blood is usually reserved for patients that are also DEA 1.1 negative.

Blood typing can be done by most diagnostic laboratories, but should also be available in most emergency and critical care settings, as blood administration may be required urgently. Commercially available blood-typing kits for dogs and cats have facilitated on-site blood typing and enable clinicians to use blood products expediently (**184**).

CROSS-MATCHING

While the administration of type-specific blood cells minimizes immediate and acute transfusion reactions, it does not prevent the sensitization of

Table 53 Cross-matching procedure

1. EDTA-anticoagulated blood is obtained from recipient and samples of anticoagulated blood from the proposed donors

2. Both donor and recipient blood samples centrifuged for 5 min at 1000 × g

3. Plasma removed using pipettes and saved in separate labeled tubes

4. Red blood cells resuspended by adding 3–4 ml of 0.9% saline (wash)

5. Reds cells–saline suspension centrifuged for 5 min at 1000 × g. Saline pipetted off, and discarded

6. Washing procedure repeated (steps 4 and 5) twice

7. 4% red blood cell suspension prepared by adding 0.2 ml of washed pRBC and adding 4.8 ml of 0.9% saline

8. For each potential donor, two drops of recipient plasma and one drop of donor red cell suspension mixed *gently* in a labeled tube for the major cross-match

9. For each potential donor, two drops of donor plasma and one drop of recipient red cell suspension mixed *gently* in a labeled tube for the minor cross-match

10. Tubes incubated at room temperature for 15 min

11. Tubes centrifuged for 15 s at 1000 × g

12. Tubes observed for hemolysis

13. Cells resuspended by shaking gently and cells evaluated for agglutination

14. Compatible units produce no hemolysis or agglutination. In cases where all potential units produce some reaction, the least reactive should be used

Administration

Before the administration of any blood product, careful inspection of the product is absolutely critical. Unusual discoloration should prompt close inspection and, as a precautionary measure, the product should be discarded. The observation of a white or pink layer within whole blood or pRBC is indicative of lipemia and this is safe for administration. The presence of blood clots does not necessarily preclude the product from being administered as clots are removed by the filter. Frozen units of plasma should be inspected for cracks in the packaging which may occur during thawing.

The most common route of administration of blood products is via an intravenous catheter. In neonates, transfusion of blood products can be safely given through an intraosseous catheter or even directly into the peritoneal cavity. Preferably, blood should be administered through a short catheter because these have low resistance. The use of intravenous sets designed for blood transfusions is necessary as the embedded filters remove macro- and microscopic blood clots and debris. The filter size typically used in veterinary medicine is 170 µm.

The recommended initial rate of blood delivery ranges from 1 to 4 ml/kg/hour and should be completed within 4 hours. Plasma transfusions may be administered at 4–6 ml/kg/hour. Blood products can be administered through some infusion pumps that have been approved specifically for blood transfusions.

Animals experiencing life-threatening hemorrhage and believed to be in imminent danger of undergoing cardiac arrest, can be rapidly administered several units of blood as boluses. This is considered a salvage procedure whereby the consequences of delaying the transfusion outweigh the risks of transfusion reactions. Oxyglobin® can also be administered in similar fashion in such situations. The practice of autotransfusion, whereby hemorrhaged blood from the patient is salvaged from a cavity (thorax or abdomen) utilizing special auto-transfusion equipment (185) should be reserved for catastrophic situations, where no other alternative is available. This has been described in open-chest CPR situations and in hemorrhaging intraoperative patients.

MONITORING AND COMPLICATIONS

During the administration of blood products, close patient monitoring is essential. Minimally, heart rate, respiration rate, and temperature should be measured at the onset of the transfusion, every 15 minutes for the first hour and then on an hourly basis until transfusion is complete. The occurrence of vomiting, diarrhea, urticaria, tachycardia, respiratory distress, or acute alteration in mentation is indicative of a transfusion reaction. Transfusion reactions occur as a result of both immunological and nonimmunological processes. There are four classes of transfusion reactions described; these include acute and delayed forms of both immunological and nonimmunological reactions. Acute transfusion reactions occur soon after commencing or soon after completion of the transfusion, while delayed transfusion reactions are noted hours after completion of the transfusion. Manifestations of transfusion reactions and their classifications are listed in *Table 54.*

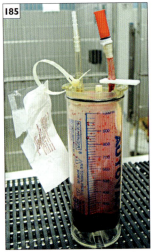

185 Auto-transfusion canister.

Table 54 Classification of transfusion reactions

Acute immunological

Acute hemolytic reactions

Febrile nonhemolytic reactions

Urticaria

Delayed immunological

Delayed hemolytic reactions (shortened red cell lifespan)

Post-transfusion purpura

Acute nonimmunological

Dilutional coagulopathy

Hypocalcemia (citrate toxicity)

Embolism (air, blood clot)

Circulatory overload

Endotoxic shock

Delayed nonimmunological

Infectious disease transmission

Sepsis

Immunological reactions

Of all transfusion reactions, acute immunological reactions are the most devastating and may result in hemolysis, shock, and death. Less severe manifestations include fever, urticaria, restlessness, and vomiting. Efforts to reduce the risks of life-threatening acute immunological reactions include administration of type-specific blood and performing cross-matching procedures when indicated. Fortunately, the most common forms of transfusion reactions are not life-threatening, especially if identified early. With frequent and adequate monitoring these complications can be dealt with and minimized. Any increase in body temperature should prompt immediate evaluation of vital parameters including heart rate, pulse quality, respiration rate and effort, blood pressure, and neurological status. If all other parameters are normal, the rate of infusion can be slowed and the patient should be closely monitored. In the event of other abnormalities or the progression of fever, the transfusion should be discontinued and the unit evaluated for possible contamination (bacterial culture, Gram stain, etc). The patient is also evaluated for evidence of hemolysis and treated aggressively with supportive measures, including resuscitative efforts and short-acting corticosteroids. The use of corticosteroids is controversial because of the lack of efficacy information, however, their use is widely recommended. The development of urticaria is usually treated with short-acting corticosteroids and antihistamines. The practice of administering antihistamines before blood transfusions has not been shown to effectively prevent transfusion reactions, but could exacerbate hypotension in critically ill patients. Therefore, this practice is not recommended. Delayed immunological reactions include shortened red blood cell lifespan and immunosuppression. These reactions are probably more common than currently recognized and merit further investigation. No treatment or preventative measures are currently known.

Nonimmunological processes

Nonimmunological reactions or processes include dilutional coagulopathy, hypocalcemia (citrate toxicity), embolic disease, hyperammonemia, infectious disease transmission, and sepsis from blood contamination. Some of these processes are prevented by close inspection of blood products, and adherence to good blood-banking practices. Dilutional coagulopathy and citrate toxicity are disorders caused by administering massive amounts of blood products, often exceeding the animal's entire blood volume within a 24-hour period. Patients receiving multiple units of pRBC (often concurrently with massive crystalloid and colloid fluid therapy) are at risk of developing dilutional coagulopathy. These patients require monitoring of clotting times and usually require plasma transfusions to correct coagulopathies. Ionized calcium concentrations should be evaluated in patients receiving large quantities of blood products and hypocalcemia should be promptly corrected if noted. Small animals, weighing <3 kg, and patients with pre-existing hypocalcemia are at increased risk for citrate toxicity.

CHAPTER 17

Nutritional support of the critically ill patient

- **Nutritional assessment**

- **Goals of nutritional support**

- **Nutritional plan**

- **Enteral nutrition**

- **Parenteral nutrition**

- **Monitoring and reassessment**

- **Special nutrients**

- **Summary**

Critically ill animals undergo several metabolic alterations which put them at high risk for the development of malnutrition and its subsequent complications. During periods of nutrient deprivation, a healthy animal will primarily lose fat. However, sick or traumatized patients will catabolize lean body mass when they are not provided with sufficient calories. This loss of lean body mass reduces the animal's strength, immune function, wound healing, and overall survival. Inadequate calorie intake is commonly due to a loss of appetite, an inability to eat or tolerate feelings, vomiting, or dehydration; these accompany many diseases processes. Because malnutrition can occur quickly in these animals, it is important to provide nutritional support by either enteral or parenteral nutrition if oral intake is not adequate. The goals of nutritional support are to treat malnutrition when present but, just as importantly, to prevent malnutrition in patients at risk. Whenever possible, the enteral route should be used because it is the safest, most convenient, and most physiologically sound method of nutritional support. However, when patients are unable to tolerate enteral feeding or are unable to utilize nutrients administered enterally, parenteral nutrition should be considered. Ensuring the successful nutritional management of critically ill patients involves selecting the right patient, making an appropriate nutritional assessment, and implementing a feasible nutritional plan. Photocopiable worksheets are supplied on pages 253–255.

Nutritional assessment

As with any medical intervention, there are always risks of complications. Minimizing such risks depends on patient selection and assessment. The first step in designing a nutritional strategy for a patient involves making a systematic evaluation of the patient, and this is termed *nutritional assessment*. Nutritional assessment identifies malnourished patients that require immediate nutritional support and also identifies patients at risk for developing malnutrition in which nutritional support will help to *prevent* malnutrition.

Indicators of overt malnutrition include recent weight loss of at least 10% of body weight, poor haircoat, muscle wasting, signs of poor wound healing, hypoalbuminemia, lymphopenia, and coagulopathies. However, these abnormalities are not specific to malnutrition and are not present early in the process. In addition, fluid shifts may mask weight loss in critically ill patients. Factors that predispose a patient to malnutrition include anorexia lasting longer than 3 days, serious underlying disease (e.g. trauma, sepsis, peritonitis, pancreatitis, and GI surgery), and large protein losses (e.g. protracted vomiting, diarrhea, or draining wounds). Nutritional assessment also identifies factors that can impact on the nutritional plan, such as cardiovascular instability, electrolyte abnormalities, hyperglycemia, and hypertriglyceridemia, or concurrent conditions, such as renal or hepatic disease, that will impact on the nutritional plan. Appropriate laboratory analysis should be performed in all patients to assess these parameters. Before implementation of any nutritional plan, the patient must be cardiovascularly stable, with major electrolyte, fluid, and acid–base abnormalities corrected.

Goals of nutritional support

Even in patients with severe malnutrition, the immediate goals of therapy should focus on resuscitation, stabilization, and identification of the primary disease process. As steps are made to address the primary disease, formulation of a nutritional plan should strive to prevent (or correct) overt nutritional deficiencies and imbalances. By providing adequate energy substrates, protein, essential fatty acids, and micronutrients, the body can support wound healing, immune function, and tissue repair. A major goal of nutritional support is to minimize metabolic derangements and catabolism of lean body tissue. During hospitalization, repletion of body weight is not a priority as this will only occur when the animal is recovering from a state of critical illness. The ultimate goal of nutritional support is to have the patient eating adequate amounts of food in its own environment.

Nutritional plan

Proper diagnosis and treatment of the underlying disease are key to the success of nutritional support. Based on the nutritional assessment, a plan is formulated to meet energy and other nutritional requirements of the patient and, at the same time, address any concurrent condition requiring adjustments to the nutritional plan. The anticipated duration of nutritional support should be determined and factored into the plan. This will largely depend on clinical familiarity with the specific disease process and sound clinical judgment. For each patient, the best route of nutrition should be determined – enteral versus parenteral nutrition. This decision should be based on the underlying disease and the patient's clinical signs. Whenever possible, the enteral route should be considered first. If enteral feedings are not tolerated or the GI tract must be bypassed, however, parenteral nutrition should be considered. Nutritional support should be introduced gradually and reach target levels in 48–72 hours.

CALCULATING NUTRITIONAL REQUIREMENTS

The patient's RER is the number of calories required for maintaining homeostasis while the animal rests quietly. The RER is calculated using the following formula:

$$RER = 70 \times (body\ weight\ in\ kg)^{0.75}$$

For animals weighing between 2 kg and 30 kg, the following linear formula gives a good approximation of energy needs:

$$RER = (30 \times body\ weight\ in\ kg) + 70$$

Traditionally, the RER was then multiplied by an illness factor, between 1.0 and 1.5, to account for increases in metabolism associated with different conditions and injuries. Recently, there has been less emphasis on these subjective illness factors and current recommendations are to use more conservative energy estimates in order to avoid overfeeding. Overfeeding can result in metabolic and GI complications, hepatic dysfunction increased CO_2 production, and weaken respiratory muscles. Of the metabolic complications, the development of hyperglycemia is most common, and possibly the most detrimental.

Currently, the RER is used as an initial estimate of a critically ill patient's energy requirements. It should be emphasized that these general guidelines should be used as starting points, and animals receiving nutritional support should be closely monitored for tolerance of nutritional interventions. Continued decline in body weight or body condition should prompt the clinician to reassess and perhaps modify the nutritional plan (e.g. increasing the number of calories provided by 25%).

While definitive studies determining the actual nutritional requirements of critically ill animals have not been performed, general recommendations can be made. Currently, it is generally accepted that hospitalized dogs should be supported with 4–6 g of protein/100 kcal (15–25% of total energy requirements), while cats are usually supported with 6 g (or more) of protein/100 kcal (25–35% of total energy requirements). Patients with protein intolerance, such as those with hepatic encephalopathy or severe azotemia, should receive reduced amounts of protein. Similarly, patients with hyperglycemia or hyperlipidemia may also require decreased amounts of dextrose and lipids, respectively. Other nutritional requirements will depend upon the patient's underlying disease, clinical signs, and laboratory parameters.

Enteral nutrition

The enteral route of nutritional support is usually the preferable route. Enteral nutrition is safer and less expensive than parenteral nutrition, and helps to maintain intestinal structure and function. Even with the use of feeding tubes, patients can easily be discharged for home care with good owner compliance. Complications with feeding tubes include tube occlusion and localized irritation at the tube exit site. More serious complications include infection at the exit site or, rarely, complete tube dislodgement and peritonitis if the tube was a gastrostomy or jejunostomy tube. Complications can be avoided by using the appropriate tube, proper food selection and preparation, and careful monitoring.

Although the enteral route should be utilized if at all possible there are contraindications to its use. Contraindications include persistent vomiting, severe malabsorptive conditions, and an inability to guard the airway. If the enteral route is chosen for nutritional support, the next step is selecting the type of feeding tube to be used (*Table 55*). Feeding tubes commonly used in dogs and cats include nasoesophageal, esophagostomy, gastrostomy (**186, 187**), and jejunostomy tubes. Once the desired feeding tube is placed, radiography or fluoroscopy should be used to confirm satisfactory tube placement.

Based on the type of feeding tube chosen and the disease process being treated, an appropriate diet should be selected. This will also depend upon the animal's clinical parameters and laboratory results. The amount of food is then calculated and a specific feeding plan devised (see *Worksheet 1*, page 253). Generally, feedings are administered every 4–6 hours and feeding tubes should be flushed with 5–10 ml of water after each feeding to minimize clogging of the tube. By the time of discharge, however, the number of feedings should be reduced to three to four times per day to facilitate owner compliance. Commercially available veterinary liquid diets should be used for nasoesophageal and jejunostomy tube feedings. Jejunostomy tubes are primarily for in-hospital use because they require administration of a liquid diet by CRI and this technique also requires more vigilant monitoring. Esophagostomy and gastrostomy tubes are generally larger (>12 Fr) and allow more calorifically dense, blenderized diets to be given. This decreases the volume of food necessary for each feeding. These tubes can be used for long-term enteral feeding. Mastering the placement of esophagostomy feeding tubes is essential in the management of critically ill animals and this technique should be adopted in almost all practices; a step-by-step description is outlined in Chapter 18. A volume of 5–10 ml/kg per individual feeding is generally

Table 55 Feeding tube selection			
Feeding tube	**Duration**	**Advantages**	**Disadvantages**
Nasoesophageal	Short term (<5 days)	Inexpensive; easy to place; no anesthesia required	Requires liquid diet; some animals will not eat with a nasoesophageal tube in place
Esophagostomy	Long term	Inexpensive; easy to place; can use calorifically dense diets	Requires anesthesia; cellulitis can occur if tube is removed early
Gastrostomy*			
Percutaneous endoscopically guided (PEG)	Long term	Easy to place; can use calorifically dense diets	Requires anesthesia and endoscope
Surgically placed	Long term	Can use calorifically dense diets	Requires anesthesia and laparotomy
Jejunostomy	Long term	By-passes stomach and pancreas; can be used in patients with pancreatitis	Requires anesthesia and laparotomy; for in-hospital use; requires continuous rate infusion (CRI); requires liquid diet; peritonitis can occur if tube is removed prematurely

* For all the gastrostomy tubes, peritonitis is a possible complication if the tube leaks or is removed early.

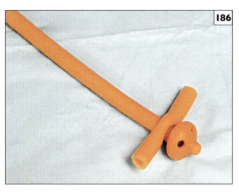

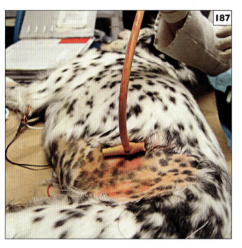

186, 187 A percutaneous gastrostomy (PEG) tube. The tube may be home-made (as displayed here) or purchased as a kit in order to provide enteral nutrition.

well tolerated but this may vary with the individual patient. In patients that are generally healthy but cannot consume food orally, such as a patient with a jaw fracture, larger volumes of food per feeding (15–20 ml/kg) may be tolerated. As enteral diets are mostly composed of water (most canned foods are already >75% water) the amounts of fluids administered parenterally should be adjusted accordingly to avoid volume overload. Prevention of premature removal of tubes can be accomplished by using an Elizabethan collar and by wrapping the tube securely. Care should be taken to avoid wrapping too tightly as this could lead to patient discomfort and even compromise proper ventilation.

Parenteral nutrition

Parenteral nutrition is more expensive than enteral nutrition and is only for in-hospital use. Indications for parenteral nutrition include vomiting, acute pancreatitis, severe malabsorptive disorders, and severe ileus. While terminology of parenteral nutrition can be confusing there are two major types. TPN is typically delivered via a central venous (jugular) catheter and provides all of the energy requirements of the patient. With PPN only a portion of the animal's energy requirements are met (40–70%) but, because of the lower osmolarity of the solution, they can usually be administered through a large peripheral vein such as the lateral saphenous vein in dogs and femoral vein in cats. Because PPN only provides a portion of the patient's requirements, it is only intended for short-term use in a nondebilitated patient with average nutritional requirements. Regardless of the exact form of parenteral nutrition, intravenous nutrition requires a dedicated catheter that is placed using aseptic technique. Long catheters composed of silicone, polyurethane, or tetrafluoroethylene are recommended for use with parenteral nutrition to reduce the risk of thrombophlebitis. Multi-lumen cathethers are often recommended for parenteral nutrition because they can remain in place for longer periods of time than normal jugular catheters, and they provide other ports for blood sampling and administration of additional fluids and intravenous medications. Most parenteral nutrition solutions are composed of a carbohydrate source (dextrose), a protein source (amino acids), and a fat source (lipids). Vitamins and trace metals can also be added.

Due to the high osmolarity of the TPN solution (usually 1100–1500 mOsm/l), it must be administered through a central venous (jugular) catheter. PPN is formulated so that it can be administered through a peripheral catheter but, because it is more dilute, it can only provide a portion of the patient's energy requirements. Formulation of TPN and PPN solutions can be individualized to each patient (see *Worksheet 2* and *Worksheet 3*, pages 254, 255). TPN and PPN must be mixed under sterile conditions; in most cases, it is easiest to have a local human hospital or human home healthcare company formulate them.

Alternatively, commercial ready-to-use preparations of glucose and amino acids are available for peripheral use but these only provide approximately a third of required calories (when administered at maintenance fluid rate) and should only be used for short-term or interim nutritional support. As with enteral nutrition, parenteral nutrition should be instituted gradually over 48–72 hours. With both TPN and PPN, the animal's catheter and lines must be handled with aseptic technique to avoid complications. Other intravenous fluids should be adjusted accordingly for the amount of fluid being administered in the parenteral nutrition to avoid volume overload.

Monitoring and reassessment

Body weights should be monitored daily with both enteral and parenteral nutrition. However, the clinician should take into account fluid shifts in evaluating changes in body weight. For this reason, body condition score is important as well. Use of the RER as the patient's calorific requirement is merely a starting point. The number of calories provided may need to be increased to keep up with the patient's changing needs, typically by 25% if well tolerated. In patients unable to tolerate the prescribed amounts, the clinician should consider reducing enteral feedings and supplementing the nutritional plan with PPN.

Possible complications of enteral nutrition include mechanical complications, such as clogging of the tube or early tube removal. Metabolic complications include electrolyte disturbances, hyperglycemia, volume overload, and GI signs (e.g. vomiting, diarrhea, cramping, bloating). In critically ill patients receiving enteral nutritional support, the clinician must also be vigilant for the development of aspiration pneumonia. Monitoring parameters for patients receiving enteral nutrition include body weight, serum electrolytes, tube patency, appearance of tube exit site, GI signs (e.g. vomiting, regurgitation, diarrhea), and signs of volume overload or aspiration pneumonia.

Possible complications with parenteral nutrition include sepsis, mechanical complications of the catheter and lines, thrombophlebitis, and metabolic disturbances, such as hyperglycemia, electrolyte shifts, hyperammonemia, and hypertriglyceridemia. Avoiding serious consequences of complications associated with parenteral nutrition requires early identification of problems and prompt action. Frequent monitoring of vital signs, catheter exit sites, and routine biochemistry panels may alert the clinician to developing problems (*Table 56*). The development of persistent hyperglycemia during nutritional support may require adjustment to the nutritional plan (e.g. decreasing dextrose content in parenteral nutrition) or administration of regular insulin. This obviously necessitates more vigilant monitoring.

With continual reassessment, the clinician can determine when to change the patient from assisted feeding to voluntary consumption of food. The discontinuation of nutritional support should only begin when the patient can consume approximately its RER without much coaxing. In patients receiving TPN, changing to enteral nutrition should occur over the course of at least 12–24 hours, depending on patient tolerance of enteral nutrition.

Table 56 Monitoring parameters of patients on parenteral nutritional support

The monitoring required will depend upon the individual patient. However, at least the following should be measured daily:

Heart/respiratory rate

Catheter site

Attitude

Body weight

Temperature

Glucose, total solids (check hematocrit tubes for lipemia)

Electrolytes (especially potassium) should be monitored at least every other day

---

WORKSHEET 1 CALCULATING ENTERAL NUTRITION

---

1 Resting Energy Requirement (PER)

RER = 70 ≥ (current body weight in kg)$^{0.75}$
or, for animals weighing between 2 and 30 kg:

RER = (30 ≥ current body weight in kg) + 70   = _____ kcal required/day

2 Product selected _____

   Contains_____ kcal/ml

3 Total volume to be administered per day

$$\frac{\text{kcal required/day}}{\text{kcal/ml in diet}}$$ = _____ ml/day

4 Administration schedule

   1/2 of total requirement on Day 1   = _____ ml/day

   Total requirement on Day 2   = _____ ml/day

5 Feedings per day

   Divide total daily volume into 4–6 feedings (depending on duration of anorexia, patient tolerance)
                                         = _____ feedings/day

6 Calculate volume per feeding

$$\frac{\text{Total ml/day}}{\text{Number of feedings/day}}$$ = _____ ml/feeding (Day 1)

                                              = _____ ml/feeding (Day 2)

*Be sure to adjust the animal's intravenous fluids according

DIET OPTIONS

Esophagostomy and gastrostomy tubes

Eukanuba Maximum Calorie canned
   Supplies 2.1 kcal/ml straight from can but needs to be diluted for tubes
   1 can + 50 ml water = 1.6 kcal/ml
   1 can + 25 ml water = 1.8 kcal/ml (for larger tubes)

Hill's a/d canned
   Supplies 1.3 kcal/ml straight from can but needs to be diluted for tubes
   1 can + 50 ml water = 1.0 kcal/ml
   1 can + 25 ml water = 1.1 kcal/ml (for larger tubes)

Royal Canin Instant Canine/Feline Convalescence Support (Europe only)
   Supplies 1.2 kcal/ml if reconstituted by adding 3 mls of water per gram of powdered diet
   Calculate amount to feed (in grams) by dividing prescribed calories/4.73 and reconstitute as above

Royal Canin Canine/Feline Recovery RS
   Supplies 1 kcal/ml straight from can but needs to be diluted for tubes
   1 can + 25 ml water = 0.9 kcal/ml

Royal Canin low fat canine diet canned
   When a low fat enteral diet is required
   1 can blenderized with 360 ml water, then strained = 0.8 kcal/ml

Nasoesphogeal and jejunostomy tubes

Veterinary liquid diets
   CliniCare Canine/Feline liquid diet (1.0 kcal/ml) (Abbott Animal Health–USA)
   CliniCare RF Feline Liquid diet (1.0 kcal/ml) (Abbott Animal Health–USA)
   Fortal C + Complete Liquid Feed (1 kcal/ml) (Arnolds Veterinary Products Ltd–UK)

Human enteral products
   Most provide 1.0 kcal/ml but do not meet canine or feline requirements as is (must be supplemented)

WORKSHEET 2 CALCULATING TOTAL PARENTERAL NUTRITION (TPN)

1 Resting energy requirement

RER = 70 × (current body weight in kg)$^{0.75}$ or,
for animals weighing between 2 and 30 kg:

RER = (30 × current body weight in kg) + 70   = _____ kcal/day

2 Protein requirements

	Canine	Feline
Standard	4–5g/100 kcal	6g/100 kcal
Decreased (hepatic/renal failure)	2–3g/100 kcal	3–4g/100 kcal
Increased (protein-losing conditions)	6g/100 kcal	6g/100 kcal

(RER ÷ 100) × _____ g/100kcal (protein req)   = _____ g protein required/day

3 Volume of nutrient solutions

a 8.5% amino acid solution (0.085 g protein/ml)

_____ g protein required/day ÷ 0.085 g/ml   =_____ ml/day of amino acids

b Non-protein calories:

The calories supplied by protein (4 kcal/g) are subtracted from the total calories needed to get total non-protein calories needed:

_____ g protein required/day × 4 kcal/g   = _____ kcal from protein

_____ total kcal required/day – kcals from protein   = _____ total non-protein kcal needed/day

c Non-protein calories are usually provided as a 50:50 mixture of lipid and dextrose

This ratio may need to be adjusted if the animal is hyperglycemic or hypertriglyceridemic

20% lipid solution (2 kcal/ml)

To supply 50% of non-protein calories

_____ lipid kcal required ÷ 2 kcal/ml   = _____ ml of lipid

50% dextrose solution (1.7 kcal/ml)

To supply 50% of non-protein calories

_____ dextrose kcal required ÷ 1.7 kcal/ml   = _____ ml of dextrose

4 Total daily requirements

_____ ml 8.5% amino acid solution

_____ ml 20% lipid solution

_____ ml 50% dextrose solution (use half on first day)

_____ ml total volume of TPN solution ÷ 24 hours   =_____ ml/hr infusion rate

5 Using standard amino acids (which contain potassium), TPN made according to this worksheet will provide potassium at higher than maintenance levels (from 25 mmol/l (25 mEq/l) potassium at 3 g protein/100 kcal to 38 mmol/l (38 mEq/l) potassium at 6 g protein/100 kcal). Therefore, it may not be necessary to supplement potassium in any other fluids the patient is receiving. If the patient is hypo- or hyperkalemic, adjustment of the TPN formula may be indicated (e.g. potassium can be supplemented for hypokalemia, and amino acids without electrolytes can be used for hyperkalemia)

The animal's other intravenous fluids must be adjusted according to on-going needs

WORKSHEET 3 CALCULATING PERIPHERAL OR PARTIAL PARENTERAL NUTRITION (PPN)

1 Resting energy requirement
RER = 70 × (current body weight in kg)$^{0.75}$ or,
for animals weighing between 2 kg and 30 kg:
RER = (30 × current body weight in kg) + 70   = RER = _____ kcal/day

2 Partial energy requirement
To supply 70% of the patient's RER
PER = RER × 0.70   = PER = _____ kcal/day

3 Nutrient requirements
(Note: For animals ≤3 kg, the formulation will provide a fluid rate higher than maintenance fluid requirements.
It is important to be sure that the animal can tolerate this volume of fluids.)
a Cats and dogs 3–5 kg:

PER × 0.20 =_____ kcal/day from carbohydrate

PER × 0.20 =_____ kcal/day from protein

PER × 0.60 =_____ kcal/day from lipid

b Cats and dogs 6–10 kg:

PER × 0.25 =_____ kcal/day from carbohydrate

PER × 0.25 =_____ kcal/day from protein

PER × 0.50 =_____ kcal/day from lipid

c Dogs 11–30 kg:

PER x 0.33 =_____ kcal/day from carbohydrate

PER x 0.33 =_____ kcal/day from protein

PER x 0.33 =_____ kcal/day from lipid

d Dogs >30 kg:

PER × 0.50 =_____ kcal/day from carbohydrate

PER × 0.25 =_____ kcal/day from protein

PER × 0.25 =_____ kcal/day from lipid

4 Volume of nutrient solutions
5% dextrose (0.17 kcal/ml)
_____ kcal/day from dextrose ÷ 0.17 kcal/ml   = _____ ml/day
8.5% amino acids (0.34 kcal/ml)
_____ kcal/day from amino acids ÷ 0.34 kcal/ml   = _____ ml/day
20% lipid (2 kcal/ml)
_____ kcal/day from lipid ÷ 2 kcal/ml   = _____ ml/day

5 Total daily requirements
_____ ml 5% dextrose
_____ ml 8.5% amino acids
_____ ml 20% lipid
_____ ml total volume of PPN solution ÷ 24 hours   =_____ ml/hr infusion rate

The standard amino acids used in PPN contain potassium. For animals <35 kg, the PPN solution made according
to this worksheet will provide approximate maintenance levels of potassium. For animals >35 kg, the PPN
solution will contain approximately 12 mmol/l (12 mEq/l) of potassium. Therefore, adjustment of the PPN formula
may be indicated

This calculation should approximate a patient's maintenance fluid requirements. The animal's other intravenous
fluids must be adjusted according to on-going needs. The volume may be higher than maintenance fluid
requirements for very small animals (<3 kg) or in animals with cardiac disease

Special nutrients

In recent years, there has been particular focus on the pharmacological role of nutrients in modulating disease in people. 'Immune-enhancing' diets often include nutrients such as glutamine, arginine, omega-3 fatty acids, antioxidants, and nucleotides. In certain populations of critically ill human patients, these strategies (singly or in combination cocktails) are significantly beneficial in reducing complications and even decreasing mortality. Unfortunately, no such benefits have been documented in veterinary patients. While such nutrients may indeed confer health benefits on veterinary patients, studies confirming these benefits are unlikely to be forthcoming. As the majority of veterinary patients are only hospitalized for a short term (a relatively low percentage is hospitalized for >10 days), pharmacological effects of nutrients will be difficult to discern. While the risk of side effects from these therapies is likely low, the added cost of such supplements in the face of little supporting evidence in veterinary patients may make use of such products unwarranted at this time. As nutrient requirements vary considerably among species, it is likely that the same holds true in respect of the pharmacological effects of nutrients. Determination of minimal dosages for each nutrient necessary to achieve desired biological effects may be warranted as the next step.

Summary

While critically ill patients are often not regarded as in urgent need of nutritional support given their more pressing problems, the severity of their injuries, altered metabolic condition, and necessity of frequent fasting place these patients at high risk of becoming malnourished during their hospitalization. Proper identification of these patients and careful planning and execution of a nutritional plan can be key factors in the successful recovery of these patients.

CHAPTER 18

Techniques

- **Vascular access**

- **Urinary catheterization**

- **Supplemental oxygen**

- **Thoracocentesis**

- **Thoracostomy tube placement**

- **Pericardiocentesis**

- **Abdominocentesis**

- **Tracheostomy**

- **Transtracheal aspirate**

- **Epidural analgesia**

- **Esophagostomy tube placement**

- **Robert Jones bandage**

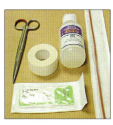
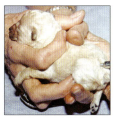
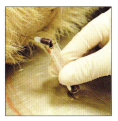
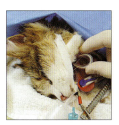

In the field of emergency medicine and critical care, it is essential that the clinician and technician be well versed in a variety of procedures. The following chapter reviews the techniques associated with some common procedures. As with any technique, inexperienced operators are advised to seek direct guidance in learning newer or more complex skills.

Vascular access

INTRAVENOUS CATHETERS

Placement of intravenous catheters is essential to the management of critically ill or injured animals. Large-bore, short catheters permit more rapid fluid delivery. In most cats, a 20 ga catheter can be successfully placed in the cephalic vein, while in larger dogs 14 ga or 16 ga catheters are appropriate. **188–190** depict placement of short over-the-needle catheters, and **191–196** illustrate long through-the-needle catheters and their placement.

Short over-the-needle catheter

188 The fur covering the desired site of venipuncture is liberally shaved. The assistant occludes the vein and restrains the patient. The site is prepared by gently scrubbing the anticipated venipuncture site with either Betadine® or chlorhexidine.

189 Successful venipuncture is confirmed by a flash of blood in the hub. The catheter is advanced into the vessel with care taken not to prematurely withdraw the stylet.

190 The catheter is secured in place with tape. Any blood is cleaned from the surface prior to taping to prevent the tape from sliding.

Short over-the-needle catheter

Long through-the-needle catheter

191 A through-the-needle catheter or multi-lumen catheter is desirable for placement of a jugular catheter. Kits are widely available for multi-lumen catheters. Catheters from Arrow® or Mila® are particularly popular.

192 The patient is restrained in lateral recumbency. The anticipated venipuncture site is clipped and prepped. Local anesthetic or sedation may be beneficial in some patients. The jugular vein should be either visualized or successfully palpated prior to attempts to place a catheter.

Long through-the-needle catheter

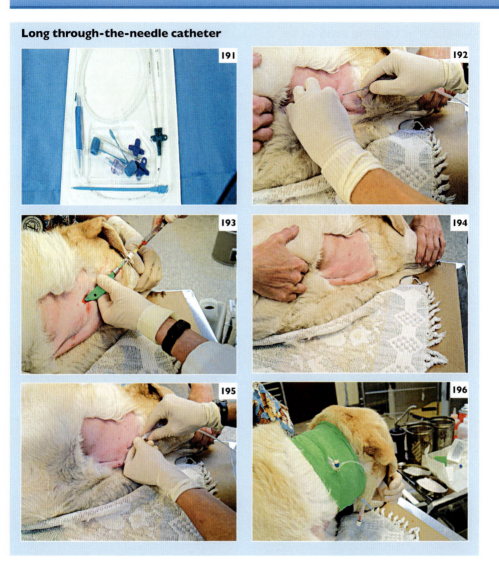

193 The skin is tented and the catheter is inserted through the skin. Usually, it is easier to place the catheter through the skin first prior to attempting venipuncture.

194 The catheter is advanced through the needle. The catheter should advance easily.

195 The catheter should be advanced completely. Blood should be able to be freely aspirated.

196 The catheter should be secured with either suture or tape and gauze. It is prudent to stop and confirm that the catheter both flushes freely and aspirates blood easily at several points during the placement of the wrap, as it is easy for the catheter to become kinked and then nonfunctional.

SMALL OR NEONATAL ANIMALS

Other options for vascular access in small or neonatal animals include the intraosseous catheter (**197**, **198**) and, for resuscitation of neonates, an umbilical vein catheter (**199**). The operator is reminded that it is often quite easy to place jugular catheters in neonates.

Intraosseous and umbilical vein catheters

197 An intraosseous catheter is placed into any long bone. In small patients, the femur often represents the best option. The area surrounding the planned site of catheterization is clipped and routinely prepped.

Intraosseous and umbilical vein catheters

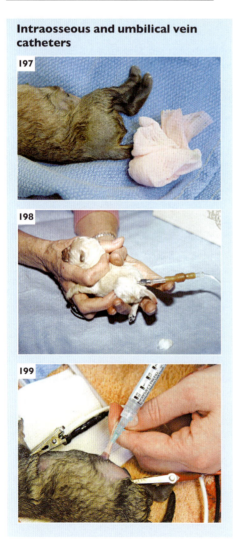

197

198

199

198 A 22 ga or 20 ga 25 mm (1 inch) needle is most commonly used. The needle is inserted into the long axis of the femur. The greater trochanter is palpated and the needle is inserted medial to that site. In neonates, the bone is very soft and minimal pressure is required. In older animals, a force similar to that for a bone marrow aspirate is required. The operator should *not* be able to palpate the tip of the needle on the medial surface of the leg and gentle motion of the needle should result in movement of the entire limb. The intraosseous catheter may be capped with an injection cap or connected directly to a fluid administration set. The catheter is considered a 'central line' and, as such, any drug may be infused through it. Flow rates may be lowered, as over-zealous boluses may dislodge the catheter. Intraosseous catheters should be removed as soon as practical as they are considered painful and may promote osteomyelitis.

199 Catheterization of the umbilical vessels is quite easy and is facilitated by leaving a longer umbilical remnant. The authors' practice has found these catheters particularly useful for reviving neonates following C-sections. The umbilical vein is thinner walled than the artery, so care should be taken during placement to avoid inadvertent penetration of the wall. One should start as far distal to the neonate as possible to allow for errors while perfecting this technique.

ARTERIAL CATHETERS

Arterial catheters are useful for directly (invasively) monitoring blood pressure and for permitting repeated arterial sampling. Most commonly, in critically ill dogs, a catheter will be placed in the metatarsal (dorsal pedal) artery. Catheters may also be placed at other sites.

Cats and very small dogs are often very difficult to catheterize successfully. Additionally, arterial catheterization is challenging, as the vessel has a thick wall and a tendency to spasm (or vasoconstrict) if puncture is not successful. Anatomically, the artery lies between the metatarsal bones, so if the puncture is not accurate, there may be burring or damage to the catheter.

An 18–24 ga catheter is used. As the mean arterial blood pressure is usually greater than 80 mmHg, the gauge is less important than for venous catheter placement.

Arterial catheter

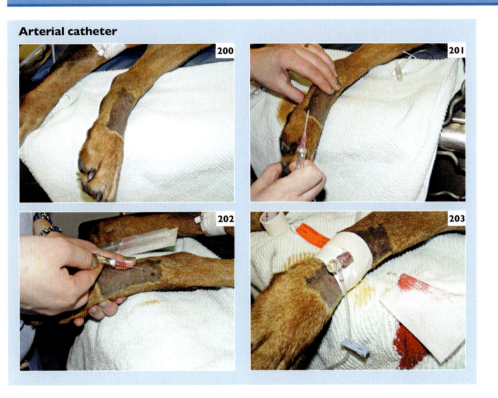

Most often, fully conscious dogs are intolerant of the procedure. Sedation or local anesthesia may be warranted. The clinician should attempt to combine placement of the arterial catheter with other procedures requiring sedation or analgesia. The dog is restrained in lateral recumbency. The foot of the *down* leg is used. The area over the proposed site is clipped and gently prepped. Over-zealous scrubbing should be avoided. The pulse should be strongly palpable. Catheterization should not be attempted too close to the hock joint.

The initial insertion should be directly into the artery, but going in at a steeper angle than for venipuncture (**200**). The catheter is advanced until blood is flowing freely (**201**), then fed into the artery. In all but cardiovascularly collapsed pets, blood will pump from the artery in a pulsatile fashion (**202**). The catheter should then be secured (**203**). It is common for catheters to kink at the site of insertion, so prior to removing a nonfunctional catheter, the catheter and the site should be closely inspected.

Arterial catheter

200 For placement of an arterial catheter, the fur covering the dorsal pedal artery is clipped and the site is gently prepped. It is often easiest to place a catheter in the down leg of a pet lying in lateral recumbency.

201 The pulse should be palpated prior to attempted placement of the catheter.

202 The catheter is inserted at approximately a 30–45° angle. Arterial catheters have a tendency to burr, especially in dogs with tough skin or if the metatarsal bone is inadvertently hit. Blood should pump freely and in a pulsatile fashion following successful placement.

203 The catheter should be taped securely and labeled as an arterial catheter.

Urinary catheter

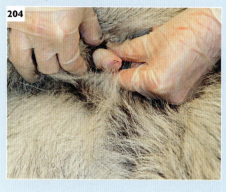

204

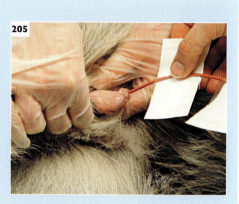

205

Urinary catheterization

A urinary catheter may be placed for urine sampling, for measurement of urine production in order to balance 'ins' and 'outs', for relief of a urinary obstruction, or for hygiene purposes. Catheters should be placed aseptically. Unless otherwise indicated, prophylactic antibiotics are not warranted following placement of a urinary catheter, due to the potential for colonization or infection with resistant bacteria. Catheters in female dogs are most commonly placed digitally, with palpation of the urethral papilla and then subsequent catheterization. Occasionally, some operators find the use of an otoscope helpful for direct visualization. Catheters in female cats are surprisingly easy to place, and usually slide into the bladder. 'Tomcat' catheters, due to their stiffness, are particularly easy to pass in female cats. Urinary catheters in male animals are usually much more straightforward to pass (**204, 205**), although sedation or analgesia may be required.

Urinary catheter

204 The penis is extruded from the prepuce.

205 The operator, having pre-measured the correct anticipated distance to the bladder, passes the catheter. The operator may choose to wear sterile gloves, or, as shown, may keep a piece of the sterilization bag free to permit manipulation without touching the catheter. The catheter is passed until urine is flowing freely. It is then secured in placed with either a Chinese finger trap suture or by a 'tape butterfly' to the prepuce. The entire system is kept closed, by connecting the catheter to a collection system. Most commonly, this collection system is a standard fluid administration set and a clean used fluid bag. The urine production should be quantified every 4–6 hr or as indicated clinically.

Supplemental oxygen

The equipment and technique for administration of supplemental oxygen via a nasal catheter are illustrated in **206–209**.

Nasal catheter
206 Supplies needed for placement of a catheter for delivery of supplemental oxygen (or nasal oxygen). These include scissors, white tape, suture material (2–3 metric [2-0 or 3-0] nylon), red rubber catheter, and lubricant. Lidocaine gel is particularly useful as it provides analgesia for the nasal passage. Catheter size used depends on the size of the patient, but usually an 8 Fr is adequate. Thought should be given to placing nasal oxygen *prior* to anesthesia recovery. Nasal oxygen is particularly beneficial for larger dogs that are not panting heavily. Panting changes the breathing strategy and decreases the concentration of oxygen (FiO_2).

207 The catheter is measured so that the tip is level with the medial canthus of the eye. A pre-placed piece of tape serves to mark the location on the tube.

208 The catheter is placed in the nasal cavity to the pre-marked piece of tape.

209 Using the white tape as an anchor, the catheter is sutured in place. The suture should be placed as close as possible to the nares. Another tacking suture may be placed to hold the catheter to the top of the head. Humidified oxygen may be delivered at flow rates of approximately 100 ml/kg/min.

Nasal catheter

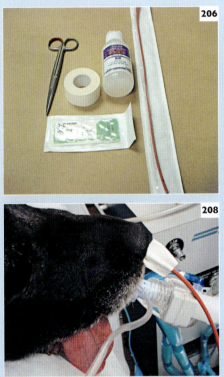

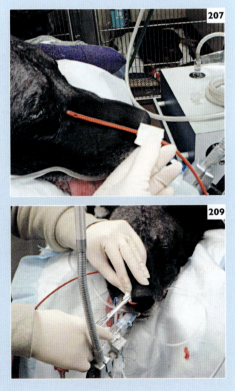

Thoracocentesis

Thoracocentesis is indicated for diagnostic and therapeutic reasons. Supplies needed for thoracocentesis depend on the size of the pet. In most cats and small dogs, a butterfly catheter is of sufficient length to reach the thoracic cavity. In obese or big cats, and in larger dogs, a 37–50mm (1.5–2 inch) needle may be used instead. The needle is connected to an extension set. A three-way stopcock is placed between the end of the butterfly catheter or extension set and a syringe. Usually a 10 or 20 ml syringe is adequate. In animals with a very large volume of effusion (e.g. >1500 ml), it is often worthwhile to place a local block to permit the use of a larger gauge catheter (e.g. 14 or 16 ga) to remove the fluid more rapidly. The preferred site of thoracocentesis is between the seventh and ninth rib spaces (**210–213**).

Thoracocentesis

210 The midventral aspect of the thorax is clipped and prepared for thoracocentesis. The intercostal vessels run caudal to the ribs. The preferred site of thoracocentesis is between the seventh and ninth rib spaces. Sterile gloves are donned to permit palpation of the desired site.

211 The needle is advanced carefully into the thoracic cavity. Upon entry of the thoracic cavity, a gentle 'pop' is often felt by the experienced operator.

212 A second operator should aspirate the fluid and provide feedback as to if the fluid is still flowing adequately.

213 An aliquot of the fluid should be retained for cytological examination and, if warranted, bacterial culture and sensitivity testing.

Thoracocentesis

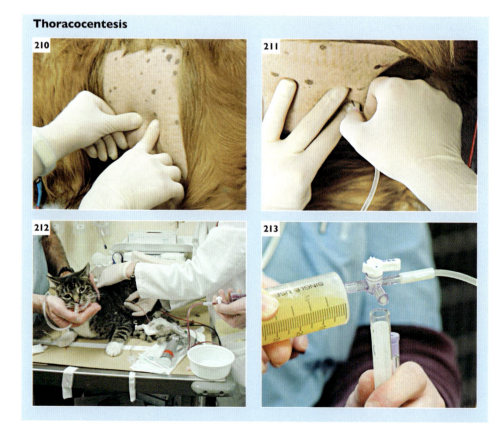

Thoracostomy tube placement

A thoracostomy (chest) tube should be placed when a significant amount of pleural effusion or pneumothorax is present. Usually, the tube is placed under general anesthesia, although, in rare cases, local anesthesia may be adequate. The patient may be placed in either sternal or lateral recumbency. The technique is illustrated in **214–217**.

Thoracostomy tube placement

214 The entire hemithorax should be clipped and draped for thoracostomy, being careful to include the 13th rib in the field so it may serve as a landmark. In this picture, the red circle represents the site of the skin incision, while the red X marks the site of intended pleural space puncture.

215 The skin is pulled cranially by an assistant. This allows the initial incision to be directly over the site of the pleural penetration. The green line represents the last rib. This line is more visible in this picture than in **214** because the skin has been pulled forward.

216 A combination of blunt and sharp dissection permits placement of the thoracostomy tube into the chest cavity with minimal force. The operator should avoid 'slamming' or 'hitting' the chest tube into place, as underlying cardiopulmonary tissues may be damaged.

217 The chest tube should be secured with a finger trap suture.

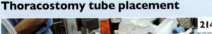

Thoracostomy tube placement

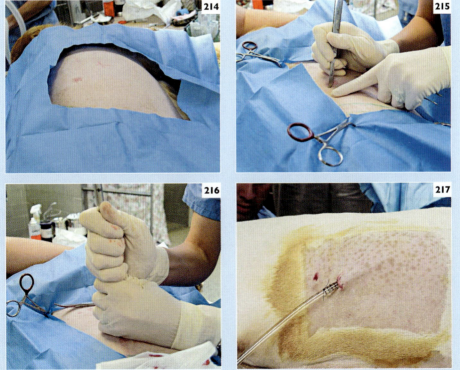

Pericardiocentesis

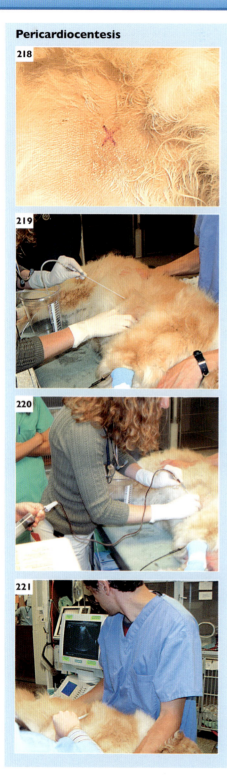

Pericardiocentesis

Pericardiocentesis (**218–221**) can be performed in sternal recumbency or left lateral recumbency, but it is recommended that the procedure be performed from the right side of the thorax to reduce the risk of coronary artery laceration. If possible, a complete echocardiogram should be performed *before* pericardiocentesis as the pericardial fluid may help to highlight any mass lesions. The right side of the thorax is clipped and aseptically prepared. A continuous ECG is monitored for arrhythmia as ventricular ectopy is common. Lidocaine (2 mg/kg) may be prepared in the event of hemodynamically significant ventricular ectopy. Echocardiography is useful to identify a good window for the tap, but, alternatively, a successful tap can be performed by selecting the fourth or fifth intercostal site approximately halfway between the sternum and the costochondral junction. Local anesthesia is usually adequate, though sedation may be used if needed. Oxymorphone should be avoided due to the tendency of dogs to pant following administration.

Pericardiocentesis
218 The intended site is marked and local anesthesia is infused.

219 The site is palpated. A small nick in the skin with a #11 blade may be made. In large dogs, a 5.25 inch 14 or 16 gauge catheter is used, while in smaller dogs a 2" 18 gauge catheter is typically adequate.

220 Fluid is carefully withdrawn while simultaneously monitoring the EKG. If arrhythmia is detected, the catheter should be retracted 0.25 to 1 cm. If severe ectopy occurs, the catheter should be withdrawn and lidocaine administered. The effusion frequently has a hemorrhagic "port wine" appearance. In some cases, a clear or serosanguineous pleural effusion is encountered first. In most dogs, a significant decline in heart rate occurs during the procedure, which is a sign of resolution of the tamponade.

221 Echocardiography maybe used to confirm that the pericardial sac has been emptied. Following pericardiocentesis serial monitoring is advisable to watch for ongoing bleeding into the thorax, recurrent pericardial effusion, or the development of cardiac arrhythmias.

Abdominocentesis

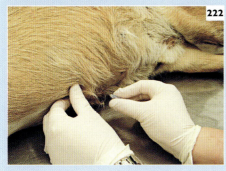
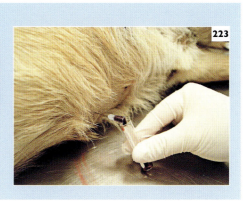

Abdominocentesis

Abdominocentesis is commonly performed in the emergency room for diagnostic and therapeutic purposes. In many cases, simple single needle abdominocentesis is successful (**222**, **223**). In other cases, where no fluid is returned despite clinical suspicion of fluid, the following options may be performed:

- Complete volume resuscitation. In animals with hemorrhage or sepsis, the depleted intravascular volume may limit the development of fluid. Repeat abdomino-centesis 30–90 min later is often successful.
- Two to four needles may be placed simultaneously in the abdomen. This technique appears to permit smaller volumes of fluid to be detected.
- Abdominal ultrasonography is useful to identify pockets of fluid. Fluid is easily recognized by most operators upon ultrasonography.

- DPL may be performed. First the patient's bladder is emptied, then, following a local anesthestic, a long 13 cm (5.25 inch) 12–14 ga catheter with additional side holes cut is inserted into the abdomen. Warmed saline (22 ml/kg) is then infused into the abdomen and the fluid allowed to drain back out again. An aliquot of the fluid is reserved for biochemical and cytological examination. It is common to retrieve only a small portion of the fluid infused.

Abdominocentesis
222 A 22 ga 25–37 mm (1–1.5 inch) needle is inserted into the abdomen. The left cranial quadrant should be avoided if only a single needle insertion is planned, due to the presence of the highly vascular spleen.

---

223 Fluid collected by abdominocentesis may be permitted to fall freely into tubes for cytology (EDTA) and culture or may be aspirated by attaching a syringe to the needle. The intended site of pericardiocentesis is marked and local anesthesia is infused.

(*221 continued*) Hospitalization is advised and vital parameters, PCV, and total solids should be routinely checked 2–6 hr after pericardiocentesis to help monitor for ongoing bleeding. ECG monitoring is indicated for animals noted to have significant arrhythmia before or after pericardiocentesis.

Tracheostomy

Trachestomy in a controlled situation is preferable; however, if needed a slash tracheostomy may be performed in < 30 seconds. In life-threatening situations, attention to sterility and anatomy may be abandoned in order to secure an airway. Tracheostomies are indicated most commonly for bypassing the upper airway, due to masses, swelling, or other dysfunction, in order to permit oral surgery or long-term mechanical ventilation. The patient is anesthetized, intubated, and placed in dorsal recumbency. The technique is illustrated in **224–229**.

Tracheostomy

224 The tracheostomy site is prepared and a location approximately at the third to fifth tracheal rings is chosen. The site should be distal enough to avoid the larynx but not too close to the thoracic inlet.

225 The site is draped and an incision is made along the midline.

226 The midline cervical muscles ('strap' muscles) are bluntly dissected and the trachea is isolated. 'Stay' sutures of large suture material (3.5–4 metric [1-0 or 0]) are placed cranial and caudal to the anticipated site of the tracheostomy. These sutures are essential should the tracheostomy tube dislodge from the patient.

227 The cuff of the orally placed endotracheal tube should be deflated and the tube gently removed. Rarely, it is possible to pierce the cuff or the tube itself with the stay sutures. However, the surgeon and the assistant should be alert as to this possible complication.

Tracheostomy

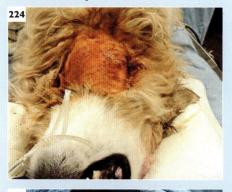

224

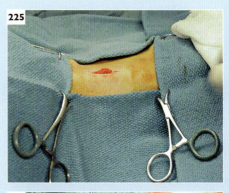

225

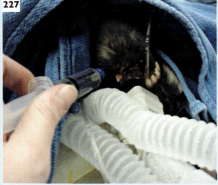

227

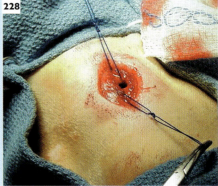

228

228 The stay sutures should be used to help lift the trachea toward the incision, and, with gentle traction, the desired stoma can be visualized.

229 The tracheostomy tube is placed via the stoma, and connected to the anesthetic circuit to permit patient recovery. Unless mechanical ventilation is pursued, the cuff should *not* be inflated.

Transtracheal aspirate

A transtracheal aspirate is performed for diagnosis of some respiratory conditions, e.g. pneumonia or allergic pulmonary disease, in dogs weighing >10 kg. Supplies needed include sterile prep and gloves, local anesthetic, a through-the-needle catheter, three to five aliquots of sterile 3–10 ml saline in syringes, EDTA tube for cytology, and culturettes or red top tubes for culture. The technique is illustrated in **230–235**.

Transtracheal aspirate
230 The ventral aspect of the neck is clipped and prepped for transtracheal aspiration.

231 The tracheal rings are palpated and local anesthetic is injected. Alternatively, a puncture may be made through the cricothyroid membrane.

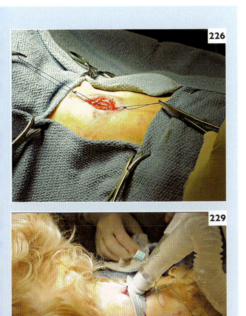

226

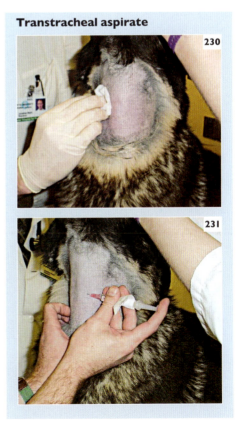

Transtracheal aspirate

230

229

231

232 The catheter is inserted through the skin and then directed into the tracheal lumen.

233 The catheter is fed in for its entire length. Most dogs will cough or swallow heavily when the catheter is within the tracheal lumen. The operator should be able to aspirate air freely as the tip of the catheter is located within the trachea.

234 Saline is injected through the catheter and then rapidly re-aspirated through the catheter for collection of the samples for cytology and culture. It is not uncommon to retrieve <20% of the saline injected. Remaining saline will be rapidly reabsorbed and is not problematic.

235 Productive transtracheal wash samples will appear cloudy and may have clumps of mucus or other debris.

Transtracheal aspirate *(continued)*

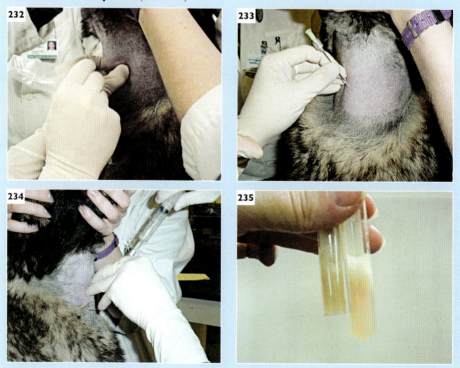

Epidural analgesia

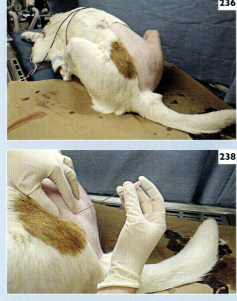

Epidural analgesia

Epidural analgesics are very useful to control post-operative pain and to limit the amount of intra-operative anesthetic agents required. Epidural catheters may also be used to provide repeated dosing. The technique is illustrated in **236–240** (photographs courtesy of Dr C. Blaze).

236 The patient to undergo epidural analgesia is placed in sternal recumbency with the legs pulled forward.

237 The site is surgically prepped. Wearing sterile gloves, the operator palpates for the landmarks for proper injection into the lumbo-sacral space. These landmarks include the cranial aspect of the ilial wings (palpated with the thumb and middle finger) and then the index finger may be used to locate the lumbosacral space.

238 Using a specially designed needle, the lumbosacral space is penetrated. A 'pop' is felt upon successful puncture.

239 Following successful needle placement, the correct placement in the epidural space may be assured by using the 'drop technique', when a drop of saline placed on the hub of the needle will be sucked into the epidural space. If, after removing the stylet, CSF is encountered, this means that the subarachnoid space has been penetrated and the dose should be reduced by 50%. If blood returns, a vessel has been penetrated and the needle should be withdrawn without injection.

240 The desired drug may be slowly injected into the epidural space.

Esophagostomy tube placement

The placement of an esophagostomy feeding tube is one of the simplest and most effective ways of providing nutritional support to critically ill patients. These tubes are well tolerated by the patient and easy for the owner to use. The placement of such tubes requires an endotracheal tube, a mouth gag, a curved carmalt, a surgical blade, and a feeding tube. The procedure is illustrated in **241–254**.

Esophagostomy tube placement

241 Proper placement of an esophagostomy feeding tube requires the distal tip to be placed in the distal esophagus at a level no further than the ninth intercostal space. The tube may need to be premeasured. Rather than cutting the tip and creating a sharp edge, the exit side hole should be elongated using a small blade.

242 The patient should be anesthetized and preferably intubated. While in right lateral recumbency, the left side of the neck should be clipped and a routine surgical scrub performed.

243 A drape is placed, and a curved Rochester carmalt is placed into the mouth and down the esophagus to the midcervical region.

244, 245 The jugular vein should be identified and avoided. The tip of the carmalt is then pushed dorsally, pushing the esophagus towards the skin. The tip of the carmalt is palpated over the skin to confirm its location and a stab incision is made through the skin and into the esophagus. The mucosa of the esophagus is relatively more difficult to incise than the skin.

246, 247 The tip of the carmalt is then forced through the incision, which can be slightly enlarged with the blade. The carmalt is opened and the tip of the tube is placed within the jaws of the instrument.

248 The carmalt is then clamped closed and pulled from the oral cavity.

249, 250 The jaws of the carmalt are disengaged and the tip of the esophagostomy tube is curled back into the mouth and fed into the esophagus.

Esophagostomy tube placement

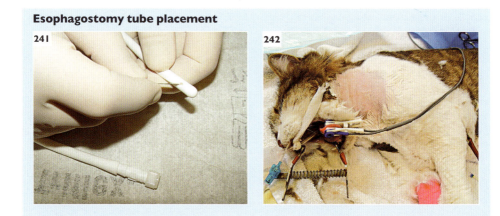

241 · 242

Esophagostomy tube placement *(continued)*

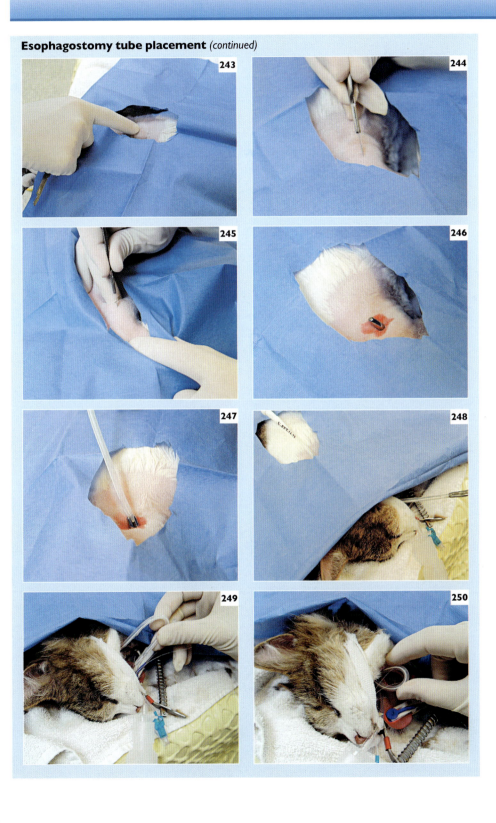

Esophagostomy tube placement *continued*

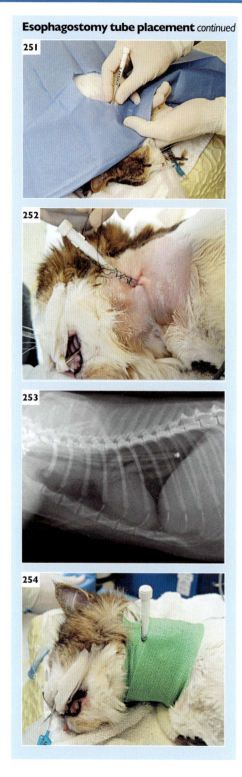

251 As the curled tube is pushed into the esophagus, the proximal end is gently pulled simultaneously. This will result in a subtle 'flip' as the tube is redirected within the esophagus. This is by the far the most difficult step – getting the tube to straighten within the larynx. If successful, the tube should easily slide back and forth a few millimeters, confirming that the tube has straightened. The tube will now naturally rest rostrally. The oropharynx is inspected visually to confirm that the tube is no longer present within the oropharynx.

252 The incision site should be briefly re-scrubbed before suturing the tube. A purse-string suture is placed followed by a 'Chinese finger trap', further securing the tube in place.

253 A thoracic radiograph is taken to confirm correct placement. The tip of the tube should be in the distal esophagus and not within the stomach.

254 After correct placement is confirmed, antibiotic ointment is applied to the exit site and a light wrap placed.

Robert Jones bandage

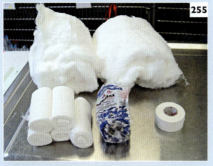

255

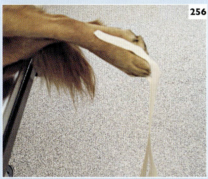

256

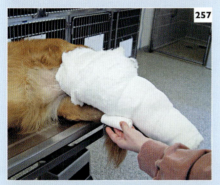

257

Robert Jones bandage

A Robert Jones bandage is a large pressure bandage used to create stability and reduce swelling and tissue edema, e.g. for initial treatment of limb fractures below the elbow or stifle. The technique is illustrated in **255–259**.

Robert Jones bandage

255 Supplies needed for placement of a Robert Jones bandage. Roll cotton may be torn in half prior to application for easier handing.

256 Tape stirrups are applied to the foot and tarsus to help keep the bandage in place.

257 Roll cotton is applied, starting at the bottom of the leg and extending upwards to above the stifle. The cotton should be applied firmly but not tightly. Next, roll gauze is placed over the cotton. This layer may be tightened, as the protective cotton layer should prevent too much pressure from being put on the leg.

258 The tape stirrups are applied to the bandage and then the entire bandage is covered with a conforming bandage. A well placed Robert Jones will 'thump' like a ripe watermelon.

259 The finished product. Some dogs may need an Elizabethan collar to prevent premature removal of the bandage.

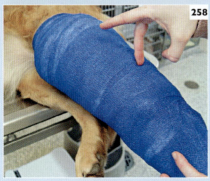

258

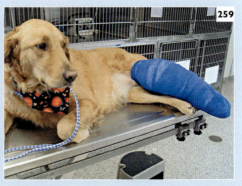

259

Appendices

1 Conversion tables

WEIGHT EQUIVALENTS
1 lb   = 453.6 g   = 0.4536 kg = 16 oz
1 oz   = 28.35 g
1 kg   = 2.2046 lb
1 mg   = 1,000 µg   = 0.001 g
1 µg   = 0.001 mg   = 0.000001 g
1 ppm   = 1 mg per kg

BODY WEIGHT (KG) TO BODY SURFACE (M²) CONVERSION
Approximate surface area in m² (dog):
$[10.1 \times (\text{weight in grams})^{0.66}]/10,000$
Approximate surface area in m² (cat):
$[10.0 \times (\text{weight in grams})^{0.66}]/10,000$

VOLUME EQUIVALENTS
Household		Metric
1 drop	=	0.06 ml
15 drops	=	1 ml (1 cc)
1 teaspoon	=	5 ml
1 tablespoon	=	15 ml
1 oz	=	30 ml
1 cup	=	240 ml (½ pint)
2 cups	=	500 ml (1 pint)

TEMPERATURE CONVERSION
°Celsius to °Fahrenheit: $([°C \times 9]/5) + 32$
°Fahrenheit to °Celsius: $([°F - 32] \times 5)/9$

CONVERSION OF UNITS FOR DOGS

Conversion table for dogs

Kilogram	m²	Kilogram	m²	Kilogram	m²	Kilogram	m²
0.5	0.06	17.0	0.66	34.0	1.05	51.0	1.38
1.0	0.10	18.0	0.69	35.0	1.07	52.0	1.40
2.0	0.15	19.0	0.71	36.0	1.09	53.0	1.41
3.0	0.20	20.0	0.74	37.0	1.11	54.0	1.43
4.0	0.25	21.0	0.76	38.0	1.13	55.0	1.45
5.0	0.29	22.0	0.78	39.0	1.15	56.0	1.47
6.0	0.33	23.0	0.81	40.0	1.17	57.0	1.48
7.0	0.36	24.0	0.83	41.0	1.19	58.0	1.50
8.0	0.40	25.0	0.85	42.0	1.21	59.0	1.52
9.0	0.43	26.0	0.88	43.0	1.23	60.0	1.54
10.0	0.46	27.0	0.90	44.0	1.25	61.0	1.55
11.0	0.49	28.0	0.92	45.0	1.28	62.0	1.57
12.0	0.52	29.0	0.94	46.0	1.30		
13.0	0.55	30.0	0.96	47.0	1.32		
14.0	0.58	31.0	0.99	48.0	1.32		
15.0	0.60	32.0	1.01	49.0	1.34		
16.0	0.63	33.0	1.03	50.0	1.36		

CONVERSION OF UNITS FOR CATS

Conversion table for cats							
Kilogram	**m^2**	**Kilogram**	**m^2**	**Kilogram**	**m^2**	**Kilogram**	**m^2**
1.0	0.100	4.0	0.252	7.0	0.366	10.0	0.464
1.5	0.131	4.5	0.273	7.5	0.383	10.5	0.480
2.0	0.159	5.0	0.292	8.0	0.400	11.0	0.495
2.5	0.184	5.5	0.311	8.5	0.416	11.5	0.510
3.0	0.208	6.0	0.330	9.0	0.432	12.0	0.524
3.5	0.231	6.5	0.348	9.5	0.449	12.5	0.540

CONVERSION OF UNITS FOR LABORATORY TESTS

Laboratory conversion table – traditional US units to SI units			
Parameter	**US units**	**Multiply by**	**To get SI units**
ALP	U/l	1.0	U/l
AST (SGOT)	U/l	1.0	U/l
ALT (SGPT)	U/l	1.0	U/l
Albumin	g/dl	10	g/l
Ammonia	µg/dl	0.554	µmol/l
Amylase	U/l	1.0	U/l
Base excess	mEq/l	1	mmol/l
Bicarbonate	mM	1	mmol/l
Bile acids	mg/dl	10	mg/l
Bilirubin	mg/dl	17.1	µmol/l
Bromide	mg/dl	0.125	mmol/l
BUN	mg/dl	0.357	mmol/l
Calcium	mg/dl	0.25	mmol/l
CO_2	mM	1	mmol/l
CO_2 partial pressure	mmHg	0.133	kPa
Chloride	mEq/l	1	mmol/l
Cholesterol	mg/dl	0.026	mmol/l
Citrate	mg/dl	52	µmol/l
Copper	µg/dl	0.157	µmol/l
Cortisol	µg/dl	27.6	nmol/l
Creatinine	mg/dl	88.4	µmol/l
Creatinine clearance	ml/min	0.0167	ml/s
Fibrinogen	mg/dl	0.01	mmol/l
Folate	ng/dl	2.27	nmol/l
Gamma globulin	g/dl	10	g/l
Globulin	g/dl	10	g/l
Glucose	mg/dl	0.055	mmol/l
GGT	IU/l	1.0	U/l
Glutathione	mg/dl	0.032	mmol/l

Laboratory conversion table – traditional US units to SI units *(continued)*

Parameter	US units	Multiply by	To get SI units
Immunoglobulins	mg/dl	0.01	g/l
Insulin	µIU/ml	0.0417	µg/l
Iron	µg/dl	0.179	µmol/l
Iron binding capacity	µg/dl	0.179	µmol/l
Lactate	mg/dl	0.111	mmol/l
LDH	U/l	1	U/l
Lead	µg/dl	0.048	µmol/l
Lipase	U/l	1.0	U/l
Lipids	mg/dl	0.01	g/l
Magnesium	mEq/l	0.5	mmol/l
Methemoglobin	g/dl	10	g/l
O_2 partial pressure	mmHg	0.133	kPa
Phosphorus	mg/dl	0.323	mmol/l
Potassium	mEq/l	1	mmol/l
Protein (total)	g/dl	10	g/l
Sodium	mEq/l	1	mmol/l
Thyroxine (T4)	µg/dl	13.0	nmol/l
Total CO_2	mM	1	mmol/l
Triglycerides	mg/dl	0.011	mmol/l
Vitamin B_{12}	pg/ml	0.74	pmol/l
Zinc	µg/dl	0.153	µmol/l

2 Calculation of a continuous rate infusion

Administration of medications as a CRI is useful to help to maintain constant blood concentrations or for medications that are so rapidly metabolized that intermittent re-dosing is impractical. Fluid pumps and syringe pumps are very useful in the delivery of CRIs and are mandatory for the use of vasoactive and otherwise potent medications. The following examples illustrate how CRIs may be easily formulated.

In order to calculate a CRI, the following variables must be known:

- Desired infusion rate. This is usually in the order of µg/kg/min. Some drugs are listed as mg/kg/hr or mg/kg/day. Some of the more frequently used drugs are listed in *Table 60*.
- The concentration of the drug. For drugs listed in percentages, multiplying the percentage by a factor of 10 yields the mg/ml concentration. For example, 2% lidocaine is 20 mg/ml.
- The desired fluid rate. For animals in heart failure, low rates of fluid should be used (one eighth to one quarter of maintenance needs). For other animals, the drug may be added to their hourly fluid, or infused as a separate infusion at a nominal fluid rate (e.g. 10–15 ml/hr).
- The size of the fluid bag to be used for the infusion (e.g. 150, 250, 500, or 1000 ml). For some drugs delivered at low infusion rates, medications may be added to a syringe with saline and infused using a syringe pump.

Table 60 Medications commonly administered as CRIs. A pharmacology text or other resource must be consulted prior to use of an unfamiliar medication

Drug	Dose range	Notes
Lidocaine *	40–80 µg/kg/min	Higher doses may cause vomiting or seizures
Dopamine *	1–20 µg/kg/min	Higher doses are used for inotropic and vasopressor effects
Dobutamine *	1–10 µg/kg/min	Higher doses (particularly in cats) may cause seizures or vomiting
Metaclopramine	1–2 mg/kg/day	Higher doses may cause neurological signs
Morphine	0.1–1 mg/kg/hr	Initiate at lower end and titrate to effect
Ketamine	0.1–0.6 mg/kg/hr	Can be used in conjunction with other analgesics
Propofol *	0.2–0.7 mg/kg/min	For seizure control, can initiate at lower end and titrate to effect. May cause severe cardiorespiratory depression
Nitroprusside sodium	1–7 mg/kg/min	May cause profound hypotension, must be titrated to effect. Requires frequent blood pressure measurements

*Requires continuous ECG monitoring

EXAMPLE 1 ADMINISTERING A LIDOCAINE CRI TO A 40 KG DOG AT 50 µG/KG/MIN

- Variable 1: lidocaine infusion at 50 µg/kg/min.
- Variable 2: lidocaine is available as a 2% solution and therefore the concentration is 20 mg/ml.
- Variable 3: it is decided to infuse at 50 ml/hr.
- Variable 4: it is decided to use a 1 liter bag of 0.9% saline.

At the chosen rate of fluid infusion (50 ml/hr), 1 liter of 0.9% saline will last 20 hours (1000 ml divided by 50 ml/hr). For this dog, the infusion rate of 50 µg/kg/min is first multiplied by the weight in kilograms and then by 60 min for a total of 20 hours to yield 2,400,000 µg (40 × 50 × 60 × 20 = 2,400,000). This is divided by 1000 to convert it into milligrams (2,400 mg). This is finally divided by the drug concentration (20 mg/ml) to yield the total volume in milliliters to add to make 1 liter solution, which in this case is 120 ml of 2% lidocaine.

Thus, by adding 120ml of 2% lidocaine to 880 ml of 0.9% saline (for a total of 1 liter) and setting the infusion pump at 50 ml/hr, the dog will be administered a lidocaine CRI of 50 µg/kg/min.

When the volume of medication to be added is small (<10 ml), there is no need to subtract a corresponding volume from the bag of fluid. However, because the volume of lidocaine is typically quite significant, it is prudent to subtract an equivalent volume, explaining the 880 ml of saline in this example.

EXAMPLE 2 ADMINISTERING A DOPAMINE CRI FOR A 5 KG CAT AT 7 µG/KG/MIN

- Variable 1: dopamine to be administered at 7 µg/kg/min.
- Variable 2: dopamine is available as 40 mg/ml.
- Variable 3: it is decided to infuse at 5 ml/hr.
- Variable 4: a bag of 250 ml of 0.9% saline is chosen.

Using the above variables, the 250 ml bag of 0.9% saline will last 50 hours (250 divided by 5). For this cat, the infusion rate of 7 µg/kg/min is multiplied by 5 kg × 60 min × 50 hours to yield 105,000 µg. This is divided by 1000 to convert it to milligrams, which yields 105 mg. Dividing the total milligrams by the drug concentration of 40 mg/ml yields the milliliters to add to 250 ml, which in this case is 2.6 ml. Thus, 2.6 ml of dopamine should be added to 250 ml of 0.9% saline, which is infused at 5 ml/hr.

EXAMPLE 3 ADMINISTERING A METACLOPRAMIDE CRI FOR A 20 KG DOG AT 2 MG/KG/DAY

- Variable 1: metaclopramide at 2 mg/kg/day.
- Variable 2: metaclopramide comes in 5 mg/ml vials.
- Variable 3: it is decided to infuse at 25 ml/hr.
- Variable 4: a 500 ml bag of fluid is chosen.

A 500 ml bag of fluid delivered at 25 ml/hr will last 20 hours. Twenty hours is equal to 83.3% of a day. Multiplying 20 kg × 2 mg/kg/day and then multiplying by 0.833 (83.3% of one day) yields a total of 33.3 mg of metaclopramide. Dividing this total (33.3 mg) by the concentration of this drug (5 mg/ml) yields the volume to be added to 500 ml of the chosen fluid (6.7 ml of metaclopramide).

3 Intensive care unit drug formulary

The following is a list of drugs, their indications, and recommended dosages that may be useful in the treatment of critically ill patients and in emergency situations. While every effort has been expended to assure that the dosages and information included in this formulary are correct, errors may occur and it is suggested that the reader refer to the approved labeling information of the product. The authors/publisher shall not be held liable for any detrimental effects related to the usage of drugs listed in this formulary.

Drug Name	Class of drug	Indications	Dosages
Acepromazine	Phenothiazide tranquilizer	Anxiolytic, anesthetic	Premedication: (Dog): 0.02–0.05 mg/kg IM;
		premedication	Sedation 0.1–0.25 mg/kg IV Cat: 0.05–0.1 mg/kg IM, IV
Acetazolamide	Carbonic anhydrase inhibitor	Glaucoma	50 mg/kg IV once then 7 mg/kg PO q 8 hr; 4–8 mg/kg PO q8–12 hr
Acetylcysteine	Mucolytic, glutathione precursor	Antidote for acetaminophen (paracetamol) toxicity	Loading dose 140 mg/kg IV then 70 mg/kg IV or PO q4hr for five doses
S-Adenosylmethionine (SAMe)	Methyl donor	Liver dysfunction	20 mg/kg/day or 2–7 kg: 90 mg 7–13 kg: 180 mg 14–18 kg: 225 mg 19–34 kg: 450 mg > 35 kg: 675 mg
Albuterol	β_2 agonist	Bronchodilator	20–50 µg/kg four times/day; up to maximum of 100 µg/kg four times daily
Amikacin	Aminoglycoside antibiotic	Susceptible infections	Dog, cat: 15 mg/kg IV, IM, SQ q 24 hrs
Aminophylline	Phosphodiesterase inhibitor	Bronchodilator	Dog: 10 mg/kg PO, IM, IV q8 hr Cat: 6.6 mg/kg PO q 12 hr
Amiodarone	Antiarrhythmic (Class 3)	Atrial, ventricular unifocal or multifocal premature depolarization, atrial flutter, atrial fibrillation	15–20 mg/kg PO q 12 hr for 7 days, then reduce to 5–15 mg/kg PO q 12 hr; 1–3 mg/kg IV over 20 minutes diluted in 5DW, repeat after 15 minutes if needed
Amlodipine	Calcium channel antagonist	Hypertension	Dog: 0.1 mg/kg PO q24 hr Cat: 0.625 mg/cat/day PO initially and increase if needed to 0.625 mg/cat PO q 12 hrs
Amoxicillin trihydrate	β-lactam antibiotic	Susceptible infections	22 mg/kg PO q12 hrs
Amoxicillin/ clavulanic acid	β-lactam antibiotic	Susceptible infections	13.65 mg/kg PO q 12 hr
Ampicillin	β-lactam antibiotic	Susceptible infections	22 mg/kg IV, IM, SC q8 hr
Ampicillin + sulbactam	β-lactam antibiotic	Susceptible infections	22 mg/kg IV, IM q8 hr
Ampicillin trihydrate	β-lactam antibiotic	Susceptible infections	6.5–10 mg/kg IM, SC q12 hr
Amrinone	Inotropic vasodilator	Low cardiac output	1–3 mg/kg over 2–3 minutes IV load, then 0.003–0.1 mg/kg/min CRI
Apomorphine hydrochloride	Dopamine receptor agonist	Emetic agent	0.25 mg/kg into conjunctival sac

Drug Name	Class of drug	Indications	Dosages
Ascorbic acid (Vitamin C)	Antioxidant	Oxidative stress	100 mg/cat/day
Atenolol	β-blocker	Tachyarrhythmia; hypertrophic cardiomyopathy	Dog: 0.2–1 mg/kg PO q12 hr Cat: 6.25–12.5 mg PO **per cat** q12 hr
Atipamezole	α_2 antagonist	Medetomidine reversal agent	Administer same volume as medetomidine
Atracurium	Non-depolarizing paralyzing agent	Controlled paralysis	0.2 mg/kg IV initially, then 0.15 mg/kg q30 min (or IV infusion at 3–8μg/kg/min)
Atropine	Anticholinergic	Bradyarrhythmias; organophosphate and carbamate toxicosis	0.02–0.04 mg/kg IV, IM; 0.2–0.5 mg/kg (as needed) for organophosphate toxicosis
Azathioprine	Thiopurine analog	Immunosuppressive agent	Dog: 2 mg/kg PO q24 hr for ten days, then 2 mg/kg q 48 hr
Azithromycin	Macrolide antibiotic	Susceptible infections	Dog: 10 mg/kg PO once every 5 days or 3.3 mg/kg q24 hr for 3 days
			Cat: 5 mg/kg PO q48 hr
Benazepril	Angiotensin converting enzyme inhibitor	Hypertension	Dog,cat: 0.25–0.5 mg/kg PO q 12–24 hr
Bupivacaine	Local analgesic	Thoracostomy tube analgesia	Dog: 1.5 mg/kg diluted with saline up to 25 ml total, infuse into thorax q 4–6 hr; Cat: 0.5 mg/kg diluted with saline up to 10 ml total, infuse into
Buprenorphine	Opioid agonist/antagonist	Mild to moderate pain	Dog: 0.006–0.02 mg/kg IM, SC q4–8 hr Cat: 0.005–0.01 mg/kg IV, IM q4–8 hr
Butorphanol	Opioid agonist/antagonist	Mild pain; antitussive	Dog: 0.2–0.4 mg/kg IV, IM, SC q2–4 hr or 0.55–1.1 mg/kg PO q 6–12 hr; Antitussive: 0.55 mg/kg PO q 4–6 hr
Calcitonin	Calcium regulating hormone	Hypercalcemia	4–8 U/kg q 12–24 hr IV, IM, SC
Calcium chloride	Calcium supplement	Hypocalcemia; cardioprotection from hyperkalemia	Using 10% solution: 0.1–0.3 ml/kg IV slowly
Calcium gluconate	Calcium supplement	Hypocalcemia; hyperkalemia	Using 10% solution: 0.1–0.3 ml/kg IV slowly
Carprofen	NSAID	Inflammation	Dog: 2.2 mg/kg PO, SQ q 12 hrs
Carvedilol	Non selective beta blocker with alpha-1 blocking activity	Arrhythmias	0.625–1.25 mg/kg PO q 12 hr
Cefaclor (Ceclor)	2nd generation cephalosporin	Susceptible infections	4–20 mg/kg PO q 8hr
Cefadroxil (Cefa-Tabs)	1st generation cephalosporin	Susceptible infections	Dog: 22–30 mg/kg PO q 12 hr; Cat: 22 mg/kg PO q 24 hr

Continued

Drug Name	Class of drug	Indications	Dosages
Cefazolin sodium	1st generation cephalosporin	Susceptible infections	22 mg/kg IV, IM q 8 hr
Cefixime (Suprax)	3rd generation cephalosporin	Susceptible infections	10 mg/kg PO q 12 hr
Cefotaxime (Claforan)	3rd generation cephalosporin	Susceptible infections	Dog: 50 mg/kg IV, IM, SC q 12 hr; Cat: 20–80 mg/kg IV, IM, q 6 hr
Cefotetan (Cefotan)	3rd generation cephalosporin	Susceptible infections	30 mg/kg IV, SC q 8 hr
Cefoxitin sodium (Mefoxin)	2nd generation cephalosporin	Susceptible infections	30 mg/kg IV q6–8 hr
Cefpodoxime (Simplicef)	3rd generation cephalosporin	Susceptible infections	5–10 mg/kg PO q 24 hr
Ceftiofur (Naxcel)	3rd generation cephalosporin	Susceptible infections	2.2–4.4 mg/kg SC q 24 hr
Cephalexin (Keflex)	1st generation cephalosporin	Susceptible infections	22 mg/kg PO q8 hr
Cephalothin sodium (Keflin)	1st generation cephalosporin	Susceptible infections	22 mg/kg IV, IM q 4–8 hr
Charcoal, activated	Toxin binder	Toxin ingestion	6–12 mg/kg
Chloramphenicol	Antibiotic	Susceptible infections	Dog: 40–50 mg/kg PO q8 hr Cat: 12.5–20 mg/kg PO q12 hr
Chlorpromazine	Dopamine receptor antagonist	Vomiting	0.5 mg/kg IM, SC q6–8 hr
Cimetidine	H_2 antagonist	Gastroprotectant	10 mg/kg IV, IM, PO q6–8 hr
Ciprofloxacin	Fluoroquinolone antibiotic	Susceptible infections	5–20 mg/kg PO, IV q 12–24 hr
Cisapride	Prokinetic	Ileus	Dog: 0.1–0.5 mg/kg PO q8–12hr; Cat: 2.5–5 mg/cat PO q8–12 hr [not widely available]
Clindamycin	Macrolide antibiotic	Susceptible infections; anaerobes	Dog: 11 mg/kg PO, IM q12 hr or 22 mg/kg PO q24 hr
			Cat: 5.5 mg/kg PO, IM q 12 hr or 22 mg/kg q 24 hr
Codeine	Opioid analgesic	Moderate to severe pain; antitussive	Analgesia: 0.5–1 mg/kg PO q 4–6 hr Antitussive: 0.1–0.3 mg/kg PO q 4–6
Cosyntropin (Cortrosyn)	ACTH analog	ACTH Stimulation test	Response test: (dog): collect pre-ACTH sample and inject 5 µg/kg IV, collect post-ACTH sample in 1 hr. (cat): collect pre-ACTH sample and inject 0.125 mg IV, IM, collect post-ACTH sample in 30 min and 1 hour p
Cyanocobalamin (Vitamin B$_{12}$)	Vitamin	Deficiency	Dog: 100–200 µg/day SC Cat: 50–100 µg/day SC
Cyclophosphamide (Cytoxan)	Immunosuppression	Immune-mediated disease	50 mg/m^2 PO q 48 hr or 2.2 mg/kg PO q 24 hr for 4 days/wk
Cyclosporine (Neoral; Sandimmune)	Immunosuppression	Immune-mediated disease	Dog: 10 mg/kg PO q 24 hr (adjust dos by monitoring blood concentrations) Cat: 4–6 mg/kg PO q 12 hr
Dantrolene	Calcium channel antagonist	Malignant hyperthermia	2–3 mg/kg IV
Deferoxamine	Iron chelator	Iron toxicosis, oxidative stress	10 mg/kg IV, IM q 2 hr for 2 doses, the 10 mg/kg q 8 hr for 24 hrs
Deracoxib	NSAID	Anti-inflammatory	3–4 mg/kg/day
Desmopressin acetate (DDAVP)	Vasopressin analog	Diabetes insipidus; von Willebrand's disease	DI: 2–4 drops (2 µg) q 12–24 hr in ey vWD: 1 µg/kg (0.01 mg/kg) SC

Drug Name	Class of drug	Indications	Dosages
Desoxycorticosterone pivalate (DOCP)	Mineralocorticoid	Replacement therapy	1.5–2.2 mg/kg IM q 25 days
Diazepam	Sedative	Pre-anesthetic; sedative; anticonvulsant	Adjunct pre-anesthetic: 0.1–0.2 mg/kg IV
			Seizures: 0.2 mg/kg IV, up to four times for status epilepticus or seizure clusters
Diazoxide (Proglycem)	Insulin release inhibitor	Insulinoma	10–40 mg/kg/day divided q 8–12 hrs
Digoxin	Digitalis antiarrhythmic	Arrhythmias	Dog: 0.005 mg/kg PO q 12 hrs Cat: 0.08–0.01 mg/kg PO q 48 hr
Dihydrotachysterol (Hytakerol)	Vitamin D	Hypocalcemia	0.01 mg/kg/day PO; for acute treatment administer 0.02 mg/kg initially, then 0.01–0.02 mg/kg PO q24–48 hr thereafter
Diltiazem (Cardizem)	Digitalis antiarrhythmic	Ventricular tachyarrhythmias	Dog: 0.5–1.5 mg/kg PO q8 hr; 0.25 mg/kg over 2 min IV (repeat if necessary). For sustained release products use 5–10 mg/kg PO q 12–24 hrs. Cat: 1.75–2.4 mg/kg PO q8 hr
Diphenhydramine (Benadryl)	Antihistamine	Pruritis; urticaria	2–4 mg/kg PO q 6–8 hr or 1–2 mg/kg IM, IV
Dobutamine	Inotrope	Inotropic support	Dog: 3–20 µg/kg/min IV infusion; use with caution in cats
Dolasetron (Anzemet)	5HT$_3$ antagonist	Anti-emetic	0.6–1 mg/kg IV, IM, SC q 24 hr
Dopamine	Inotrope	Inotropic support, hypotension	Dog, cat: 2–20 µg/kg/min IV
Doxapram (Dopram)	Respiratory center stimulant	Respiratory depression	1–2 mg/kg IV; manual ventilation recommended Neonate: 1–5 mg SC, sublingual, or via umbilical vein
Doxycycline	Antibiotic	Susceptible infections	3–5 mg/kg PO, IV q 12 hr or 10 mg/kg PO q 24 hr
Edrophonium (Tensilon)	Anticholinesterase	Myasthenia gravis	Dog: 0.11–0.22 mg/kg IV
Enalapril (Enacard, Vasotec)	Angiotensin converting enzyme inhibitor	Hypertension; proteinuria	Dog: 0.5 mg/kg PO q 12–24 hr
Enrofloxacin	Fluoroquinolone antibiotic	Susceptible infections	Dog: 10–20 mg/kg PO, IV, IM q 12–24 hr Cat: 5 mg/kg PO, IV, IM, q 24 hr (Use with caution, associated with blindness)
Epinephrine	Catecholamine	Vasopressor; cardiac arrest	Low dose for CPR: 0.02 mg/kg; High dose for CPR: 0.2 mg/kg
			1:1,000 injection: 10–20 µg/kg IV, 200 µg/kg intratracheally diluted with sterile water
			Anaphylaxis: 2.5–5 µg/kg IV or 50 µg/kg intratracheally
Ergocalciferol (Calciferol)	Vitamin D2	Hypocalcemia	500–2,000 U/kg PO

Continued

Drug Name	Class of drug	Indications	Dosages
Erythromycin	Macrolide antibiotic	Susceptible infections; Prokinetic	Antibacterial dose: 10–20 mg/kg PO q8–12 hr
			Prokinetic: 0.5–1.0 mg/kg PO q8 hr
Erythropoietin (Epogen)	Erythropoetic hormone	Anemia	35–50 U/kg three times/wk to 400 U/kg/wk IV, SC
Esmolol (Brevibloc)	β-blocker	Tachyarrhythmia	50–200 µg/kg/min infusion
Etodolac (Etogesic)	NSAID	Inflammation	Dog: 10–15 mg/kg PO q 24 hr
Etomidate	Hypnotic anesthetic	Anesthetic induction	Dog: 0.5–2.0mg/kg
Famotidine (Pepcid)	H$_2$ blocker	Gastroprotectant	0.5 mg/kg IM, SC, PO, IV q12–24 hr
Felbamate	Anticonvulsive	Seizures	Dog: Start with 15 mg/kg PO q 8 hr and increase gradually to maximum of 65 mg/kg q 8 hr
Fentanyl	Opioid agonist	Analgesic; anesthetic	0.5–8.0µg/kg/hr IV
			CRI: 0.2–0.7 µg/kg/min
Fentanyl transdermal	Opioid agonist	Analgesic	Cats and dogs < 10 kg: 25 µg/hr patch
			Dogs 10–30 kg: 50 µg/hr patch
			Dogs > 30 kg: 75 µg/hr patch
Fluconazole (Diflucan)	Antifungal	Susceptible infections	Dog: 10–12 mg/kg/day PO Cat: 50 mg/cat PO q 12 hr or 50 mg/cat/day PO
Fludrocortisone (Florinef)	Mineralocorticoid	Replacement therapy	Dog: 0.015–0.02 mg/kg/day PO q 24 hr (13–23 µg/kg) Cat: 0.1–0.2 mg/cat PO q 24 hr
Flumazenil (Romazicon)	Benzodiazepine reversal agent	Benzodiazepine overdose	0.2 mg (total dose) IV as needed
Fluticasone (Flovent)	Inhalant corticosteroid	Asthma	1 actuation (110µg) q 12 hr with 1 mg/kg prednisone PO q 12 hrs, then taper
Furosemide	Loop diuretic	Fluid overload	Dog: 2–6mg/kg IV, IM, SC, PO q 4–12 hr (or as needed) Cat: 1–4mg/kg IV, IM, SC, PO q 8–24 hr (or as needed)
Gabapentin (Neurontin)	Anticonvulsive	Seizures; Neuropathic pain	Anticonvulsive: 5–15 mg/kg divided q 8 hr Neuropathic pain: 3–5 mg/kg PO divided q 8 hr
Gentamicin	Aminoglycoside antibiotic	Susceptible infections	Dog, cat: 5–7 mg/kg IV, IM, SC q 24 hr
Glucagon	Insulin antagonizing hormone	Insulin overdose; insulinoma	0.03 mg/kg IV, IM. CRI 5–10 ng/kg/min
Glycopyrrolate	Anticholinergic	Bradycardia	0.005–0.01 mg/kg IV, IM, SC
Granulocyte-colony-stimulating factor (GSF)	Cytokine	Neutropenia	2.5 µg/kg SC q 12 hr
Heparin sodium (unfractionated)	Anticoagulant	Hypercoagulable state; hypertriglyceridemia	200 units/kg IV loading dose, then 100–300 units/kg SC q 6–8 hr (target is to prolong PTT by 1.5 x baseline). CRI: 10–25 IU/kg/hr

Drug Name	Class of drug	Indications	Dosages
Heparin, low-molecular weight (fractionated) (Dalteprin–Fragmin)	Anticoagulant	Hypercoagulable state	Dog: 100–200 U/kg SC q 12–24 hr Cat: 100 U/kg SC q 12 hr
Hydralazine	α-1 antagonist	Hypertension	Dog: 0.5 mg/kg (initial dose); titrate to 0.5–2 mg/kg PO q 12 hr Cat: 2.5 mg/cat PO q 12–24 hr
Hydrochlorothiazide	Thiazide diuretic	Fluid overload	2–4 mg/kg PO q 12–24 hr
Hydrocodone bitartrate (Hycodan)	Opioid	Antitussive	Dog: 0.22 mg/kg PO q 4–8 hr
Hydrocortisone (Cortef)	Corticosteroid	Inflammation; replacement therapy	Replacement therapy: 1–2 mg/kg PO q 12 hr Anti-inflammatory: 2.5–5 mg/kg PO q 12 hr
Hydrocortisone sodium succinate (Solu-Cortef)	Corticosteroid	Replacement therapy	Anti-inflammatory: 5 mg/kg IV q 12 hr
Hydromorphone	Pure opioid agonist	Moderate to severe pain	Dog, cat: 0.05–0.1 mg/kg IV, IM, SC q 4–6 hr
Imipenem (Primaxin)	Potentiated penicillin	Susceptible infections	3–10 mg/kg IV, IM, q 6–8 hr
Insulin, regular crystalline	Glucose regulating hormone	Diabetes mellitus, DKA	Intermittent IM technique: Initial dose 0.2 U/kg IM; repeat IM doses of 0.1 U/kg hourly, guided by blood glucose. CRI: Initially give regular insulin at a rate of 0.05–0.1 U/kg/hr. Adjust infusion rate based upon glucose levels
Insulin, NPH	Glucose regulating hormone	Diabetes mellitus	0.25 U/kg SC q 12 hr
Isoproterenol	Sympathomimetic	Bradyarrhythmias	10 μg/kg IM, SC q 6 hr; or dilute 1 mg in 500 ml of 5DW and infuse IV 0.5–1 ml/min (1–2 μg/min) to effect
Ketamine	Dissociative anesthetic	Adjunct anesthetic, analgesic	Dog: 5 mg/kg IV, IM Cat: 2–5 mg/kg IV, IM Analgesic (CRI): 0.3–0.6 mg/kg/hr
Ketoprofen	NSAID	Inflammation	2 mg/kg IV, IM, SC single dose
Lactulose	Disaccharide	Stool softener; hyperammoniemia	Constipation: 1 ml/ 5 kg PO q 8 hr (to effect) Hepatic encephalopathy: dog: 0.5 ml/kg PO q 8 hr; cat: 2–5 ml/cat PO q 8 hr
Lansoprazole (Prevacid)	Proton pump inhibitor	Gastroprotectant	0.7 mg/kg IV diluted over 30 minutes. Administer through filter
Lidocaine	Sodium channel blocker	Antiarrhythmic; adjunct analgesic; local anesthetic; prokinetic	Dog antiarrhythmic: 2–4 mg/kg IV (max dose of 8 mg/kg over 10 minute period); If responsive, 50–75 μg/kg/min IV CRI; Analgesic/ Prokinetic: 50 μg/kg/min
Mannitol	Osmotic diuretic	Cerebral edema, glaucoma	Diuretic: 0.5–1 g/kg IV over 20–30 min. For glaucoma, may use up to 2 g/kg
Medetomidine	α-2 agonist	Moderate to severe pain	Dog: CRI: 3 μg/kg/hr
Meperidine	Opioid	Moderate pain	Dog: 5–10 mg/kg IV, IM, as often as q 2–3 hr (or as needed) Cat: 3–5 mg/kg IV, IM, q 2–4 hr (or as needed)

Continued

Drug Name	Class of drug	Indications	Dosages
Methocarbamol	Muscle relaxant	Tremorgenic mycotoxin, muscle spasms (IVDD), tetanus, strychnine toxicosis	Tremorgenic mycotoxin: 55–220 mg/k IV; muscle spasms:15–20 mg/kg PO q 8 hr; tetanus, strychnine toxicosis: 55–220 mg/kg IV, do not exceed 330 mg/kg/day
Methylprednisolone (Medrol)	Corticosteroid	Spinal injury, anti-inflammatory	0.22–0.44 mg/kg PO q 12–24 hr
Methylprednisolone (Depo-Medrol)	Long lasting corticosteroid	Asthma; inflammatory bowel disease	Dog: 1 mg/kg (or 20–40 mg/dog) IM q 1–3 wk Cat: 10–20 mg per cat IM q 1–3 wk
Methyprednisolone sodium succinate (Solu-Medrol)	Corticosteroid	Spinal injury	30 mg/kg IV and repeat at 15 mg/kg IV in 2–6 hr; 30 mg/kg IV followed 2 hr later with CRI of 5.4 mg/kg/hr for 24–48 hr
4-Methylpyrazole (Fomepizole, Antizol-Vet)	Alcohol dehydrogenase inhibitor	Ethylene glycol toxicosis	Dog: 20 mg/kg initially, then 15 mg/k at 12- and 24-hr intervals, then 5 mg/kg at 36 hr Cat: 125 mg/kg slow IV; at 12, 24, 36 hrs give 31.25 mg/kg IV
Metoclopramide	Dopamine antagonist	Anti-emetic; prokinetic	1–2 mg/kg/day CRI; 0.2–0.5 mg/kg IM, PO q 6–8 hr
Metoprolol tartrate	β-blocker	Antiarrhythmic	Dog, cat: 0.2–0.8 mg/kg PO q 8–12 hr
Metronidazole	Antibiotic	Susceptible infections	Dog, cat: 10 mg/kg IV q 8 hr
Mexilitine	Sodium channel blocker	Antiarrhythmic	Dog: 5–8 mg/kg PO q 8 hr (use cautiously)
Meloxicam	NSAID	Inflammation	Dog: 0.2 mg/kg PO, IV, SQ loading dos then 0.1 mg/kg q 24 hrs Cat: 0.05 mg/kg PO, SQ q 24–48 hrs
Midazolam	Benzodiazepine	Pre-anesthetic, sedative	0.1–0.25 mg/kg IV, IM
Misoprostol (Cytotec)	Prostaglandin E_2 analog	Gastroprotectant	Dog: 2–5 µg/kg PO q 6–8 hr
Morphine	Opioid	Analgesic, anesthetic, epidural	Dog: 0.5–1 mg/kg IV, IM, SC; epidural: 0.1 mg/kg CRI: 0.1–0.5 mg/kg/hr Cat: 0.1 mg/kg q 3–6 hr IM, SC (or as needed)
Naloxone	Opioid reversal agent	Opioid overdose, complication	0.01–0.04 mg/kg IV, IM, SC administered slowly to effect
Neomycin	Antibiotic	Hepatic encephalopathy	10–20 mg/kg PO q 6–12 hr
Neostigmine bromide (Prostigmin)	Acetylcholinesterase inhibitor	Myasthenia gravis; reversal agent for nondepolarizing neuromuscular blocker	2 mg/kg PO divided doses to effect Injection: 10 µg/kg IM, SC, as needed; Antidote for nondepolarizing neuromuscular blocker: 40 µg/kg IM, Diagnostic aid for myasthenia gravis: 40 µg/kg IM or 20 µg/kg IV
Nitroglycerin ointment	Nitrate	Congestive heart failure	Dog: 1/4 to 1/2 inch ointment transcutaneously per 3–6 kg BW q 6– BW q 6–8 hr Cat: 2–4 mg topically q 12 hr (or 1/4 inch of ointment per cat)

Drug Name	Class of drug	Indications	Dosages
Nitroprusside	Vasodilator	Severe heart failure	1–5, up to a max of 10 µg/kg/min CRI
Norepinephrine	Vasopressor	Septic shock	0.5–10 µg/kg/min
Omeprazole	Proton pump inhibitor	Esophagitis, gastric ulceration	Dog: 20 mg/dog PO once daily or 0.7 mg/kg q 24 hr
Ondansetron (Zofran)	$5HT_3$ antagonist	Anti-emetic	0.5–1 mg/kg IV, PO q 24 hr
Oxymorphone	Opioid	Moderate to severe pain	0.05–0.1 mg/kg IV, SC, IM q 4–6 hr
Oxytetracycline (Terramycin)	Tetracycline antibiotic	Susceptible infections	7.5–10 mg/kg IV q 12 hr; 20 mg/kg PO q 12 hr
Oxytocin	Sodium channel modulator	Uterine inertia	Dog: 1–10 U/dog IM, two doses 30 minutes apart Cat: 3–5 U/cat IM (repeat every 30 minutes up to 3 times)
Pamidronate (Aredia)	Bisphosphonate	Hypercalcemia	1.3–2 mg/kg diluted in 150 ml saline administered over 2 hr
Pancuronium bromide	Nondepolarizing neuromuscular blocker	Controlled paralysis	0.1 mg/kg IV or start with 0.01 mg/kg and additional 0.01 mg/kg doses every 30 min
D-Penicillamine (Cuprimine)	Lead chelator	Lead toxicosis	10–15 mg/kg PO q 12 hr
Penicillin G potassium or sodium	Penicillin antibiotic	Susceptible infections	20, 000–40, 000 U/kg IV, IM q 6–8 hr
Penicillin G procaine	Penicillin antibiotic	Susceptible infections	20, 000–40, 000 U/kg IM q 12–24 hr
Penicillin V	Penicillin antibiotic	Susceptible infections	10 mg/kg PO q 8 hr
Pentobarbital	Barbiturate	Anesthesia	25–30 mg/kg IV CRI: 1–2 mg/kg/hr
Phenobarbital	Barbiturate	Anticonvulsant	Dog: 2–8 mg/kg PO q 12 hr Cat: 2–4 mg/kg PO q 12 hr
Phenoxybenzamine	α-1 antagonist	Urethral spasm; pheochromocytoma	Dog: 0.25 mg/kg PO q 8–12 hr or 0.5 mg/kg q 24 hr Cat: 2.5 mg/cat q 8–12 hr
Phenylephrine	α-1 agonist sympatho-mimetic	Vasopressor	Vasopressor: 1–3 µg/kg/min IV
Physostigmine (Antilirium)	Long acting acetylcho-linesterase inhibitor	Myasthenia gravis	0.02 mg/kg IV q 12 hr
Pimobendan	Calcium sensitizer	Congestive heart failure	0.25 mg/kg PO q 12 hr
Piperacillin	Penicillin + β-lactamase inhibitor	Susceptible infections	40 mg/kg IV or IM q 6 hr
Potassium bromide	Anticonvulsive	Seizures	Dog: 25–50 mg/kg PO q 24 hr Loading dose of 400 mg/kg divided over 3 days. Not recommended in cats
Potassium citrate	Potassium supplement	Hypokalemia	2.2 mEq/100 kcal of food/day or 40–75 mg/kg PO q 12 hr
Potassium gluconate (Tumil-K)	Potassium supplement	Hypokalemia	Dog: 0.5 mEq/kg PO q 12–24 hr Cat: 2–8 mEq/day PO divided twice daily

Continued

Drug Name	Class of drug	Indications	Dosages
Pralidoxime chloride (2-PAM)	Cholinergic antidote	Organophosphate toxicosis	20 mg/kg q 8–12 hr IV slowly
Prazosin (Minipress)	Antihypertensive	Urethral spasm	0.5–2 mg/animal (1 mg/15 kg) PO q 8–12 hr
Prednisolone sodium succinate (Solu-Delta-Cortef)	Fast-acting glucocorticoid	Upper airway obstruction; anaphylaxis; Addisonian crisis	15 mg/kg IV slowly
Prednisone 2.2–6.6 mg/kg/day	Glucocorticoid	Anti-inflammatory; immunosuppressive	Anti-inflammatory: 0.5–1 mg/kg PO q 12 hr, then taper to q 48 hr; Immunosuppressive: PO then taper to 2–4 mg/kg q 48 hr
Primor (ormetoprim + sulfadimethoxine)	Antibiotic	Susceptible infections	27 mg/kg on first day, then 13.5 mg/kg PO q 24 hr
Procainamide	Antiarrhythmic (Class 1)	Ventricular tachycardia, ventricular premature complexes	Dog: 10–30 mg/kg PO q 6 hr (to a maximum dose of 40 mg/kg), 8–20 mg/kg IV, IM; 25–50 µg/kg/min CRI Cat: 3–8 mg/kg IM, PO q 6–8 hr
Prochlorperazine (Compazine)	Phenothiazide derivative	Anti-emetic	0.1–0.5 mg/kg IM, SC q 6–8 hr
Propantheline bromide (Pro-Banthine)	Anticholinergic	Bradyarrhythmia	0.25–0.5 mg/kg PO q 8–12 hr
Propofol	Anesthetic	Anesthetic; Status epilepticus	2–6 mg/kg IV slowly over 1 minute; CRI: 0.1–0.6 mg/kg/min
Propranolol	Beta-blocker	Tachyarrhythmia	Dog: 20–60 µg/kg over 5–10 min IV; 0.2–1 mg/kg PO q 8 hr (titrate dose to effect) Cat: 0.4–1.2 mg/kg (2.5–5 mg/cat) PO q 8 hr
Pyridostigmine bromide (Mestinon)	Anticholinesterase	Myasthenia gravis	0.02–0.04 mg/kg IV q 2 hr or 0.5–3 mg/kg PO q 8–12 hr
Ranidine (Zantac)	Weak H_2 antagonist	Gastroprotectant, prokinetic	Dog: 2 mg/kg IV, PO q 8 hr Cat: 2.5 mg/kg IV q 12 hr, 3.5 mg/kg PO q 12 hr
Sodium bicarbonate	Buffer	Severe metabolic acidosis	Correct deficit: 0.3(kg x base deficit). Administer 1/2 calculated dose IV then add to fluids
Sotalol (Betapace)	β-blocker antiarrhythmic	Tachyarrhythmias	Dog: 1–2 mg/kg PO q 12 hr Cat: 1–2 mg/kg PO q 12 hr
Spironolactone (Aldactone)	Diuretic, aldosterone antagonist	Fluid overload, ascites	1–2 mg/kg PO q 12–24 hr
Succimer	Lead chelator	Lead toxicosis	10 mg/kg PO q 8 hr for 5 days, then 10 mg/kg PO q 12 hr for 2 more weeks
Sucrafate (Carafate)	Gastroprotectant	Gastric ulcer	0.5–1 g/dog PO q 8 hr. Cat: 0.25 g/cat PO q 8 hr
Sufentanil citrate	Opioid	Analgesic	2 µg/kg IV, up to a maximum dose of 5 µg/kg
Tepoxali (Zubrin)	NSAID	Inflammation	10–20 mg/kg PO first day then 10 mg/kg per day

Drug Name	Class of drug	Indications	Dosages
Terbutaline (Brethine)	Short acting β-2 agonists–bronchodilator	Asthma	Dog: 1.25–5 mg/dog PO q 8 hr Cat: 0.1–0.2 mg/kg PO q 12 hr (or 0.625 mg/cat)
Theophylline	Bronchodilator	Asthma	Dog: 9 mg/kg PO q 6–8 hr Cat: 4 mg/kg PO q 8–12 hr
Theophylline sustained release (Inwood Laboratories)	Bronchodilator	Asthma	Dog: 10 mg/kg PO q 12 hr Cat: 15–20 mg/kg PO q 24 hr at night
Thiamine (Vitamin B1)	Vitamin	Thiamine deficiency	Dog: 100–250 mg/dog/day SC q 12 hr until regression of signs Cat: 200 mg/cat/day SC q 12 hr until regression of signs
Thiopental sodium (Pentothal)	Barbiturate	Anesthetic; seizures	Dog: 10–25 mg/kg IV (to effect) Cat: 5–10 mg/kg IV (to effect)
Ticarcillin	Potentiated penicillin	Susceptible infections	33–50 mg/kg IV, IM q 4–6 hr
Ticarcillin + clavulanate (Timentin)	Potentiated penicillin	Susceptible infections	33–50 mg/kg IV, IM q 4–6 hr
Tramadol	Opioid-like drug	Analgesic	2–5 mg/kg PO q 8–12 hr
Trimethoprim + sulfonamide (Tribrissen)	Antibiotic	Susceptible infections	15 mg/kg PO q 12 hr or 30 mg/kg PO q 12–24 hr
Ursodiol (Actigall)	Choleretic	Biliary disease	10–15 mg/kg PO q 24 hr
Vancomycin	Antibiotic	Susceptible infections	Dog: 15 mg/kg IV q 6–8 hr Cat: 12–15 mg/kg IV q 8 hr
Vasopressin, arginine	Vasopressor	CPR; septic shock	CPR: 0.8 U/kg IV Vasopressor: CRI: 0.0006 U/kg/min
Vincristine	Tubulin inhibitor	Thrombocytopenia	0.02 mg/kg IV
Vitamin K	Vitamin	Vitamin K antagonism, coagulopathy	For anticoagulant rodenticide: 3–5 mg/kg SC, PO q 24 hr For liver-disease associated coagulopathy: 0.5 mg/kg SC q 24 hr
Warfarin (Coumadin)	Vitamin K antagonist	Anticoagulant	Dog: 0.1–0.2 mg/kg PO Cat: 0.5 mg/cat/day Therapy guided via PT clotting times
Xylazine	α-2 agonist	Emetic agent	Cat: 0.44–1.1 mg/kg IM
Zafirlukast (Accolate)	Leukotriene inhibitor	Chronic asthma	1–2 mg/kg PO q 12–24 hr; 2.5–5 mg/cat PO q 12 hr

Index

W

X